AIR FRYER COOKBOOK FOR BEGINNERS

625 Budget Friendly, Quick & Easy, Healthy Air Fryer Recipes for Beginners

AUTHOR

Ton Poon

TABLE OF CONTENTS

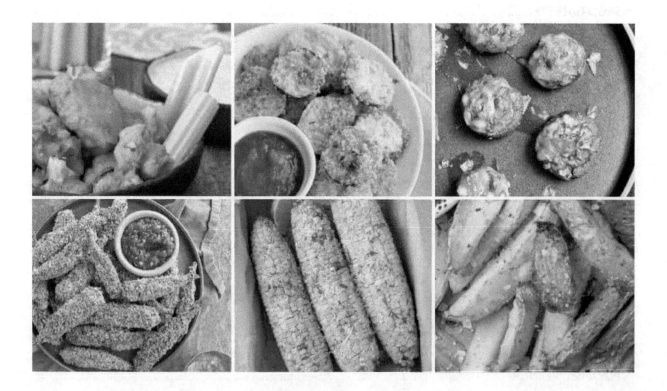

INTRODUCTION TO AIR-FRYER

An air-fryer is a kitchen apparatus that cooks by coursing hot air around the food utilizing the convection instrument.

An air fryer fundamentally utilizes hot air to cook and fresh the food. The heat is typically created by either an incandescent light or a heating component.

The heat is produced by a fan rapidly circling the hot air all around the food.

This is called Rapid Air Technology.

On account of the heat and the speed, the food will be singed equitably and rapidly, bringing about a firm outside and delicious inside.

An air fryer is a cutting edge kitchen cooker that cooks food by flowing hot air around it as opposed to utilizing oil. It offers a low-fat form of foods that would generally be cooked in a profound fryer. Thus, for the most part, meals, for example, French fries, seared chicken, and the onion-rings are prepared with no oil or up to 80 percent less fat substance contrasted with regular cooking strategies. The Air Fryer gives more beneficial seared foods and meals, empowering you to be freed of the calories that accompany eating singed foods while as yet giving you that crunchiness, surface, and quality that you want.

This family unit apparatus works by coursing exceptionally hot air (up to 400°F) uniformly and rapidly around a food fixing that is put in an encased space. The heat makes the food fixing firm and dries outwardly, however delicate and damp within. The air fryer can be utilized on practically everything. Other than searing, you can flame broil, prepare, and cook. Its assortment of cooking alternatives makes it simpler to set up any sort of meal whenever of the day.

An air fryer is an extraordinary method to set up your preferred seared foods without the extra calories you get from profound fricasseeing those foods in oil. You can set aside to 70% on oil contrasted with the profound fryer. By and large, all you need is a tablespoon of oil.

So it's significantly more beneficial than profound browning.

Less Energy = Lower Electricity Bill

Another explanation behind utilizing an air fryer is that it utilizes less energy than a profound fryer or an ordinary oven. This is on the grounds that more heat can be created and moved all through a little space.

How an Air Fryer Works

Air fryers recreate the customary browning of foods by coursing hot air around food as opposed to submerging the food in oil. Similarly, as with searing, appropriately arranged foods are fresh, succulent, brilliant dark-colored, and delightful.

Air fryers work because of the Maillard response, a logical guideline which alludes to what we ordinarily call "cooking." A Maillard response happens when the outside of a food thing structures a covering because of lack of hydration, and the extraordinary heat separates proteins, starches, and strands. That is the thing that gives seared, cooked, and prepared foods, their heavenly, complex flavors.

An air-fryer cooker or appliances is a convection oven in smaller than expected – a conservative round and hollow ledge convection oven, to be accurate (have a go at saying that multiple times quick).

Fundamentally, convection is the inclination of gases (or fluids) to move past one another when heated. Hot air ascends, for instance, at the same time driving cooler air to sink. Convection impacts the climate; it is even grinding away in the liquid stone that causes volcanic ejections. Yet, what, you may ask, does this have to do with your kitchen cookers?

Air fryers utilize convection to rapidly and productively cook fresh foods. A heating component inside the air fryer super-heats the air, creating common convection flows. A fan inside the cooker helps in air development, circling it much more rapidly. Apertures or gaps in the cooking bin permit the hot air to stream unreservedly around the food. This air development builds heat to move from the air to the food. In this manner, your supper completes quicker.

Air Fryer And The Use Of Radiation

Not at all like microwaves, which utilize a type of electromagnetic radiation called microwaves to energize water particles, they are subsequently heating the food because of grinding, and air fryers don't utilize any type of radiation. Rather, air fryers utilize a heating component like that found on any oven, toaster, or stovetop. The heating component works by changing over an electrical flow into heat.

Do Air Fryers Really Work?

At the point when utilized as planned and with quality plans, air fryers accomplish work. You can make fresh French fries, delicious cooked poultry, air seared veggies, and the sky is the limit from there. You may wish to counsel our air fryer cooking graphs to become familiar with the best temperature at which to cook your preferred foods and to what extent.

Why Use It

Low-Fat Meals: Unarguably, the most basic advantage of the air fryer is its utilization of hot-air course to cook food fixings from all edges, consequently taking out the requirement for oil use. This makes it feasible for individuals on low-fat eating routine to serenely get ready wonderfully sound meals.

More advantageous Foods& Environment: Air fryers are intended to work without swelling oils and to create more advantageous foods with up to 80 percent less fat. This makes it simpler to shed pounds since you can at present eat your seared dishes while moderating the calories and soaked fat. Doing that change to a more advantageous life is progressively reachable by utilizing this cooker. Your house is additionally freed of the smell that accompanies broiled foods that regularly remains around the environment even a few hours after profound searing.

Multipurpose Use: The air fryer empowers you to perform various tasks as it can set up numerous dishes on the double. It is your everything in-one apparatus that can flame broil, prepare, fry, and meal those dishes that you love! You never again need different apparatuses for different occupations. It can do different employments separate cookers will do. It can barbecue meat, broil veggies, and heat baked goods. It fills in as a compelling substitution for your oven, profound fryer, and stovetop.

Amazingly Safe: Remember how extra cautious you must be while tossing chicken or some different fixings into the profound fryer? You need to guarantee that the hot oil doesn't spill and consume your skin since it's in every case exceptionally hot. With your air-fryer, you wouldn't have to stress over brunt skin from hot oil spillage. It does all the broiling and is totally sheltered. By and by, use cooking gloves while repositioning your fryer to stay away from perils from the heat. Also, keep the air fryer cooker out of youngsters' scope.

Simple Clean Up: The Air Fryer leaves no oil and, in this manner, no chaos. Tidy up time is pleasant since their oils spill to clean on dividers and floors, and no rejecting or scouring of the skillet. There is no reason to invest in energy, guaranteeing that everything is immaculate. The Air fryer apparatus parts are made of non-stick material, which keeps food from adhering to surfaces, in this way making it difficult to clean. These parts are anything but difficult to clean and keep up. They are removable and dishwasher-sheltered also.

Spare Valuable Time: People who are on tight timetables can utilize the quickness of the air fryer to make delectable meals. For occurrences, you can make French fries in under 15 minutes and heat a cake inside 25 minutes. Inside minutes as well, you can appreciate firm chicken strips or brilliant fries. If you are consistently in a hurry, the air fryer is perfect for you since you will spend

Less time in the kitchen. It empowers you to deal with your tumultuous and occupied day by day life, filling your heart with joy increasingly reasonable.

Basic Parts, Accessories and Their Importance

Set up your fixings and put it into the bin, and afterward set your clock. The hot air from the air fryer goes to work, and when its work is finished, the clock goes off with a ding sound, showing that your food is finished. You may even check your food to perceive how it's advancing without disturbing the set time. When you pull out the skillet, the fryer will delay; when you place back the container, heating will continue.

The Air-Fryer is a direct apparatus, with no gathering required and no inconveniences. It consists of three principal things; the cooking bushel, the skillet, and the fundamental fryer unit.

The Cooking Basket is the place you put your food. It has a crate handle where you place your hand when taking care of the cooker and cooked food to forestall consumes or wounds when the air fryer is turned on. The crate fits superbly into the dish. The Pan gathers the food remainders and abundance oil and fits flawlessly into the Air-Fryer& then produces the Main Fryer Unit, which consists of numerous parts. There are other helpful parts that incorporate a rack, twofold flame broil layer, container, and food separators that make it conceivable to set up various dishes on the double.

The Tips For Using Air fryer

Keep It Clean and Dry: Pat dry foods before cooking, particularly marinated foods. Doing this will forestall overabundance smoke and splattering. Foods that contain high-fat substances, for example, chicken bosom and wings, for the most part, store fat when cooking.

Consequently, ensure you void the kept fat from the base of the air fryer every so often.

Space Your Foods: Overcrowding is a no-no with the air fryer. In the event that you need your food to cook well, give it a lot of room with the goal that air can flow well.

You need to appreciate the firmness of your meals, correct? Congestion keeps air from flowing over the foods. So make certain to space foods out.

Shake Foods Around: Open the Air Fryer like clockwork of cooking and shake around foods in the bin. Chips, French fries, and other littler foods can pack yet shaking around forestalls that. Pivot foods each 5 to 10 minutes to empower them to cook and shape well.

Shower Foods. You will require your cooking shower when utilizing the air fryer cooker as it assists with keeping foods from adhering to the bushel. Shower foods gently, or you could simply include a tad of oil.

Cook in Batches: The air fryer has a little cooking limit. In the event that you are cooking for an enormous number of individuals, you should cook in bunches.

Pre-heat the air-fryer when it has not been utilized for some time. Preheat for 3-5 minutes to permit it to heat up appropriately.

Presently you can utilize the air fryer cooker to set up the deliberately chosen sound and delicious plans beneath. Just adhere to the directions and appreciate even meals for you and your family.

TYPES OF AIR-FRYER

1. Ninja Air Fryer

Pros:

- Holds as much as two pounds of fries

- Low fan speed for browning

- Can likewise be utilized to broil food

Cons:

- Doesn't accompany a formula book

- Slightly constrained limit with regards to families and bigger gatherings

- Not the most reduced plan

The four-quart Ninja Air Fryer can hold as much as two pounds of fries one after another. A temperature scope of 105 to 400 degrees Fahrenheit makes it simple to prepare your preferred tidbits. Hot air is circled rather than oil, which fries foods in a lot more advantageous way while holding that equivalent scrumptious fresh surface. A few racks are incorporated for fricasseeing a bigger bunch, or a couple of your preferred foods, without a moment's delay. A portion of the parts is dishwasher, alright for quicker and simpler cleaning.

2. GoWISE Electric Air Fryer

Pros:

- Temperature scope of 175 to 400 degrees Fahrenheit
- User-accommodating touchscreen
- Includes worked in keen projects with well-known foods.

Cons:

- does exclude a rack for layers

- Can take for a spell to learn best cooking occasions and temperatures

- Frying bin can be difficult to embed

This electric air fryer, presently in its fourth era, has a flexible temperature scope of 175 to 400 degrees Fahrenheit and can cook a wide range of kinds of food inside 30 minutes. A 3.7-quart and 1400 watts of intensity settle on this air fryer a commonsense decision for littler family units and for any individual who doesn't have to cook enormous amounts on the double.

The touchscreen is effectively open and has seven worked in brilliant projects. You can browse well-known menu things, for example, chips, chicken, fish, and meat, with the goal that the fryer removes the mystery from the condition. There's likewise a 30-minute clock that changes to reserve mode when the time is up. A nonstick dishwasher-safe container is additionally included.

3. Philips XL Air-Fryer

Pros:

- Family-sized 3.5-quart limit

- Starfish configuration advances even and careful cooking.

- Adjustable temperatures up to 390 degrees

Cons:

- Can smoke a piece when cooking meat

- The initial expectation to absorb information

- Pricey

Its bigger limit settles on this air fryer a strong decision for families and any individual who needs to broil greater amounts without a moment's delay. An unmistakable starfish configuration permits hot air to flow equitably around the unit, bringing about a fresh outside and delicate inside.

Notwithstanding fricasseeing, the Philips Air-Fryer additionally works for preparing, flame broiling, cooking, and steaming food. The segments are dishwasher-alright for easy cleanup. Different highlights incorporate flexible temperatures up to 390 degrees, an hour-long clock, and easy to understand computerized touchscreen interface. A formula book is incorporated alongside an application for access to various plans.

4. Force Air-Fryer XL

Pros:

- Cyclonic hot air activity helps cook food

- Digital touchscreen

- Cool-contact handle

Cons:

- Frying crate can be hard to push back in

- Some discover it cooks quicker or more slowly than the suggested The cooking times

- The exterior can get hot

Cyclonic hot air activity helps cook food equitably and altogether for flavorful final products without utilizing included oil. Different features incorporate an advanced touch screen, and seven presets for top choices, for example, chicken, French fries, steak, and heated merchandise. The air finds a workable pace degree for speedier outcomes. There are likewise 1500 to 1700 watts to guarantee a lot of intensity all through the cooking procedure. A simple hold handle stays cool to the touch in any event when the air fryer heats up.

5. NuWave Brio Air Fryer

Pros:

- Pre-heat work

- Won't start until fry can is safely set up.

- Temperature scope of 100 to 390 degrees Fahrenheit

Cons:

- Can take momentarily to cook food

- The nonstick covering may wear off after some time.

- Relatively little cooking limit

Regardless of whether you're lacking in time or basically need an air fryer that can deal with the rudiments for you, this fryer accompanies a few highlights to make the cooking procedure simpler. A few models incorporate a pre-heat work, which carries the fryer to the ideal cooking temperature for your food, alongside a press button contact screen.

You can utilize the computerized screen to alter the temperature in five-degree increases for consistent outcomes. For your security, the unit won't start working until the frying basin is completely set up. There's additionally a 3.5-quart bushel and a temperature run from 100 to 390 degrees Fahrenheit.

6. BLACK+DECKER PuriFry Air Fryer

Pros:

- Dual convection fans

- Variable temperature control

- Eight-cup inside

Cons:

- Some wish it had a more noteworthy cooking limit

- Very little temperature dial numbers

- Lacks a computerized show

Double convection fans help circulate the air for fast and in any event, cooking. There's likewise factor temperature control with a temperature scope of 175 to 400 degrees Fahrenheit. Pointer lights let you realize that the unit is on and when the ideal preheat temperature has been come to. An eight-cup inside limit is sufficient to cook approximately two potatoes or up to eight chicken wings one after another. This air fryer is furnished with an hour-long clock, and naturally, close off when the clock is up.

7. T-fal ActiFry Air Fryer

Pros:

- Included channel limits smell

- Nonstick removable container

- Includes an estimating spoon

Cons:

- A bit massive

- Some wish there were more highlights at the cost.

- Several clients notice an underlying plastic smell.

The trademark highlight of this air fryer is the way that it just requires one tablespoon of oil to cook your preferred foods. An estimating spoon is incorporated to assist you with apportioning the exact sum. You may even have the option to utilize not exactly a tablespoon, contingent upon what you're cooking just as your taste inclination. There's sufficient inside space to cook up to 2.2 pounds of food. The earthenware nonstick dish is removable and simple to clean. A channel keeps under control while the top is intended to fit safely for sans mess cooking. A formula book is incorporated.

8. NutriChef Electric Air Fryer

Pros:

- Slide-out singing container

- 30-minute clock

- Nonstick covering

Cons:

- Doesn't have a trickle container

- Vague guidance manual

- Some wish the dial markings were bigger.

A few varieties of this air fryer are accessible, including this spending limit, well-disposed rendition with manual handles. There's additionally one with an advanced handle and a blend air fryer and halogen oven. A slide-out singing bushel makes embeddings food and tidying up simple. Hot air courses around the food along these lines as a convection oven for even and careful cooking. A nonstick covering on the searing container guarantees food won't stall out. Different features incorporate a 30-minute clock and the most extreme cooking temperature of 400 degrees Fahrenheit.

9. BELLA Electric Hot Air Fryer

Pros:

- 1500 watt circling framework

- 60-minute clock with auto-off

- Stainless steel heating component

Cons:

- Lacks computerized controls

- does exclude a cookbook or plans

- Small singing bushel

This spending limit amicable air fryer is a strong decision in case you're searching for an essential air fryer without the additional extravagant accessories commonly found on pricier models. A 1500 watt circling framework moves air around such that it is like a convection oven. The container holds up to 2.2 pounds of food. You can control the temperature up to 400 degrees utilizing the customizable indoor regulator. Different features incorporate an auto-off hour-long clock alongside a tempered steel heating component to rapidly heat up food.

WHAT CONTAINS AN AIR FRYER?

An air fryer isn't convoluted like other cooking apparatus. It contains a dish, a divider, preparing tin, twofold barbecue layer. The divider offers you the chance to cook two foods simultaneously.

Container fits well on the apparatus. There is a bushel which is put in the skillet. The bushel has a handle which permits you to shake your food during cooking without experiencing any difficulty.

There is a heating tin likewise which permits you to prepare merchandise and desserts like cookies and biscuits. The fixings which you need to cook put within the container, which consummately fits in the skillet.

The fixings which you need to sear ought to be placed into the crate. At the point when you are going to evacuate the bushel, ensure that the dish is perched superficially on a level plane.

Air fryer accompanies non-clingy surface and tempered steel.

WHAT IS THE MAIN PART OF AIR FRYER?

Manual Temperature

Only one out of every odd food needs equivalent temperature. This cooking cooker is allowing you the chance to work temperature of your own with the goal that food won't get over scorched. There is an auto arrangement nearly in each air fryer with the goal that you can without much of a stretch cook your ideal food.

Size of Tray

The size of the plate gives you the sum that the amount you are going to cook food. The Smaller plate is sufficient for one individual; on another hand greater plate is for more than one individual.

Size of Air Fryer

The diverse air fryer has a distinctive size of its own. Some are little, and some are large enough for an entire family. Some family has bigger space in their home, and some family doesn't.

So everybody can purchase this cooker for their decision. You can discover compact air fryer, which is especially helpful for the bustling individual who voyages a great deal.

Clean Easily

Cooking instruments are particularly hard to clean due to the oil of oil. Once in a while, it leaves a stain on the instrument, and it gets harmed.

In any case, the air fryer is liberated from it since it utilizes no oil to broil or cook any food. It tends to be put in the dishwasher effectively, and it is lightweight.

In the event that you deal with the air fryer, you can utilize this fryer for quite a while.

Cost

The cost of this cooking cooker is very convenient. You can get it at a modest rate too.

There is some air fryer which you can purchase at a modest rate and have a decent nature of this convenient cooking apparatus.

In any case, you ought to pick carefully in light of the fact that modest one isn't in every case great one and satisfy your requirements.

BENEFITS OF AIR FRYER

Consider the accompanying reasons why an air fryer may be directly for you:

Sound Cooking

Everybody cherishes the flavor of southern-style foods, yet numerous individuals must keep away from these for wellbeing reasons. In case you're hoping to bring down cholesterol or get more fit, your primary care physician may thank you for utilizing an air fryer. Air-fryers use up to 75 percent less oil than profound fryers, giving a solid option without giving up the season.

Speed of Cooking

The air fryer's little convection oven preheats and cooks more rapidly than an ordinary oven. You'll have scrumptious meals in a flurry, with less pause!

Green Cooking

Have you "made strides toward environmental friendliness?" Cooking with an air fryer can help. Most air fryers are energy proficient, and shorter cook times mean less generally power utilization.

Basic and Easy

Air fryers use basic controls, commonly two handles for cook time and temperature, or simple to peruse advanced showcase. You basically hurl the food in oil (whenever wanted), place it in the crate, and the air fryer wraps up.

Tidy Up Is a Breeze

The bushels and container of most air fryers are dishwashers alright for simple cleanup. Likewise, the encased idea of the air fryer forestalls the splatters and spills related to profound searing and sautéing.

Safe

Coming up short on the huge oil tanks of conventional profound fryers, air fryers wipe out the danger of genuine consumes from spilled oil. Additionally, air fryers are structured with the goal that the outside doesn't turn out to be hazardously hot to the touch.

Other Health Benefits of Air Fryers

Air fryers are present-day cookers that utilization imaginative air dissemination and heat move innovation to sear and cook foods without oil or oil. On the off chance that this sounds unrealistic, at that point, you can settle your questions. Air fryers have reformed regular profound singing into a snappy, sound, and safe procedure. You would now be able to anticipate cooking most loved singed foods for your family without going with sentiments of blame. In the event that you've been considering putting resources into an air fryer, however, are not exactly sure, investigate the various advantages of utilizing air fryer in your kitchen.

Low Fat Healthy Cooking

One of the most significant advantages of air fryers is that we can appreciate delectable, dried up, fresh seared foods without going with oil, oil, and fat. The little oil makes a reviving appear differently in relation to the colossal puddles of oil that you'd have to use for profound fricasseeing foods. The manual will contain data about the various sorts of oils that can be utilized with the air fryer model being referred to. When all is said in done, air fryers use about 80% less oil (contrasted with traditional profound browning). For instance, 300 g of generally singed food will contain 37 g of fat while the equivalent 300 g of food will contain just 9 grams of fat when cooked in an air fryer.

It's totally brilliant to have the option to eat a more advantageous rendition of singed foods. Air singing lessens fat-loaded calories and subsequently diminishes inborn wellbeing dangers, including stoutness and so forth. Best of all, you're ready to eliminate the fat substance without settling on taste, surface, and flavor. Foods taste a lot of equivalent to they do on the off chance that they are expectedly pan-fried – you get the crunch, the searing, and the tempting smell too.

Quick Cooking: You can spare important time

The air fryer can be utilized for crunchy fries or firm chicken in practically no time. In contrast to convection ovens (numerous convection ovens take in any event 10 minutes to heat up to the craving temperature and afterward start the cooking procedure), the gadget needn't bother with time to heat up before beginning to broil food. Because of the high heat force, the viability of heat radiation is high, and foods begin cooking a lot quicker. The outside structures' prior and planning times are considerably quicker. French fries, for instance, can cook in as meager as 12 minutes and you can broil fish in a short time.

You can move solidified foods like chunks, potato wedges, and fries directly from the cooler into the fryer without sitting around idly on preheating. Nuts take around 10 minutes to become crunchy, toasty and fragrant. Furthermore, you can likewise reheat foods rapidly in air fryers – it takes around 10 minutes all things considered. This is a greatly improved choice of purchasing calorie-plagued prepared foods at the general store. Air fryers are especially helpful for cooking littler bits of food rapidly and no problem at all.

On the off chance that you have hungry children sitting tight for a meal, an air fryer can assist you with planning tasty foods truly quick! Additionally, the procedure is perfect and non-muddled on the grounds that all the browning occurs inside the fryer; no oil splatters to wipe up and clean. Regular stovetops accompany an uncovered surface and result in sleek fume beads that get kept on the ledge or in any event, roof. The cooker is ideal for individuals who need to cook in a hurry and eliminates time spent in the kitchen. All you have to clean is the trickle plate and cooking skillet, and you never again need to dispose of a huge amount of utilized oil. The flame broil, container, and bushel are completely worked to be dishwasher agreeable and made of non-stick material. It's a smart thought to drench them for quite a while before cleaning.

All things considered, the last we need is to remain around tidying up the kitchen when we have to race to work in a rush.

Basic and Easy to Use

Air fryers are anything but difficult to utilize and don't include any confounded dealing with. There are basically two kinds of air fryers accessible in the market: The bowl and mixing paddle model and the work base on the dribble plate model. Most air fryers utilize the work crate structure. The flexible temperature controls permit you to utilize various settings for various foods, and you can essentially adjust the cooking dish properly and overlap down the handle. You can utilize the blending oar to flip the food once in a short time to guarantee in any event, cooking. Truth be told, not normal for customary stove or gas cooking, you don't need to keep up a cautious watch over the container. At the point when you pull out the prospect (the food), the clock will naturally delay. At the point when you slide back the dish, the heating will continue from the latest relevant point of interest.

The main two fastens that you have to press the clock and the temperature, in any case, the procedure is, for the most part, programmed that requires negligible information. Indeed, a few models of air fryers even accompany customized settings for various foods. In the event that you're uncertain of the time or temperature, essentially press the right setting for the food that you're cooking. For your data, air fryers are worked to a meal, flame broil, and heat foods also. It offers adaptability and is easy to understand simultaneously. Actually, it resembles owning an oven, a barbecue, a skillet just as a toaster in a solitary gadget.

Numerous models of air fryers are planned with food separators so you can cook product meals on the double. You can spare a great deal of time without agonizing over the flavors getting stirred up. It's a smart thought to cook foods that require comparative temperature settings to cook simultaneously.

Safe to utilize

Not at all like traditional profound broiling that is laden with dangers of fire and spillage of hot oil, air fryers offer phenomenal security. The food cooks inside securely, and there is no risk of tipping over a dish of hot oil onto the floor. In addition, most models come outfitted with a programmed shutdown component that switches off the cooker when the food is cooked. This significantly lessens the danger of consuming or overheating food (Leaving hot oil on the stove or gas is hazardous as the oil may burst into flames). Air fryer cookers likewise have – non-slip feet' that forestall coincidental sliding and slipping. You can be certain that your fryer will never slide off the kitchen counter. Furthermore, the encased food chamber configuration guarantees that we appreciate a without splatter cooking encounter and don't need to fear getting burnt by hot oil.

Reserve funds regarding time and cash

Since air fryers work quickly and utilize next to no oil, you can anticipate reserve funds regarding time just as cash. You save money on power use just as oil consumption. In addition, since the gadget closes itself down, there is no danger of energy wastage. Truth be told, you can even consider utilizing natural oils (they're typically progressively expensive contrasted with customary oils) since you need to utilize only a smidgen for cooking foods (pretty much a tablespoon full).

No Pollution

Numerous stoves, gas cookers, and so forth naturally include some type of ecological contamination. Air fryers come outfitted with cooling frameworks that keep the cooker liberated from pollution. The heated air in the air-fryer is cooled and separated before being discharged into the air. The air channel likewise keeps the wet smell of oil from spreading around the kitchen. You can hope to appreciate crisp kitchen smells when cooking with an air fryer.

Scrumptious, Delicious and Even Cooking

The impartial heat move and configuration guarantee that food particles are heated uniformly. The food builds up a delicious smash superficially while the delicacy and succulence are held inside. Air fricasseeing jelly surface, flavor, and taste of foods. A touch of blending with the oar guarantees that no food is left uncooked. Oven and microwave cooked foods don't create a similar degree of crunch and freshness than an air fryer can deliver.

By and large, an air fryer is a protected, helpful, and flexible kitchen colleague which you can use to cook breakfast, lunch just as supper. Air fryers are an incredible venture for occupied guardians, wellbeing conscious individuals just as for the individuals who are consistently in a hurry.

You don't need to fear kids getting splattered with hot oil or the gadget slipping and sliding about on the kitchen counter. Above all, you presently have the alternative of getting a charge out of all-around cooked, succulent seared food without the orderly dangers of fat-loaded calories. In the present quick paced life and furious timetables, the air fryer is truly a much-needed refresher. They offer object free, quick, and solid cooking with insignificant exertion and supervision. You can cook your preferred foods without sweating over a hot, clingy stove. At whatever point you ache for singed food or feel too drained to even think about spending a large amount of time in the kitchen, you should simply turn on the air fryer cooker.

HOW TO USE AN AIR FRYER

There are four distinct stages during the utilization of any air fryer:

- Preparation Of The Food

- Preparation Of The Air Fryer

- Cooking In The Air Fryer

- Cleaning The Air Fryer

1) Preparation Of The Food

- Keeping the food from adhering to the fryer container, include absolute minimum oil.

- Let space between the food to permit the hot air to go through and cook from all sides. Utilize an aluminum foil paper as a separator.

- If you are utilizing marinated or slick fixings at that point, pat them dry. This will stay away from any splattering or overabundance smoke. Expel any oil/fat from the base of the fryer.

2) Preparation Of The Air Fryer

- Plug in the fryer and preheat it for around 5 minutes.

- Ensure that the air fryer cooker is sufficiently hot.

- Place the food things inside and abstain from congestion. Air must have the option to flow through all the sides of every food thing to cook it appropriately.

- If you are cooking pre-made foods, you can change the underlying oven temperature by 70 degrees and cut The cooking time down the middle.

3) Cooking In The Air Fryer

- While cooking little food, things like chicken wings or fries, attempt to shake the fryer around multiple times. Likewise, have a go at turning the food things at regular intervals to ensure an all-adjusted fry.

- If you are cooking high-fat food, you will find that it discharges fat in the base of the fryer. You would need to evacuate this fat in the wake of cooking.

4) Cleaning The Air Fryer

- After separating the food from the fryer, you should clean it appropriately to guarantee that the apparatus is in the top shape.

- You should clean the container and the skillet in the wake of using them. Many air fryers accompany dishwasher safe parts, which makes your work simple.

- However, if you have to physically clean the parts, at that point, absorb them hot water and include dishwashing cleanser. Following 10 minutes, clean them with a wipe while under the sink.

- This will guarantee that your fryer doesn't have any food particles obstructed in it, and your food's smell isn't caught in it.

- For cleaning the outside and within the fryer, utilize a delicate soggy fabric and dishwasher cleanser to spot clean the territory.

The air fryer will absolutely change your discernment about cooking. With its obvious quality and advantageous activity, it is unquestionably going to be one of your preferred kitchen cookers.

NORMAL MISTAKES WHICH ARE COMMITTED BY NEWBIES

Numerous purchasers lament in the wake of buying air fryer since they figure they would have purchased a superior air fryer at this cost. Once in a while, they don't purchase the air fryer, which satisfies their prerequisite.

Here are a few slip-ups which are submitted by new purchasers

Size

The vast majority of the clients buy the wrong size air fryer. They purchase excessively huge or excessively little. You should remember that for whom and why you have to purchase an air fryer.

- If it is for the little family, at that point, purchase a little one.

- If you have a major family at that point, clearly purchase the huge one, so it spares your the cooking time.

- If you are a bustling individual and ventures a great deal, at that point, purchase the convenient one.

So be cautious about the size. You will lament on the off chance that you don't.

Numerous Features

Few out of every odd air fryer has the same and all highlights. Some have numerous highlights, and some have essential highlights. In any case, you needn't bother with all the highlights regularly.

Some new purchasers get intrigued by the new and alluring highlights, and they get it without pondering it. In the wake of getting it, they think twice about it.

So before purchasing any cooking cooker must reverify the rundown of highlights that you need and that you needn't bother with.

Purchase that one which satisfies your prerequisites.

Overpaying

If you are going to require an ideal and all around ok air fryer, at that point, you can burn through cash on that. Be that as it may, if you are going to utilize it for everyday schedule, at that point, don't go for costly one.

HOW TO CLEAN AN AIR FRYER

Making new and solid food from Air fryer is very simple and less tedious when contrasted and other profound fryers. In any case, air fryers likewise must be cleaned intermittently, for the most part, in the wake of utilizing it for some time.

Since air fryers don't require a great part of the oil while getting ready food, it is a characteristic procedure to clean an air fryer. By utilizing the best possible arrangement of materials and hardware, you can rapidly clean the air fryer. Underneath right now, make stride by-step strategies on the best way to clean an air fryer.

In the underneath article, we investigate materials required for cleaning the air fryer, at that point the means on the best way to clear all through the Air fryer, after which we investigate how to clean the Air Fryer bushel and dish materials.

At that point, we talk about reinstalling the parts back to where they ought to be, and afterward, we likewise talk about precautionary measures to be taken while cleaning Air fryer. At last, we will take some normally approached questions and offer responses for them and with some snappy video manages that let you know guidelines of cleaning Air fryer.

Prior to anything, you ought to comprehend that there are these five significant parts an Air fryer is comprised of. These materials are:

- Body or shell itself

- Air Fryer Pan

- Air Fryer bushel

- Air Fryer work

- Air Fryer exhaust vents

So once you know about the pieces of Air fryer, let us get jump into the cleaning procedure straightforwardly.

Materials Required for Cleaning Air Fryer:

Before realizing how to clean an air fryer, let us investigate what are the materials required for cleaning an air fryer accurately.

Miniaturized scale Fiber fabric: Depending upon to what extent it has been that you have cleaned the air fryer cooker, the decision of material from assortments of Microfiber material can be chosen. There are numerous small scale fiber garments accessible in various bundles. It is encouraged to utilize microfiber fabric on the grounds that while cleaning the different pieces of Air fryer like work, container, and bin, there shouldn't be any smears or scratches framed on the outside of these materials. Between the medium to thin thickness will be sufficient to clear off the earth from the different components of Air fryer.

Non-rough scrubber wipes: The name may confound you a piece. However, yes, there are non-grating scrubber wipes accessible in the closest store, which has scrubber on one side and wipe on another side of them. The scrubber side is really to evacuate on the off chance that you have a greater amount of oil or oil adhered to the dish and isn't effortlessly expelled off. Wipe side is the thing that prescribed for cleaning the different pieces of the Air Fryer. These wipes joined with certain beads of fluid cleaner can try to please zones of Air fryer.

Cleaning Liquid: Again, the cleaning fluid is the one which really changes over that strong oil or food wastage was gentler and expels them from the Air dryer parts rapidly. This fluid, for the most part, consists of vinegar that assists with battling against those intense materials patched up broadcasting in real-time fryer parts.

Container brush: While choosing the skillet brush to clean the air fryer cooker, there are two things you should remember. One is that the fibers of the brush ought not to be that difficult that it might make scratches over the outside of the Air Fryer. Also is the length of the brush. It should go through each corner through the inward bit of the Air fryer rapidly. This will help you, whimsically, which will be depicted later in the article.

Paper clothes: These are again fundamental to spotless or dry the pieces of Air Fryer. Paper garments or tissue papers with no mellow abrasiveness can be utilized to clean the inward surfaces of Air fryer. You don't need to independently buy the paper towels in the event that you are as of now spending a great deal on purchasing wet non-rough garments.

Heating Powder: This is a discretionary decision. In the event that you think, there is a lot of smudgy parts inside the Air fryer and needs profound cleaning and drenching then you have to have preparing powder side by you to such an extent this can work productively and expel every one of those from those pieces of Air fryer totally.

Cleaning the In and Out of the Air-Fryer:

So we should begin directly with the cleaning of the Air Fryer. To begin with, we will clear off within and outside of the Air Fryer first since they are very simpler to clean contrasted with the bushel and dish of the Air Fryer relying upon span, after which you are cleaning the Air Fryer. The following are the quite basic strides to clean inside and outside of the Air fryer.

1) Unplug the Air fryer power supply.

2) Remove the bin and dish portions of the Air Fryer tenderly with care.

3) Once you expel the container and dish from the Air Fryer, you may see that there could be earth or buildup or oil of food aggregated. Nothing to stress, since this is very normal and can be handily expelled.

4) Now flip around the Air fryer.

5) With the assistance of cleaner you have bought or by making a Baking powder arrangement (3 gms. of preparing powder to 100ml of water), splash tenderly over the internal territories of the Air fryer.

6) Let the arrangement enter through the buildup for 1 to 2 minutes

7) Turn the Air Fryer topsy turvy once more, in this manner carrying it to the ordinary position.

8) Wait for 30 minutes in the interim you can take a taste of espresso or complete some other pending works.

9) After 30 minutes, rehash the means 4 to 8.

10) Now put the container and bushel again into the Air Fryer at their separate positions.

11) Fill the container with about 400ml of water so that in the following barely any means it can gather the buildups or soil from inside and furthermore give dampness.

12) Connect the Air Fryer to the force source.

13) Now work the Air Fryer at 200-degree celsius for around 20 minutes.

14) After 20 minutes, you can expel the container and crate from the Air Fryer and mood killer the force supply, subsequently letting the Air Fryer chill off.

15) Again flip around the Air Fryer when it is in tepid condition.

16) You can expel the buildup of soil at the base of the Air Fryer with the assistance of wet garments or paper towels, as we recommended before. At that point, you can toss the water from the bushel or container gathered.

17) Finally, when everything is done, you can unplug the Air Fryer from the force supply, and with the assistance of smaller scale fiber garments, you can clean the external surface.

18) You can likewise utilize the cleaning arrangement or heating arrangement and shower it over the surface in the event that you feel it looks monstrous or has scratches. In any case, remember to clear off the earth again with a material.

Cleaning the Air Fryer Basket and Pan:

Presently we come to generally significant or, on certain occasions, the most monotonous undertaking of all. The Air Fryer's most urgent parts are its crate and dish where you place all your tasty food things like Chicken or French fries or some other such stuff to cook. Since these parts are the person who is, for the most part, getting presented to the food things and the heat radiations from Air Fryer, it bodes well that these things will get filthy after some time and appropriate cleaning and upkeep of these materials now and again are very basic.

You can clean the Air Fryer crate and skillet first and afterward clean within and outside of the Air Fryer or the other way around whichever you are open to cleaning first.

1) The initial step is to take out both container and work out from the Air fryer

2) Then fill the Air fryer skillet with hot water once to which you can likewise include the cleaning arrangement, or the heating arrangement arranged dependent on its earth or oil to it.

3) After filling the dish with water, let the bushel absorb the search for gold at least 10 minutes. This will help the materials connected to the container get disintegrated at the base of the dish.

4) After a couple of moments, take the brush or non-rough wipe and clean all the sides of the container.

5) Turn the bin topsy turvy and wipe the base piece of it tenderly with a non-rough brush or wipe

6) After that, keep aside the crate and clean all the sides of a skillet with a non-grating brush.

7) Finally, rub the surfaces of both containers and bin with paper towels or clammy material. You can likewise keep all the parts in a cold and dry spot for them to get dried totally.

Reinstalling all the Parts and Check the Air Fryer Functioning:

Subsequent to cleaning all the pieces of Air fryer, next comes the reinstallation of parts and checking the air fryer working so as to be certain that it is working appropriately as it was previously.

When all the parts are dry, check for any of the rest of the buildups or the water forgot about on them and on the off chance that not, at that point, place all the parts in their separate positions. Additionally, ensure the electric string associating the air fryer to the force supply is perfect and isn't harmed.

At that point, place the Air Fryer to its unique position, which is upstanding on a level surface before you could begin cooking. There are vents accessible, which should remove the heat from the Air Fryer, subsequently keep up a protected good ways from the divider. Ensure the vents are looking towards an open region with the end goal that the heat can escape out rapidly.

At last, before beginning setting up your food in the air fryer in the wake of reinstalling all the parts, ensure that all the segments are in acceptable working condition and if at all they are harmed, contact the maker promptly and get them supplanted.

Signs for Next Maintenance:

The following support or cleaning of the air fryer ought to be done promptly when you think it is looking foul, or it's been too long that you have utilized the air fryer. Beneath are some genuine considerations wherein you should hop in immediately to clean the pieces of Air Fryer.

1. At the point when you smell awful scent:

Air fryers are the freshest type of advancements in the field of cooking food. One may feel that profound fryers are better than air fryers as they are high on upkeep, however clearly, that isn't the situation. On the off chance that legitimate cleaning is done at a suitable time, air fryers could be your best accomplices while cooking food.

If you are utilizing an air fryer after quite a while and abruptly, you understand that an awful scent or foul smell is leaving the Air fryer when you take out the parts. At that point, that is your prompt first sign to clean the air fryer.

2. The white vapor leaving the air smoke:

Unquestionably, there are chances that you notice white smoke turning out from the vents of the air fryer when you turn it on. This could be a result of the accompanying reasons.

- You would have arranged greasy meals or greasy wiener meals and left the air fryer simply like that.

- You may have utilized over the top of oil for cooking a dish that isn't planned. Consequently, ensure you read the proprietor's manual and utilize the fitting measure of oil for planning singular dishes.

- Mostly, the low-fat materials are anything but difficult to cook through air fryer and inevitably are anything but difficult to get crispier. Thus while buying the crude materials or tidbits, ensure you look at the fat rate in them.

- If at all you can't avoid buying foods that are high in fat since you are kicking the bucket to set up that delectable dish, no stresses! Notwithstanding, ensure you clean the container and bin following use by the strategies referenced previously.

By following these straightforward advances, you can maintain a strategic distance from cost on upkeep and furthermore increment the solidness of air fryer.

3. Air pockets or Peeling Inside the Air Fryer:

There could be chances that before finding a good pace, grating materials shouldn't be utilized for cleaning reason; you may have used to the bin or dish portions of the air fryer. So since you have utilized them, you may see gurgling or stripping of the layer from the crate some portion of the air fryer.

Since there is the non-clingy covering over the container, thus there is nothing to stress over the food you admission. Nonetheless, the best suggestion is to contact the maker to the most punctual and get the issue settled.

4. Trouble in sliding the dish:

Once more, this may sound excess, yet there are chances that in the event that you haven't cleaned the air fryer in a drawn-out period of time and you are cooking through Air Fryer consecutive, at that point the aggregation of food or oil over within zone of the air fryer may happen.

The basic answer for this is to before you begin cooking for your next meal, clean the air fryer accurately as referenced above, and afterward feel free to cook your tasty dishes. Cleaning right now helps diminish your weight further.

Insurances to be Taken While Cleaning Air Fryer:

Cleaning anything isn't a simple assignment, and when you are cleaning an air fryer on which you have contributed a considerable amount, you would prefer not to take any dangers or risks while cleaning it. Thus beneath are some basic precautionary measures taken while or in the wake of cleaning air fryer.

- When you are cleaning the pieces of Air fryer, make sure to deal with the parts with delicate consideration. Try not to hurry into things accordingly. Your closure of harm any of the parts.

- Use the preparing arrangement, when there is a great deal of soil living inside the air fryer or even on the crate and dish regions.

- Before and in the wake of cleaning the parts, ensure you check the ropes, all the pieces of the air fryer aren't harmed in any which ways.

- Never utilize the steel wire brush or scrubber to clean the pieces of the air fryer.

- Read the guidance manual or proprietor's manual appropriately before planning food.

- Don't utilize unnecessary oil for cooking food and attempt to cook the ideal amount of food without a moment's delay in an air fryer.

- Make sure that you clean the air fryer after each utilization with the goal that you don't need to burn through a lot of energy when it gets foul.

- Never submerge the parts which come in contact (Eg: Dashboard) to control supply in water. Utilize a soggy material to clean them appropriately.

THE DEEP FRYER AND THE AIR FRYER

A profound fryer is a cooking cooker that gives a generally sheltered approach to submerge food in the hot oil without the cook getting scorched. Cooking with a lot of oil can be perilous, as it will, in general, splatter and can cause genuine consumption. Oil is regularly heated to temperatures moving toward 280° to 400°F (140° to 200°C). As opposed to heat oil in a pot, it's a lot more secure to utilize a fryer to cook such foods.

This apparatus is comprised of an enormous tank, into which the oil is poured, and a container, which can be securely submerged into the oil after it has gotten hot enough. There are both business and home models. Business fryers are regular in drive-through eateries and are utilized to get ready French fries and different foods. A profound fryer isn't one of the most widely recognized home cooking apparatuses. However, it tends to be utilized to get ready singed foods at home.

When utilizing a profound fryer, the oil can normally be reused on various occasions, frequently upwards of 10 or 15. Either corn oil or vegetable oil are acceptable decisions; olive oil is commonly too costly to even consider using since a considerable amount of oil is required. Cooks can even keep the oil in the tank, as long as it will be kept in a cool spot and will be reused inside half a month.

There are numerous sorts of food that can be cooked in a fryer. Numerous individuals appreciate rotisserie French fries, sweet potato fries, mozzarella sticks, seared chicken, onion rings, potato tots, and numerous different kinds of food. A few gourmet experts guarantee that the ideal approach to cook a Thanksgiving turkey is to fry it profoundly. In profound fricasseeing, however, the food is submerged in oil, it doesn't commonly turn out to be excessively oily. Rather, the oil just infiltrates the food's surface, making it firm, while steaming within. Foods cooked along these lines frequently have numerous calories, be that as it may, in light of the fact that the outside or breading holds a great deal of the oil from cooking.

One of the most well-known dishes made in a profound fryer is the pan-fried Twinkie™, a development where a bite cake is dunked in hitter and southern style, with the goal that within liquefies and the outside is firm. This food may be scrumptious, yet very unfortunate. In any case, this treat would now be able to be found at numerous event congregations and different places all through the world, alongside pan-fried cookies and pieces of candy.

THE DIFFERENCES BETWEEN THE AIR FRYER AND THE DEEP FRYER

From the outset, profound fryers and air fryers appear to be very comparative. Both give customary food, (for example, veggies or bits of meat) a delectable taste and crunchy outside. Be that as it may, the technique a profound fryer utilizes (dunking food into a lot of hot oil) is vastly different from that of an air fryer, which covers the food with a tad of oil at that point shoots it with hot air.

On the off chance that you love conventional singed food, the profound fryer could be your most solid option. In case you're more wellbeing conscious and need to accomplish comparable outcomes without altogether surrendering that unmistakable seared taste and surface, an air fryer could be the ideal decision. You may even be pondering: Do air fryers fill in just as profound fryers? In case you're willing to surrender a slight measure of flavor and even surface to appreciate more advantageous singed foods, consider putting resources into an air fryer.

Regardless of whether you're looking for a profound fryer or an air fryer, you've most likely chosen a spending limit. You may likewise have considered certain highlights, for example, simple versatility or programmed temperature control. Looking at highlights, dependability after some time, general strength, and different components can assist you with narrowing down the accessible profound fryers and air fryers to locate what's directly for you.

1. Profound Fryers versus Air Fryers: Features

For certain consumers, a fryer's highlights (or absence of highlights) can be an integral factor. One element rich fryer we like is the Secura Triple Basket Electric Deep Fryer. This specific fryer incorporates a removable oil tank, an additional oil channel, flexible heat controls, a see-through window in the top, and a programmed clock.

As a rule, the two sorts of fryers share a few similitudes regarding highlights, especially with regards to advanced screens, flexible temperatures, and easy to use controls. Right now, banter about whether to get an air fryer versus profound fryer may boil down to only a couple of must-have highlights. The pricier the fryer, the more highlights it's probably going to have. For instance, you can locate a well-outfitted fryer with movable temperature control and a clock with a prepared sign and programmed shut-off. A few fryers even accompany cooking pre-sets to remove the mystery from The cooking time.

In the event that you acknowledge accommodation, you'll need to consider an air fryer with a straightforward touch activity and a helpful on/off switch. In case you're the sort to disregard food when it's cooking, a fryer with an advanced commencement clock and signal can be an incredible decision. Different highlights to consider incorporate simple to clean materials or fryers that accompany a formula book.

Southern-style food smells flavorful when it's cooking, yet it can likewise abandon a horrendous fragrance, particularly if it's been overcooked or consumed. In the event that you'd preferably stay away from this unsavory experience, search for a profound fryer with sufficient scent control (particularly ones with charcoal channels). Since cooking with all that oil can likewise be unwieldy — particularly when it's an ideal opportunity to tidy up — you may likewise consider a removable compartment with an oil pouring spout.

Other helpful highlights are cool-contact or collapsible handles and a computerized clock with an effectively discernible presentation screen. In the event that you need to remain in charge of your food all through the cooking procedure, search for a profound fryer with a customizable indoor regulator. A few units accompany show windows incorporated with their covers to let you take a look without opening up the top. Another component to consider is the unit's general force. A 1,600-watt power fryer probably won't appear that vastly different from a 1,800-watt dryer from the outset, yet the more impressive unit regularly heats and cooks food quicker.

2. Profound Fryers versus Air Fryers: The cooking time and Capacity

Perhaps the greatest contrast among air and profound fryers is their general size. Most air fryers are altogether littler than profound fryers, as their substance doesn't should be dunked into a lot of oil for profound searing. One model that has an incredible limit is the AIGEREK Digital Electric 3.2L air fryer. This ought to be adequate space for most home cooks.

In case you're searching for a fryer that is bound to fit on your counter, the air fryer is your most logical option. Try not to let the littler size moron you, however, as most air fryers have a lot of room for a better than average measure of food. You can, without much of a stretch, discover an air fryer with a 1.5 to 2-pound limit, which is all that anyone could need space to take care of two to four individuals. If you need the air fryer for an incidental bite or little meal, you can pull off a lower food limit, yet it's ideal for locating a bigger unit in case you're keen on making meals with the fryer.

Except if you plan on making the periodic broiled side dish, you'll need a profound fryer with enough ability to hold any food you want to cook. The Generally, the range is 2 to 12 cups, in spite of the fact that most of the profound fryers fall someplace in the center. While the serving size will shift dependent on singular needs, a 6 cup fryer is frequently enough for an OK measure of food for two individuals.

A few fryers accompany two huge bins or a blend of enormous and little bushels in the event that you want to make a little sum. Numerous profound fryers available today are enormous, requiring assigned counter space or capacity zone. Profound fryers are basic in café settings, but on the other hand, they're getting progressively famous among property holders.

The two sorts of fryers require some The cooking time to get your food pleasant and firm. In spite of the fact that they will, in general, be littler, air fryers commonly take longer in light of the fact that the food is cooked by hot air instead of oil. In a profound fryer, the hot oil heats up food quicker, bringing about speedier The cooking time.

3. Profound Fryers versus Air Fryers: Healthiness

Let's be honest — fryers aren't the most beneficial cooking cooker around. Another consideration as you're discussing an air fryer versus a profound fryer is calories. It's difficult to get those mouth-watering results (and the perfect measure of freshness) without utilizing oil, which implies more calories. Profound fryers work by utilizing a lot of oil, which the food is then dove into and expelled from. Then again, air fryers don't dunk food into hot tanks of oil. Despite the fact that you will place your food into a container with the air fryer, it's covered with a modest quantity of oil. The air fryer at that point blows hot air over it to cook the food.

If you're in the market for a dry fryer, which depends on heat as opposed to oil to cook food, you might need to consider one with Rapid Air Technology. This sort of innovation is fairly new available, and by and large, requires an insignificant measure of oil. A portion of the top air fryers available with this innovation utilizes something like 70 percent less oil than customary fryers.

In the event that you need a profound fryer rather, the Hamilton Beach 35034 Professional-Style Deep Fryer is pleasant in light of the fact that it has twofold crates with snares for simple depleting, so you get each and every drop of abundance oil off the outside of your food.

4. Profound Fryers versus Air Fryers: Maintenance and Reliability

If you don't care for high upkeep apparatuses, you'll be very content with a profound or air fryer. The two sorts of fryers normally keep going for quite a while absent a lot of exertion on your end. One choice that may speak to you is the GoWISE USA GW22621 Electric Air Fryer, which delivers an assortment of firm foods utilizing next to zero oil and won't use up every last cent.

The greatest protest among clients of the two sorts of fryers is that the plastic parts, for example, handles or even dishes to get overabundance oil, can sever or wear out after some time. In any case, these issues (on the off chance that they do happen by any stretch of the imagination) appear to collect following a couple of long periods of consistent use. The ideal approach to keep up the two sorts of fryers is to routinely investigate them, clean the units at customary interims, and intermittently check for indications of mileage. Most fryers (the two sorts) likewise require the oil to be depleted or sifted.

5. Profound Fryers versus Air Fryers: Price

You, by and large, get a great deal of value for your money with the two kinds of fryers. You'll pay more forthright for it is possible that one, yet the general dependability, low support after some time, and consistently flavorful outcomes make a fryer an incredible venture. It may appear as though profound fryers are more costly in light of the fact that they're a lot greater than air fryers. Be that as it may, most air fryers will, in general, cost more, particularly on the off chance that they're utilizing forefront innovation or inventive browning frameworks. A fair value run for a top-notch profound fryer is by and large somewhere in the range of $50 and $100. You can locate a balanced fryer for less, however, particularly on the off chance that it has a progressively minimized size.

Air fryers, then again, will, in general, range somewhere in the range of $100 and $200. In contrast to profound fryers, it's the particular innovation that the air fryer utilizes — as opposed to estimate — that directs the last cost. Most pricier models have Rapid Air innovation for quicker and increasingly proficient cooking (also less oil use when cooking). These units are additionally well-outfitted with highlights that numerous consumers find very valuable, from programmable settings to scent control and splendidly lit showcase screens with commencement clocks and alerts. If you're on a strict spending plan. However, this doesn't imply that you can't discover a consummately decent air fryer at a somewhat increasingly moderate cost. One ease alternative you may like is the VonShef Stainless Steel Deep Fryer, which just expenses $39.99.

THE SIMILARITIES BETWEEN THE AIR FRYER AND THE DEEP FRYER

Air Fryer versus Deep Fryer

Here we have set aside the effort to plunge into the subject of how air fryers and profound fryers analyze. What are their likenesses? What are the benefits of an air fryer? Does the profound fryer have a few favorable circumstances as well? We trust this article responds to every one of your inquiries on the clash of the air fryer versus profound fryer.

From the outset, air fryers and profound fryers could be viewed as being very comparable, and they are both after totally intended to cook food that is both scrumptious and has that seared food crunch. The strategy for how this outcome is accomplished is the place the air fryer and profound fryer contrast. The customary profound fryer includes sinking food into a pool of hot oil, oil that contains a great deal of fat. Air fryers attempt to decrease the oil required, some of the time to zero, to cook food, yet giving the ideal taste and surface. The air fryer expects to accomplish this by shooting the food with rapidly coursing hot air. Those with an eye on smart dieting will take note of the decrease in oil required is a significant advantage of the air fryer technique.

Both air fryers and profound fryers provide food for a scope of spending plans.

1.   Air Fryer versus The Deep Fryer: Features

Here we'll lay out some key highlights you ought to consider during the way toward concluding which to purchase, an air fryer or profound fryer.

In the same way, like other kitchen apparatuses, both air fryers and profound fryers share some fundamental highlights, to be specific, digital screens, advanced or straightforward temperature controls, and an ergonomic structure. Air fryers go a lot in cost, and for the most part, the more costly, the more highlights it has. A few fryers even accompany cooking pre-sets for various food types.

Thinks to consider incorporate, does it have a clock with auto-shutdown? How simple are the materials to clean? Support of an air fryer is fairly basic, see our guide on the best way to think about the air fryer cooker here.

Profound fryers require various highlights, and as I would see it, the most significant interesting point when buying a profound fryer is smell control, search for one with a charcoal channel. Along these lines to the air fryer, you ought to consider that it is so natural to clean and keep up the profound fryer. Given the huge amounts of oil, cleaning, and care is additional tedious with a profound fryer.

Wellbeing is likewise of essential worry with a profound fryer, consider fryers that have cool-touch handles and a showcase window in the top.

2.   Air Fryer versus Deep Fryer: Size and Cooking Capacity

We have recently expounded on the sizes and limits of air fryers accessible; see it here to enable you to choose what size you'll require.

This is one of the vast dividers in the skirmish of the air fryer versus profound fryer. Air fryers do regularly have a littler cooking limit, however, produces are tending to this issue with some presently propelling XXL ranges. Likewise, the way that the apparatus doesn't have to hold a huge sum of oil implies air fryers are commonly littler in size, occupying less counter room contrasted with a profound fryer.

We would prescribe going for the biggest air fryer your spending will permit as you'll presumably utilize it more than you anticipate. If you know you'll just utilize it for the odd little tidbit, there are a lot of littler ones available.

A 6 cup (size) profound fryer is commonly large enough for two individuals. Anyway, profound fryers do go in size from 2 to 12 cups. The bigger ones regularly accompanying 2 huge containers, instead of only one. Profound fryers are commonly less convenient than air fryers, so ensure you have enough counter space to forget about it fall time.

3.   Air Fryer versus Deep Fryer: Health

Profound fryers aren't considered the most beneficial approach to cook your food, yet the vast majority of us are suckers for the food they produce. Air fryer makers guarantee that air cooking uses 80% less oil versus profound broiling. Clients of air fryers guarantee that the measure of oil required is even less; a few clients cook with no oil by any means. The huge decrease in oil utilized is the place the air fryer gets its a medical advantage over the profound fryer.

4.   Air Fryer versus Deep Fryer: Maintenance and Reliability

Air fryers and profound fryers are both, for the most part, low kept up and solid. The fundamental consideration is how simple either is to clean, and this fluctuates by brand and model, get your work done on your picked model.

Both apparatus structures are all around tried now, and both ordinarily have a decent life expectancy, which is dependant on how frequently you use it, and how you care for it.

5.   Air Fryer versus Deep Fryer: Price

Slicing directly to it, profound fryers simply win here, and they are commonly a little less expensive than a similar air fryer. Numerous conspicuous brands have a better than average air fryer for around $70, and given the medical advantages over a profound fryer, the little expense is justified, despite all the trouble.

6.   Air Fryer versus Deep Fryer: Other considerations

Important is the air fryers flexibility, and it could be your lone home cooking cooker. You can see by the plans on our site that the air fryer can cook breakfast, lunch, and supper. Just as having the option to cook up a little treat now and once more.

AIR FRYER RECIPES

AIR FRYER BREAKFAST RECIPES

DELECTABLE BAKED EGGS

Planning time: 10 minutes The cooking time: 20 minutes The recipe servings: 4

Fixings:

4 eggs

1 pound child spinach, torn 7 ounces ham, cleaved

4 tablespoons milk

1 tablespoon of olive oil Cooking splash

Salt and dark pepper to the taste

Bearings:

1.   Heat a container with the oil over medium heat, include child spinach, mix cook for two or three minutes and take off the heat.

2.   Grease 4 ramekins with cooking splash and gap child spinach and ham in each.

3. Crack an egg in every ramekin, additionally partition milk, season with salt and pepper, place ramekins in the preheated air fryer at 350 degrees F and prepare for 20 minutes.

4. Serve heated eggs for breakfast. Appreciate!

The nutritional facts: calories 321, fat 6, fiber 8, carbs 15, protein 12

BREAKFAST EGG BOWLS

Planning time: 10 minutes

The cooking time: 20 minutes

The recipe servings: 4

Fixings:

1. 4 supper moves, finish cut off, and internal parts scooped out 4 tablespoons overwhelming cream

2. 4 eggs

3. 4 tablespoons blended chives and parsley Salt and dark pepper to the taste

4. 4 tablespoons parmesan, ground

Guidelines:

1.   Arrange supper moves on a preparing sheet and break an egg in each.

2.   Divide overwhelming cream, blended herbs in each roll and season with salt and pepper.

3.   Sprinkle parmesan on your moves, place them in the air fryer cooker, and cook at 350 Deg. Fahrenheit for about 20 minutes.

4.   Divide your bread bowls between plates and serve for breakfast. Appreciate!

Nourishment: calories 238, fat 4, fiber 7, carbs 14, protein 7

TASTY BREAKFAST SHOUFLE

The cooking time: 8 minutes

The recipe servings: 4

Fixings:

- 4 eggs, whisked

- 4 tablespoons overwhelming cream

- A touch of red bean stew pepper squashed 2 tablespoons parsley, slashed

- 2 tablespoons chives, hacked Salt and dark pepper to the taste

Guidelines:

1.   In a bowl, blend eggs in with salt, pepper, substantial cream, red bean stew pepper, parsley, and chives, mix well, and gap into 4 soufflé dishes.

2.   Arrange the dishes in the air-fryer and cook soufflés at 350 Deg. Fahrenheit for about 8 minutes.

3.   Serve them hot. Appreciate!

Sustenance: calories 300, fat 7, fiber 9, carbs 15, protein 6

AIR FRIED SANDWICH

Prep. time: multiple times

The cooking time: 6 minutes

The recipe servings: 2

Fixings:

2 English biscuits, divided 2 eggs

2 bacon strips

Salt and dark pepper to the taste

Guidelines:

1.   Crack eggs in the air fryer cooker, include bacon top, spread, and cook at 392 Deg. Fahrenheit for about 6 minutes.

2.   Heat your English biscuit parts in your microwave for a couple of moments, isolate eggs on 2 parts, include bacon top, season with salt and pepper, spread with the other 2 English biscuits, and serve for breakfast.

Enjoy the recipe!

The nutritional facts: calories 261, fat 5, fiber 8, carbs 12, protein 4

NATURAL BREAKFAST

Prep. time

The cooking time: 13 minutes

The recipe servings: 4

Fixings:

- 7   ounces child spinach

- 8   chestnuts mushrooms split 8 tomatoes, divided

- 1 garlic clove, minced 4 chipolatas

- 4 bacon cuts, hacked

- Salt and dark pepper to the taste 4 eggs

Cooking splash

Guidelines:

1. Grease a cooking dish with the oil and include tomatoes, garlic, and mushrooms.

2. Add bacon and chipolatas, additionally include spinach and break eggs toward the end.

3. Season with salt and pepper, place the dish in the cooking bushel of your air-fryer and cooking for 13 minutes at 350 degrees F.

4. Divide among plates and serve for breakfast. Enjoy the recipe!

The nutritional facts: calories 312, fat 6, fiber 8, carbs 15, protein 5

EGG MUFFINS

Prep. time: 10 minutes

The cooking time: 15 minutes The recipe servings: 4

Fixings:

- egg

- tablespoons olive oil 3 tablespoons milk

    o   ounces white flour
- 1 tablespoon heating powder 2 ounces parmesan, ground
- A sprinkle of Worcestershire sauce

Guidelines:

1.   In a bowl, blend egg in with the flour, oil, heating powder, milk, Worcestershire and parmesan, whisk well, and partition into 4 silicon biscuit cups.

2.   Arrange cups in the air fryer cooker's cooking crate, spread and cook at 392, Deg. Fahrenheit for about 15 minutes.

3.   Serve warm for breakfast. Enjoy the recipe!

The nutritional facts: calories 251, fat 6, fiber 8, carbs 9, protein 3

POLENTA BITES

Prep. time: 10 minutes

The cooking time: 20 minutes The recipe servings: 4

Fixings:

For the polenta:

- 1 tablespoon spread

- 1 cup cornmeal

- 3 cups of water

- Salt and dark pepper to the taste

For the polenta chomps:

- 2 tablespoons powdered sugar Cooking splash

Guidelines:

1. In a dish, blend water in with cornmeal, margarine, salt and pepper, mix, heat to the point of boiling over medium heat, cook for 10 minutes, take off heat, whisk once again and keep in the cooler

2. Scoop 1 tablespoon of the polenta, and shape a ball, and spot-on a working surface.

3. Repeat with the remainder of the polenta, organize all the balls in the cooking crate of the air fryer cooker, shower them with a cooking splash, spread, and cook at 380 Deg. Fahrenheit for about 8 minutes.

4. Arrange polenta chomps on plates, sprinkle sugar all finished, and serve for breakfast.

Enjoy the recipe!

The nutritional facts: calories 231, fat 7, fiber 8, carbs 12, protein 4

TASTY BREAKFAST POTATOES

Prep. time: 10 minutes

The cooking time: 35 minutes

The recipe servings: 4

Fixings:

- 2 tablespoons olive oil 3 potatoes, cubed
- 1 yellow onion, hacked 1 red ringer pepper, cleaved
- Salt and dark pepper to taste a teaspoon of garlic powder
- 1 teaspoon of the sweet paprika and 1 teaspoon onion powder

Guidelines:

1. Grease the air fryer cooker's crate with olive oil, include potatoes, hurl and season with salt and pepper.
2. Add onion, chime pepper, garlic powder, paprika, and onion powder, hurl well, spread, and cook at 370 Deg. Fahrenheit for about 30 minutes.
3. Divide potatoes blend on plates and serve for breakfast. Enjoy the recipe!

The nutritional facts: calories 214, fat 6, fiber 8, carbs 15, protein 4

DELICIOUS CINNAMON TOAST

Prep. time: 10 minutes

The cooking time: 5 minutes

The recipe servings: 6

Fixings:

- 1 stick spread, delicate 12 bread cuts

- ½ cup of sugar

- 1 and ½ teaspoon vanilla concentrate

- 1 and ½ teaspoon cinnamon powder

Guidelines:

1. In a bowl, blend delicate margarine in with sugar, vanilla, and cinnamon and whisk well.

2. Spread this on bread cuts, place them in the air fryer cooker and cook at 400 Deg. Fahrenheit for about 5 minutes,

3. Divide among plates and serve for breakfast. Enjoy the recipe!

The nutritional facts: calories 221, fat 4, fiber 7, carbs 12, protein 8

DELIGHTFUL POTATO HASH

Prep. time: 10 minutes

The cooking time: 25 minutes

The recipe servings: 4

Fixings:

- 1 and ½ potatoes, cubed 1 yellow onion, cleaved 2 teaspoons olive oil
- 1 green chime pepper, hacked Salt and dark pepper to the taste
- ½ teaspoon thyme dried 2 eggs

Guidelines:

1. Heat the air-fryer at 350 degrees F, including oil, heat it, include onion, chime pepper, salt, and pepper, mix and cook for 5 minutes.
2. Add potatoes, thyme and eggs, mix, spread and cook at 360 Deg. Fahrenheit for about 20 minutes.
3. Divide among plates and serve for breakfast. Enjoy the recipe!

The nutritional facts: calories 241, fat 4, fiber 7, carbs 12, protein 7

SWEET BREAKFAST CASSEROLE

Prep. Time: 10 minutes

The cooking time: 30 minutes

The recipe servings: 4

Fixings:

- 3 tablespoons dark colored sugar 4 tablespoons spread

- 2 tablespoons white sugar
- ½ teaspoon cinnamon powder
- ½ cup flour
- For the meal:
- 2 eggs
- 2 tablespoons of white sugar 2 and ½ cups white flour 1 teaspoon preparing pop
- teaspoon preparing powder 2 eggs
- ½ cup milk
- cups buttermilk
- tablespoons spread
- Get-up-and-go from 1 lemon, ground 1 and 2/3 cup blueberries

Guidelines:

1.   In a bowl, blend eggs in with 2 tablespoons white sugar, 2 and ½ cups white flour, heating powder, preparing pop, 2 eggs, milk, buttermilk, 4 tablespoons margarine, lemon pizzazz, and blueberries, mix and fill a skillet that accommodates the air fryer cooker.

2.   In other dishes, blend 3 tablespoons darker sugar with 2 tablespoons white sugar, 4 tablespoons margarine, ½ cup flour, and cinnamon, mix until you acquire a disintegrate and spread over blueberries blend.

3.   Place in preheated air fryer and heat at 300 Deg. Fahrenheit for about 30 minutes.

4.   Divide among plates and serve for breakfast. Enjoy the recipe!

The nutritional facts: calories 214, fat 5, fiber 8, carbs 12, protein 5

EGGS CASSEROLE

Prep. Time: 10 minutes

The cooking time: 25 minutes

The recipe servings: 6

Fixings:

- 1 pound of turkey, ground 1 tablespoon of olive oil

- ½ teaspoon bean stew powder 12 eggs

- 1 sweet potato, cubed 1 cup infant spinach

- Salt and dark pepper to the taste 2 tomatoes, cleaved for serving

Guidelines:

1. In a bowl, blend eggs in with salt, pepper, bean stew powder, potato, spinach, turkey, and sweet potato and whisk well.

2. Heat the air-fryer cooker at 350 degrees F, include oil, and heat it.

3. Add eggs blend, spread into the air fryer cooker, spread, and cook for 25 minutes.

4. Divide among plates and serve for breakfast. Enjoy the recipe!

The nutritional facts: calories 300, fat 5, fiber 8, carbs 13, protein 6

HOTDOG, EGGS AND CHEESE MIX

Prep. time: 10 minutes

The cooking time: 20 minutes

The recipe servings: 4

Fixings:

- 10 ounces hotdogs, cooked and disintegrated 1 cup cheddar, destroyed

- 1 cup mozzarella cheddar, destroyed 8 eggs, whisked

- 1 cup milk

- Salt and dark pepper to the taste Cooking splash

Guidelines:

1. In a bowl, blend hotdogs in with cheddar, mozzarella, eggs, milk, salt, and pepper and whisk well.

2. Heat-up the air-fryer at 380 deg. F, splash cooking oil, include eggs and frankfurter blend, and cook for 20 minutes.

3. Divide among plates and serve. Enjoy the recipe!

The nutritional facts: calories 320, fat 6, fiber 8, carbs 12, protein 5

CHEDDAR AIR FRIED BAKE

Prep. time: 10 minutes

The cooking time: 20 minutes

The recipe servings: 4

Fixings:

- 4 bacon cuts, cooked and disintegrated 2 cups milk

- 2 and ½ cups cheddar, destroyed

- 1 pound breakfast wiener, housings evacuated and slashed 2 eggs

- ½ teaspoon onion powder

- Salt and dark pepper to the taste 3 tablespoons parsley, cleaved Cooking shower

Guidelines:

1.	In a bowl, blend eggs in with milk, cheddar, onion powder, salt, pepper, and parsley and whisk well.

2.	Grease the air fryer cooker with cooking shower, heat it up at 320 degrees F, and include bacon and hotdog.

3.	Add eggs blend, spread, and cook for 20 minutes.

4.	Divide among plates and serve. Enjoy the recipe!

The nutritional facts: calories 214, fat 5, fiber 8, carbs 12, protein 12

ROLLS CASSEROLE

Prep. time: 10 minutes

The cooking time: 15 minutes

The recipe servings: 8

Fixings:

- 12 ounces rolls, quartered 3 tablespoons flour
- ½ pound hotdog slashed
- A touch of salt and dark pepper 2 and ½ cups milk
- Cooking splash

Guidelines:

1. Grease the air fryer cooker with a cooking splash and heat it more than 350 degrees F.
2. Add rolls on the base and blend in with frankfurter.
3. Add flour, milk, salt, and pepper, hurl a piece and cook for 15 minutes.
4. Divide among plates and serve for breakfast. Enjoy the recipe!

The nutritional facts: calories 321, fat 4, fiber 7, carbs 12, protein 5

TURKEY BURRITO

Prep. time: 10 minutes

The cooking time: 10 minutes

The recipe servings: 2

Fixings:

- 4 cuts turkey bosom previously cooked

- ½ red ringer pepper, cut 2 eggs

- small avocado, stripped, hollowed and cut 2 tablespoons salsa

- Salt and dark pepper to the taste 1/8 cup mozzarella cheddar, ground Tortillas for serving

Guidelines:

1.   In a bowl, whisk the eggs with salt and pepper to the taste, pour them in a skillet and spot it in the air fryer's bin.

2.   Cook at 400-deg. F for 5 minutes, remove skillet from the fryer and move eggs to a plate.

3.   Arrange tortillas on a working surface, isolate eggs on them, likewise partition turkey meat, chime pepper, cheddar, salsa, and avocado.

4.   Roll your burritos and spot them in the air fryer cooker after you've fixed it with some tin foil.

5.   Heat-up the burritos at 300 Deg. Fahrenheit for about 3 minutes, separate them on plates and serve.

Enjoy the recipe!

The nutritional facts: calories 349, fat 23, fiber 11, carbs 20, protein 21

TOFU SCRAMBLE

Prep. time: 5 minutes

The cooking time: 30 minutes

The recipe servings: 4

Fixings:

- 2   tablespoons soy sauce 1 tofu square, cubed

- teaspoon turmeric, ground

- tablespoons additional virgin olive oil 4 cups broccoli florets

- ½ teaspoon onion powder

- ½ teaspoon garlic powder

- and ½ cup red potatoes, cubed

- ½ cup yellow onion hacked Salt and dark pepper to the taste

Guidelines:

1.   Mix tofu with 1 tablespoon oil, salt, the pepper, the soy sauce, garlic powder, onion powder, turmeric and onion in a bowl, mix and leave aside.

2.   In a different bowl, consolidate potatoes with the remainder of the oil, a spot of salt and pepper, and hurl to cover.

3.   Place the potatoes in the air fryer at 350 degrees F and prepare for 15 minutes, shaking once.

4.   Add the tofu and its marinade to the air fryer and prepare for 15 minutes.

5.   Add the broccoli to the air-fryer and cook everything for 5 minutes more.

6.   Serve immediately. Enjoy the recipe!

The nutritional facts: calories 140, fat 4, fiber 3, carbs 10, protein 14

OATMEAL CASSEROLE

Prep. time: 10 minutes

The cooking time: 20 minutes

The recipe servings: 8

Fixings:

- 2 cups moved oats

- 1 teaspoon heating powder 1/3 cup darker sugar

- 1 teaspoon cinnamon powder

- ½ cup chocolate chips 2/3 cup blueberries

- 1 banana, stripped and squashed 2 cups milk

- 1 egg

- 2   tablespoons margarine

- 1 teaspoon vanilla concentrate Cooking shower

Guidelines:

1. In a bowl, blend sugar in with heating powder, cinnamon, chocolate chips, blueberries, and banana and mix.

2. In a different bowl, blend eggs in with vanilla concentrate and margarine and mix.

3. Heat the air-fryer cooker at 320 degrees F, oil with cooking shower, and include oats the base.

4. Add cinnamon blend and eggs blend, hurl and cook for 20 minutes.

5. Stir once again, isolate into bowls and serve for breakfast. Enjoy the recipe!

The nutritional facts: calories 300, fat 4, fiber 7, carbs 12, protein 10

HAM BREAKFAST

Prep. time: 10 minutes

The cooking time: 15 min.

The recipe servings: 6

Fixings:

- 6 cups French bread, cubed
- 4 ounces green chilies, slashed 10 ounces ham, cubed
- 4   ounces cheddar, destroyed 2 cups milk
- 5   eggs
- 1 tablespoon mustard
- Salt and dark pepper to the taste Cooking shower

Guidelines:

1. Heat the air-fryer cooker at 350 degrees F and oil it with cooking shower.

2. In a bowl, blend eggs in with milk, cheddar, mustard, salt, and pepper and mix.

3. Add bread blocks in the air fryer cooker and blend in with chilies and ham.

4. Add eggs blend, spread, and cook for 15 minutes.

5. Divide among plates and serve. Enjoy the recipe!

The nutritional facts: calories 200, fat 5, fiber 6, carbs 12, protein 14

TOMATO AND BACON BREAKFAST

Prep. time: 10 minutes

The cooking time: 30 minutes

Recipes The recipe servings: 6

Fixings:

- 1 pound white bread, cubed

- 1 pound smoked bacon, cooked and slashed

- ¼ cup olive oil

- 1 yellow onion, slashed

- 28 ounces canned tomatoes, slashed

- ½ teaspoon red pepper, squashed

- ½ pound cheddar, destroyed

- 2 tablespoons chives, slashed

- ½ pound Monterey jack destroyed 2 tablespoons stock

- Salt and dark pepper to the taste 8 eggs, whisked.

Guidelines:

1. Add oil to the air fryer and heat it up at 350 degrees F.

2. Add bread, the bacon, the onion, tomatoes, red pepper, and stock and mix.

3. Add eggs, cheese and the Monterey jack and cook everything for 20 minutes.

4. Divide among plates, sprinkle chives, and serve. Enjoy the recipe!

The nutritional facts: calories 231, fat 5, fiber 7, carbs 12, protein 4

SCRUMPTIOUS HASH

Prep. time: 10 minutes

The cooking time: 15 minutes

The recipe servings: 6

Fixings:

- 16 ounces hash tans

- ¼ cup olive oil

- ½ teaspoon paprika

- ½ teaspoon garlic powder

- Salt and dark pepper to the taste 1 egg, whisked.

- 2 tablespoon chives, slashed 1 cup cheddar, destroyed

Guidelines:

1. Add oil to the air-fryer, heat it at 350 degrees F, and include hash tans.

2. Also include paprika, garlic powder, salt, pepper, and egg, hurl, and cook for 15 minutes.

3. Add cheddar and chives, hurl, separate among plates and serve. Enjoy the recipe!

The nutritional facts: calories 213, fat 7, fiber 8, carbs 12, protein 4

CREAMY HASH BROWNS

Prep. time: 10 minutes

The cooking time: 20 minutes

The recipe servings: 6

Fixings:

- 2 pounds hash tans 1 cup entire milk

- 8 bacon cuts, hacked 9 ounces cream cheddar

- 1 yellow onion, hacked

- 1 cup cheddar, destroyed 6 green onions, hacked

- Salt and dark pepper to the taste 6 eggs

- Cooking splash

Guidelines:

1. Heat the air-fryer cooker at 350 degrees F and oil it with cooking splash.

2. In a bowl, blend eggs in with milk, cream cheddar, cheddar, bacon, onion, salt, and pepper and whisk well.

3. Add hash tans to the air fryer cooker, include eggs blend over them and cook for 20 minutes.

4. Divide among plates and serve. Enjoy the recipe!

The nutritional facts: calories 261, fat 6, fiber 9, carbs 8, protein 12

BLACKBERRY FRENCH TOAST

Prep. time: 10 minutes

The cooking time: 20 minutes

The recipe servings: 6

Fixings:

1 cup of blackberry jam, warm 12 ounces bread portion and cubed

8 ounces cream cheddar, cubed 4 eggs

1 teaspoon cinnamon powder 2 cups cream

½ cup dark colored sugar

1 teaspoon vanilla concentrate Cooking splash

Guidelines:

1.   Grease the air fryer cooker with cooking splash and heat it up at 300 degrees F.

2.   Add blueberry jam on the base, layer half of the bread shapes, at that point include cream cheddar and top with the remainder of the bread.

3.   In a bowl, blend eggs in with creamer, cinnamon, sugar and vanilla, whisk well and include over bread blend.

4.   Cook for 20 minutes, separate among plates and serve for breakfast. Enjoy the recipe!

The nutritional facts: calories 215, fat 6, fiber 9, carbs 16, protein 6

SMOKED SAUSAGE BREAKFAST MIX

Prep. time: 10 minutes

The cooking time: 30 minutes

The recipe servings: 4

Fixings:

1 and ½ pounds smoked hotdog, hacked and seared A spot of salt and dark pepper

1 and ½ cups corn meal 4 and ½ cups water

16 ounces cheddar, destroyed 1 cup milk

¼ teaspoon garlic powder

1 and ½ teaspoons thyme, hacked Cooking splash

4 eggs, whisked

Guidelines:

1.   Put the water in a pot, heat to the point of boiling over medium heat, include cornmeal, mix, spread, cook for 5 minutes, and take off the heat.

2.   Add cheddar, mix until it melts and blend in with milk, thyme, salt, pepper, garlic powder, and eggs and whisk truly well.

3.   Heat the air-fryer cooker at 300 degrees F, oil with a cooking splash, and include seared hotdog.

4.   Add cornmeal blend, spread, and cook for 25 minutes.

5.   Divide among plates and serve for breakfast. Enjoy the recipe!

The nutritional facts: calories 321, fat 6, fiber 7, carbs 17, protein 4

DELECTABLE POTATO FRITTATA

Prep. time: 10 minutes

The cooking time: 20 minutes

The recipe servings: 6

Fixings:

6 ounces jostled broiled red chime peppers, slashed 12 eggs, whisked

½ cup parmesan, ground 3 garlic cloves, minced

2 tablespoons parsley, hacked Salt and dark pepper to the taste 2 tablespoons chives, cleaved 16 potato wedges

6 tablespoons ricotta cheddar Cooking splash

Guidelines:

1.   In a bowl, blend eggs in with red peppers, garlic, parsley, salt, pepper, and ricotta and whisk well.

2.   Heat the air-fryer cooker at 300 degrees F and oil it with cooking splash.

3.   Add a portion of the potato wedges on the base and sprinkle half of the parmesan everywhere.

4.   Add a portion of the egg blend, including the remainder of the potatoes and the remainder of the parmesan.

5.   Add the remainder of the eggs blend, sprinkle chives and cook for 20 minutes.

6.   Divide among plates and serve for breakfast. Enjoy the recipe!

The nutritional facts: calories 312, fat 6, fiber 9, carbs 16, protein 5

ASPARAGUS FRITTATA

Prep. time: 10 minutes

The cooking time: 5 minutes

The recipe servings: 2

Fixings:

- 4 eggs, whisked

- 2   tablespoons parmesan, ground 4 tablespoons milk

- Salt and dark pepper to the taste 10 asparagus tips, steamed Cooking splash.

Guidelines:

1. In a bowl, blend eggs in with parmesan, milk, salt, and pepper and whisk well.

2. Heat the air-fryer at 400 degrees F and oil with cooking shower.

3. Add asparagus, include eggs blend, hurl a piece, and cook for 5 minutes.

4. Divide the frittata between the plates and then serve for breakfast. Enjoy the recipe!

The nutritional facts: calories 312, fat 5, fiber 8, carbs 14, protein 2

UNCOMMON CORN FLAKES BREAKFAST CASSEROLE

Prep. time: 10 minutes

The cooking time: 8 minutes

The recipe servings: 5

Fixings:

- 1/3 cup milk

- 3   teaspoons sugar

- 2 eggs, whisked

- ¼ teaspoon nutmeg, ground

- ¼ cup blueberries

- 4   tablespoons cream cheddar, whipped 1 and ½ cups corn drops, disintegrated

- 5   bread cuts

Guidelines:

1.   In a bowl, blend eggs in with sugar, nutmeg, and milk and whisk well.

2.   In another bowl, blend cream cheddar with blueberries and whisk well.

3.   Put corn pieces in a third bowl.

4.   Spread blueberry blend on each bread cut; at that point, dunk in eggs blend and dig in corn chips toward the end.

5.   Place bread in the air fryer cooker's bushel, heat up at 400 degrees F, and prepare for 8 minutes.

6.   Divide among plates and serve for breakfast. Enjoy the recipe!

The nutritional facts: calories 300, fat 5, fiber 7, carbs 16, protein 4

HAM BREAKFAST PIE

Prep. time: 10 minutes

The cooking time: 25 minutes

The recipe servings: 6

Fixings:

16 ounces sickle moves mixture 2 eggs, whisked

2 cups cheddar, ground 1 tablespoon parmesan, ground

2 cups ham, cooked and cleaved Salt and dark pepper to the taste Cooking splash

Guidelines:

1.   Grease the air fryer cooker's container with cooking splash and press half of the sickle moves batter on the base.

2.   In a bowl, blend eggs in with cheddar, parmesan, salt, and pepper, whisk well and include over batter.

3.   Spread ham, cut the remainder of the sickle moves batter in strips, orchestrate them over ham and cook at 300 deg. F for 25 min.

4.   Slice pie and serve for breakfast. Enjoy the recipe!

The nutritional facts: calories 400, fat 27, fiber 7, carbs 22, protein 16

BREAKFAST VEGGIE MIX

Prep. time: 10 minutes

The cooking time: 25 minutes

The recipe servings: 6

Fixings:

- 1 yellow onion, cut

- red ringer pepper, cleaved 1 gold potato, hacked

- tablespoons olive oil

- 8 ounces brie, cut and cubed 12 ounces sourdough bread, cubed 4 ounces parmesan, ground

- 8 eggs

- tablespoons mustard

- cups of milk

- Salt and dark pepper to the taste

Guidelines:

1.   Heat the air-fryer cooker at 350 degrees F, include oil, onion, potato, and ringer pepper, and cook for 5 minutes.

2.   In a bowl, blend eggs in with milk, salt, pepper, and mustard and whisk well.

3.   Add the bread and the brie to the air fryer cooker, include half of the eggs blend and include half of the parmesan also.

4.   Add the remainder of the bread and parmesan, hurl only a tad, and cook for 20 minutes.

5.   Divide among plates and serve for breakfast. Enjoy the recipe!

The nutritional facts: calories 231, fat 5, fiber 10, carbs 20, protein 12

FRIED EGGS

Prep. time: 10 minutes

The cooking time: 10 minutes

The recipe servings: 2

Fixings:

- 2 eggs

- 2 tablespoons spread

- Salt and dark pepper to the taste 1 red chime pepper, slashed.

- A touch of sweet paprika

Guidelines:

1. In a bowl, blend eggs in with salt, pepper, paprika, and red chime pepper and whisk well.

2. Heat the air-fryer cooker at 140 deg. F, including spread and dissolve it.

3. Add eggs blend, mix and cook for 10 minutes.

4. Divide fried eggs between plates and serve for breakfast. Enjoy the recipe!

The nutritional facts: calories 200, fat 4, fiber 7, carbs 10, protein 3

QUICK EGGS AND TOMATOES

Prep. time: 5 minutes

The cooking time: 10 minutes

The recipe servings: 4

Fixings:

4 eggs

2 ounces milk

2 tablespoons parmesan, ground Salt and dark pepper to the taste 8 cherry tomatoes, divided Cooking shower

Guidelines:

1.   Grease the air fryer cooker with cooking shower and heat it up at 200 degrees F.

2.   In a bowl, blend eggs in with cheddar, milk, salt, and pepper and whisk.

3.   Add this blend to the air fryer cooker and cook for 6 minutes.

4.   Add tomatoes, cook your fried eggs for 3 minutes, isolate among plates and serve.

Enjoy the recipe!

The nutritional facts: calories 200, fat 4, fiber 7, carbs 12, protein 3

AIR FRIED TOMATO BREAKFAST QUICHE

Prep. time: 10 minutes

The cooking time: 30 minutes

heTThe recipe servings: 1

Fixings:

2 tablespoons yellow onion, slashed 2 eggs

¼ cup milk

½ cup gouda cheddar, destroyed

¼ cup tomatoes, slashed

Salt and dark pepper to the taste Cooking shower

Guidelines:

1.   Grease a ramekin with cooking shower.

2.   Crack eggs include onion, milk, cheddar, tomatoes, salt, and pepper and mix.

3.   Add this in the air fryer cooker's skillet and cook at 340 Deg. Fahrenheit for about 30 minutes.

4.   Serve hot. Enjoy the recipe!

The nutritional facts: calories 241, fat 6, fiber 8, carbs 14, protein 6

BREAKFAST MUSHROOM QUICHE

Prep. time: 10 minutes

The cooking time: 10 minutes

The recipe servings: 4

Fixings:

1 tablespoon flour

1   tablespoon margarine, delicate 9 inch pie batter

2   button mushrooms, slashed 2 tablespoons ham, hacked

3   eggs

1 little yellow onion, slashed 1/3 cup overwhelming cream

A spot of nutmeg, ground

Salt and dark pepper to the taste

½ teaspoon thyme, dried

¼ cup Swiss cheddar, ground

Guidelines:

1.   Clean a working surface with the flour and roll the pie mixture.

2.   Press in on the base of the pie skillet the air fryer cooker has.

3.   In a bowl, blend margarine in with mushrooms, ham, onion, eggs, overwhelming cream, salt, pepper, thyme, and nutmeg and whisk well.

4.   Add this over pie outside layer, spread, sprinkle Swiss cheddar all finished, and spot pie dish in the air fryer cooker.

5.   Cook the quiche at 400 Deg. Fahrenheit for about 10 minutes.

6.   Slice and serve for breakfast. Enjoy the recipe!

The nutritional facts: calories 212, fat 4, fiber 6, carbs 7, protein 7

SMOKED AIR FRIED TOFU BREAKFAST

Prep. time: 10 minutes

The cooking time: 12 minutes

The recipe servings: 2

Fixings:

- 1 tofu square, squeezed and cubed Salt and dark pepper to the taste 1 tablespoon smoked paprika

- ¼ cup cornstarch Cooking shower

Guidelines:

1.   Grease the air fryer cooker's container with a cooking splash and heat the fryer at 370 degrees F.

2.   In a bowl, blend tofu in with salt, pepper, smoked paprika, and cornstarch and hurl well.

3.   Add tofu to you air fryer's bushel and cook for 12 minutes, shaking the fryer at regular intervals.

4.   Divide into bowls and serve for breakfast. Enjoy the recipe!

The nutritional facts: calories 172, fat 4, fiber 7, carbs 12, protein 4

TASTY TOFU AND MUSHROOMS

Prep. time: 10 minutes

The cooking time: 10 minutes The recipe servings: 2

Fixings:

1 tofu square, squeezed and cut into medium pieces 1 cup panko bread scraps

Salt and dark pepper to the taste

½ tablespoons flour 1 egg

1 tablespoon mushrooms, minced

Guidelines:

1.   In a bowl, blend egg in with mushrooms, flour, salt, and pepper and whisk well.

2.   Dip tofu pieces in egg blend. At that point, dig them in panko bread scraps.

3.   Serve them for breakfast immediately. Enjoy the recipe!

The nutritional facts: calories 142, fat 4, fiber 6, carbs 8, protein 3

BREAKFAST BROCCOLI QUICHE

Prep. time: 10 minutes

The cooking time: 20 minutes

The recipe servings: 2

Fixings:

- 1 broccoli head, florets isolated and steamed 1 tomato, hacked

- 3 carrots, hacked and steamed 2 ounces cheddar, ground 2 eggs

- 2 ounces milk

- teaspoon parsley, hacked 1 teaspoon thyme, cleaved

- Salt and dark pepper to the taste

Guidelines:

1.   In a bowl, blend eggs in with milk, parsley, thyme, salt, and pepper and whisk well.

2.   Put broccoli, carrots, and tomato in the air fryer cooker.

3.   Add eggs blend on top, spread cheddar, spread, and cook at 350 Deg. Fahrenheit for about 20 minutes.

4. Divide among plates and serve for breakfast. Enjoy the recipe!

The nutritional facts: calories 214, fat 4, fiber 7, carbs 12, protein 3

CREAMY EGGS

Prep. time: 10 minutes

The cooking time: 12 minutes

The recipe servings: 4

Fixings:

2 teaspoons spread, delicate 2 ham cuts

4 eggs

2 tablespoons overwhelming cream

Salt and dark pepper to the taste 3 tablespoons parmesan, ground 2 teaspoons chives, hacked.

A touch of smoked paprika

Guidelines:

1. Grease the air fryer cooker's dish with the margarine, line it with the ham and add it to the air fryer cooker's bushel.

2.	In a bowl, blend 1 egg in with overwhelming cream, salt, and pepper, whisk well, and include over ham.

3.	Crack the remainder of the eggs in the container, sprinkle parmesan and cook your blend for 12 minutes at 320 degrees F.

4.	Sprinkle paprika and chives all finished, partition among plates and serve for breakfast.

Enjoy the recipe!

The nutritional facts: calories 263, fat 5, fiber 8, carbs 12, protein 5

MUSHY BREAKFAST BREAD

Prep. time: 10 minutes

The cooking time: 8 minutes

The recipe servings: 3

Fixings:

6 bread cuts

5	tablespoons margarine, liquefied 3 garlic cloves, minced

6	teaspoons sun-dried tomato pesto 1 cup mozzarella cheddar, ground

Guidelines:

1.   Arrange bread cuts on a working surface.

2.   Spread margarine all finished, partition tomato glue, garlic, and top with ground cheddar.

3.   Add bread cuts to your heated air fryer and cook them at 350 Deg. Fahrenheit for about 8 minutes.

4.   Divide among plates and serve for breakfast. Enjoy the recipe!

The nutritional facts: calories 187, fat 5, fiber 6, carbs 8, protein 3

BREAKFAST BREAD PUDDING

Prep. time: 10 minutes

The cooking time: 22 minutes

The recipe servings: 4

Fixings:

½ pound white bread, cubed

¾ cup milk

¾ cup of water

2 teaspoons cornstarch

½ cup apple, stripped, cored and generally cleaved 5 tablespoons HONNEY

1   teaspoon vanilla concentrate

2 of teaspoons cinnamon powder 1 and 1/3 cup flour

3/5 cup dark colored sugar 3 ounces delicate margarine

Guidelines:

1.   In a bowl, blend bread in with apple, milk with water, HONNEY, cinnamon, vanilla, and cornstarch and whisk well.

2.   In a different bowl, blend flour in with sugar and margarine and mix until you get a disintegrated blend.

3.   Press portion of the disintegrate blend on the base of the air fryer cooker, include bread and apple blend, including the remainder of the disintegrate and cook everything at 350 Deg. Fahrenheit for about 22 minutes.

4.   Divide bread pudding between plates and serve. Enjoy the recipe!

The nutritional facts: calories 261, fat 7, fiber 7, carbs 8, protein 5

BUTTERMILK BREAKFAST BISCUIT

Prep. time: 10 minutes

The cooking time: 8 minutes

The recipe servings: 4

Fixings:

1 and ¼ cup white flour

½ cup self-rising flour

¼ teaspoon heating pop

½ teaspoon heating powder 1 teaspoon sugar

4   tablespoons margarine, cold and cubed+ 1 tablespoon softened spread

¾ cup buttermilk Maple syrup for serving

Guidelines:

1.   In a bowl, blend white flour in with self-rising flour, heating pop, preparing powder and sugar, and mix.

2.   Add virus spread and mix utilizing your hands.

3.   Add buttermilk, mix until you get a mixture, and move to a floured working surface.

4.   Roll your batter and cut 10 pieces utilizing a round shaper.

5.   Arrange bread rolls in the air fryer cooker's cake skillet, brush them with dissolved spread and cook at 400 Deg. Fahrenheit for about 8 minutes.

6.   Serve them for breakfast with some maple syrup on top. Enjoy the recipe!

The nutritional facts: calories 192, fat 6, fiber 9, carbs 12, protein 3

BREAKFAST BREAD ROLLS

Prep. time: 10 minutes

The cooking time: 12 minutes

The recipe servings: 4

Fixings:

- 5   potatoes, bubbled, stripped and squashed 8 bread cuts, white parts as it were

- coriander pack, slashed 2 green chilies, hacked

- small yellow onions, hacked

- ½ teaspoon turmeric powder 2 curry leaf springs

- ½ teaspoon mustard seeds 2 tablespoons olive oil

- Salt and dark pepper to the taste

Guidelines:

1. Heat up a skillet with 1 teaspoon oil, include mustard seeds, onions, curry leaves, and turmeric, mix and cook for a couple of moments.

2. Add pureed potatoes, salt, pepper, coriander, and chilies, mix well, take off the heat and chill it off.

3. Divide potatoes blend into 8 sections and shape ovals utilizing your wet hands.

4. Wet bread cuts with water, press so as to deplete overabundance water and keep one cut in your palm.

5. Add a potato oval over bread cut and fold it over it.

6. Repeat with the remainder of the potato blend and bread.

7. Heat up the air fryer cooker at 400 degrees F, including the remainder of the oil, including bread moves, cook them for 12 minutes.

8. Divide bread moves on plates and serves for breakfast. Enjoy the recipe!

The nutritional facts: calories 261, fat 6, fiber 9, carbs 12, protein 7

SPANISH OMELET

Prep. time: 10 minutes The cooking time: 10 minutes The recipe servings: 4

Fixings:

- 3   eggs

- ½ chorizo, cleaved

- 1 potato, stripped and cubed

- ½ cup of corn

- 1 tablespoon of olive oil

- 1 tablespoon parsley, cleaved

- 1 tablespoon feta cheddar, disintegrated Salt and dark pepper to the taste

Guidelines:

1.   Heat up the air fryer cooker at 350 degrees F and include oil.

2.   Add chorizo and potatoes, mix, and dark-colored them for a couple of moments.

3.   In a bowl, blend eggs in with corn, parsley, cheddar, salt, and pepper, and whisk.

4.   Pour this over chorizo and potatoes, spread, and cook for 5 minutes.

5.   Divide omelet between plates and serve for breakfast. Enjoy the recipe!

The nutritional facts: calories 300, fat 6, fiber 9, carbs 12, protein 6

EGG WHITE OMELET

Prep. time: 10 minutes

The cooking time: 15 minutes

The recipe servings: 4

Fixings:

- cup egg whites

- ¼ cup tomato, cleaved 2 tablespoons skim milk

- ¼ cup mushrooms, cleaved

- tablespoons chives, cleaved Salt and dark pepper to the taste

Guidelines:

1.   In a bowl, blend egg whites with tomato, milk, mushrooms, chives, salt, and pepper, whisk well and immerse the air fryer cooker's container.

2.   Cook at 320 deg. F for just 15 minutes, chill omelet off, cut, separate among plates and serve.

Enjoy the recipe!

The nutritional facts: calories 100, fat 3, fiber 6, carbs 7, carbs 4

ARTICHOKE FRITTATA

Prep. time: 10 minutes

The cooking time: 15 minutes

RECIPES The recipe servings: 6

Fixings:

- 3   canned artichokes hearts, depleted and hacked 2 tablespoons olive oil

- ½ teaspoon oregano, dried

- Salt and dark pepper to the taste 6 eggs, whisked.

Guidelines:

1.   In a bowl, blend artichokes in with oregano, salt, pepper, and eggs and whisk well.

2.   Add the oil to the air fryer cooker's dish, include eggs blend and cook at 320 Deg. Fahrenheit for about 15 minutes.

3.   Divide the frittata between the plates and serve for breakfast. Enjoy the recipe!

The nutritional facts: calories 136, fat 6, fiber 6, carbs 9, protein 4

ASTONISHING BREAKFAST BURGER

Prep. time: 10 minutes

The cooking time: 45 minutes

The recipe servings: 4

Fixings:

1 pound meat, ground

1 yellow onion, hacked 1 teaspoon tomato puree 1 teaspoon garlic, minced 1 teaspoon mustard

1 teaspoon basil, dried

1 teaspoon parsley, hacked

1 tablespoon cheddar, ground Salt and dark pepper to the taste

4 bread buns, for serving

Guidelines:

1.   In a bowl, blend meat in with the onion, tomato puree, garlic, mustard, basil, parsley, cheddar, salt, and pepper, mix well and shape 4 burgers out of this blend.

2. Heat the air-fryer cooker at 400 degrees F, include burgers, and cook them for 25 minutes.

3. Reduce temperature to 350 degrees F and prepare burgers for 20 minutes more.

4. Arrange the bread buns and then serve for a fast breakfast. Enjoy the recipe!

The nutritional facts: calories 234, fat 5, fiber 8, carbs 12, protein 4

ONION FRITTATA

Prep. time: 10 minutes

The cooking time: 20 minutes

The recipe servings: 6

Fixings:

- 10 eggs, whisked

- 1 tablespoon of olive oil

- pound little potatoes, slashed 2 yellow onions, hacked

- Salt and dark pepper to the taste 1-ounce cheddar, ground

- ½ cup harsh cream

Guidelines:

1.   In an enormous bowl, blend eggs in with potatoes, onions, salt, pepper, cheddar, and sharp cream and whisk well.

2.   Grease the air fryer cooker's skillet with the oil, including eggs blend, place in the air fryer and cook it for 20 min. at 320 degrees F.

3.   Slice frittata, isolate among plates and serve for breakfast. Enjoy the recipe!

The nutritional facts: calories 231, fat 5, fiber 7, carbs 8, protein 4

RINGER PEPPERS FRITTATA

Prep. time: 10 minutes

The cooking time: 20 minutes

The recipe servings: 4

Fixings:

- 2   tablespoons olive oil

- ½ pounds chicken frankfurter, housings expelled and cleaved 1 sweet onion, slashed

- 1 red ringer pepper, cleaved

- orange ringer pepper, slashed 1 green chime pepper, hacked

- Salt and dark pepper to the taste 8 eggs, whisked.

- ½ cup mozzarella cheddar, destroyed 2 teaspoons oregano, slashed

Guidelines:

1. Add 1 tablespoon oil to the air fryer cooker, including frankfurter, heat up at 320 degrees F and darker for 1 moment.

2. Add the remainder of the oil, onion, red ringer pepper, orange and green one, mix and cook for 2 minutes more.

3. Add oregano, salt, pepper, and eggs, mix and cook for 15 minutes.

4. Add mozzarella, leave frittata aside for a couple of moments, partition among plates and serve.

Enjoy the recipe!

The nutritional facts: calories 212, fat 4, fiber 6, carbs 8, protein 12

CHEDDAR SANDWICH

Prep. time: 10 minutes

The cooking time: 8 minutes

The recipe servings: 1

Fixings:

- 2   bread cuts

- 2 teaspoons margarine

- 2 cheddar cuts A spot of sweet paprika

Guidelines:

1. Spread margarine on bread cuts include cheddar one, sprinkle paprika, top with the other bread cuts, cut into 2 parts, orchestrate them in the air fryer cooker and cook at 370 Deg. Fahrenheit for about 8 minutes, flipping them once, organize on a plate and serve.

Enjoy the recipe!

The nutritional facts: calories 130, fat 3, fiber 5, carbs 9, protein 3

LONG BEANS OMELET

Prep. time: 10 minutes

The cooking time: 10 minutes

The recipe servings: 3

Fixings:

½ teaspoon of soy sauce, and 1 tablespoon of olive oil 3 eggs, whisked

A spot of salt and dark pepper 4 garlic cloves, minced

4 long beans, cut and cut

Guidelines:

1.   In a bowl, blend eggs in with a spot of salt, dark pepper, and soy sauce and whisk well.

2.   Heat the air-fryer cooker at 320 degrees F, including oil and garlic, mix and dark-colored for 1 moment.

3.   Add long beans and eggs blend, spread, and cook for 10 minutes.

4.   Divide omelet between plates and serve for breakfast. Enjoy the recipe!

The nutritional facts: calories 200, fat 3, fiber 7, carbs 9, protein 3

FRENCH BEANS AND EGG BREAKFAST MIX

Prep. time: 10 minutes

The cooking time: 10 minutes

The recipe servings: 3

Fixings:

2 eggs, whisked

½ teaspoon of soy sauce and 1 tablespoon of olive oil 4 garlic cloves, minced

3   ounces French beans, cut and cut corner to corner Salt and white pepper to the taste

Guidelines:

1.   In a bowl, blend eggs in with soy sauce, salt, and pepper and whisk well.

2.   Heat the air-fryer cooker at 320 degrees F, including oil, and heat it up also.

3.   Add garlic and dark-colored for 1 moment.

4.   Add French beans and egg blend, hurl and cook for 10 minutes.

5.   Divide among plates and serve for breakfast. Enjoy the recipe!

The nutritional facts: calories 182, fat 3, fiber 6, carbs 8, protein 3

BREAKFAST DOUGHNUTS

Prep. time: 10 minutes

The cooking time: 18 minutes The recipe servings: 6

Fixings:

4   tablespoons spread, delicate

1 and ½ teaspoon preparing powder 2 a ¼ cups white flour

½ cup of sugar

1/3 cup caster sugar

1 teaspoon cinnamon powder 2 egg yolks

½ cup sharp cream

Guidelines:

1. In a bowl, blend 2 tablespoons spread with basic sugar and egg yolks and whisk well.

2. Add a portion of the acrid cream and mix.

3. In other dishes, blend flour in with preparing powder, mix, and furthermore add to eggs blend.

4. Stir well until you acquire a batter, move it to a floured working surface, turn it out and cut large circles with little ones in the center.

5. Brush doughnuts with the remainder of the spread, the air-fryer cooker at 360 degrees F, put the doughnuts inside air fryer, and cook them for 8 minutes.

6. In a bowl, blend cinnamon in with caster sugar and mix.

7. Arrange doughnuts on plates and plunge them in cinnamon and sugar before serving.

Enjoy the recipe!

The nutritional facts: calories 182, fat 3, fiber 7, carbs 8, protein 3

CREAMY BREAKFAST TOFU

Prep. time: 15 minutes

The cooking time: 20 minutes

The recipe servings: 4

Fixings:

1   block firm tofu, squeezed and cubed 1 of teaspoon rice vinegar

2 tablespoons of the soy sauce 2 and the teaspoons sesame oil

1   tablespoon potato starch 1 cup Greek yogurt

Guidelines:

1.   In a bowl, blend solid tofu shapes with vinegar, soy sauce, and oil, hurl, and leave aside for 15 minutes.

2.   Dip tofu 3D squares in potato starch, hurl, move the air-fryer cooker, heat the at 370 degrees F, and cooking for 20 min. shaking midway.

Enjoy the recipe!

The nutritional facts: calories 110, fat 4, fiber 5, carbs 8, protein 4

VEGGIE BURRITOS

Prep. time: 10 minutes

The cooking time: 10 minutes

The recipe servings: 4

Fixings:

2   tablespoons cashew spread 2 tablespoons tamari

2 tablespoons water

2 tablespoons fluid smoke 4 rice papers

½ cup sweet potatoes, steamed and cubed

½ little broccoli head, florets isolated and steamed 7 asparagus stalks

8 broiled red peppers, slashed A bunch kale, cleaved

Guidelines:

1.   In a bowl, blend cashew spread with water, tamari, and fluid smoke and whisk well.

2.   Wet rice papers and organize them on a working surface.

3.   Divide the sweet potatoes, the broccoli, asparagus, the red peppers, and kale, wrap burritos and dunk each in cashew blend.

4.   Arrange burritos in the air-fryer cooker and cook them at 350 Deg. Fahrenheit for about 10 minutes.

5.   Divide veggie burritos between plates d serve. Enjoy!

The nutritional facts: calories 172, fat 4, fiber 7, carbs 8, protein 3

BREAKFAST FISH TACOS

Prep. time: 10 minutes

The cooking time: 13 minutes The recipe servings: 4

Fixings:

- 4 major tortillas

- 1 red ringer pepper, hacked 1 yellow onion, cleaved 1 cup corn

- 4 white fish fillets, skinless and boneless

- ½ cup of salsa

- A bunch blended romaine lettuce, spinach, and radicchio 4 tablespoon parmesan, ground

Guidelines:

1.   Place the fish fillets in the air-fryer cooker and cook at 350 Deg. Fahrenheit for about 6 minutes.

2.   Meanwhile, heat up a container over medium-high heat, include chime pepper, onion, and corn, mix and cook for 1-2 minutes.

3.   Arrange tortillas on a working surface, partition fish fillets, spread salsa over them, separate blended veggies and blended greens and spread parmesan on each toward the end.

4.   Roll your tacos, place them in the preheated air fryer and cook at 350 Deg. Fahrenheit for about 6 minutes more.

5.   Divide fish tacos between plates and serve for breakfast. Enjoy the recipe!

The nutritional facts: calories 200, fat 3, fiber 7, carbs 9, protein 5

GARLIC POTATOES WITH BACON

Prep. time: 10 minutes

The cooking time: 20 minutes

The recipe servings: 4

Fixings:

4 potatoes, stripped and cut into medium solid shapes 6 garlic cloves, minced

4 bacon cuts, cleaved

2 rosemary springs, cleaved 1 tablespoon of olive oil

Salt and dark pepper to the taste 2 eggs, whisked.

Guidelines:

1.   In the air fryer cooker's container, blend the oil in with potatoes, garlic, bacon, rosemary, salt, pepper and eggs, and whisk.

2.   Cook the potatoes at 400 Deg. Fahrenheit for about 20 minutes, isolate everything on plates, and serve for breakfast.

Enjoy the recipe!

The nutritional facts: calories 211, fat 3, fiber 5, carbs 8, protein 5

SPINACH BREAKFAST PARCELS

Prep. time: 10 minutes

The cooking time: 4 minutes

The recipe servings: 2

Fixings:

4 sheets filo cake

1 pound child spinach leaves, generally slashed

½ pound ricotta cheddar 2 tablespoons pine nuts 1 egg, whisked

Get-up-and-go from 1 lemon, ground Greek yogurt for serving

Salt and dark pepper to the taste

Guidelines:

1.   In a bowl, blend spinach in with cheddar, egg, lemon pizzazz, salt, pepper, and pine nuts and mix.

2.   Arrange filo sheets on a working surface, isolate spinach blend, overlay corner to corner to shape your packages, and spot them in your preheated air fryer at 400 degrees F.

3.   Bake packages for 4 minutes, separate them on plates, and serve them with Greek yogurt as an afterthought.

Enjoy the recipe!

The nutritional facts: calories 182, fat 4, fiber 8, carbs 9, protein 5

HAM ROLLS

Prep. time: 10 minutes

The cooking time: 10 minutes

The recipe servings: 4

Fixings:

1 sheet puff baked good

4 bunch gruyere cheddar, ground 4 teaspoons mustard

8 ham cuts, slashed

Guidelines:

1.   Roll out puff baked goods on a working surface, isolate cheddar, ham, and mustard, fold tight, and cut into medium rounds.

2.   Place all moves in an air fryer and cook for 10 minutes at 370 degrees F.

3.   Divide moves on plates and serves for breakfast. Enjoy the recipe!

The nutritional facts: calories 182, fat 4, fiber 7, carbs 9, protein 8

SHRIMP FRITTATA

Prep. time: 10 minutes

The cooking time: 15 minutes The recipe servings: 4

Fixings:

4 eggs

½ teaspoon basil, dried Cooking splash

Salt and dark pepper to the taste

½ cup of rice, cooked

½ cup shrimp, cooked, stripped, deveined and hacked

½ cup child spinach, slashed

½ cup Monterey jack cheddar, ground

Guidelines:

1.   In a bowl, blend eggs in with salt, pepper, and basil and whisk.

2.   Grease the air fryer cooker's container with cooking shower and include rice, shrimp, and spinach.

3.   Add eggs blend, sprinkle cheddar all finished and cook in the air fryer cooker at 350 Deg. Fahrenheit for about 10 minutes.

4.   Divide among plates and serve for breakfast. Enjoy the recipe!

The nutritional facts: calories 162, fat 6, fiber 5, carbs 8, protein 4

TUNA SANDWICHES

Prep. time: 10 minutes

The cooking time: 5 minutes

The recipe servings: 4

Fixings:

16 ounces of canned tuna, depleted

¼ cup mayonnaise

2 tablespoons mustard

1 tablespoon lemon juice 2 green onions, hacked 3 English biscuits, divided 3 tablespoons margarine

6 provolone cheddar

Guidelines:

1.   In a bowl, blend tuna in with mayo, lemon juice, mustard, and green onions and mix.

2.   Grease biscuit parts with the spread, place them in the preheated air fryer, and heat them at 350 Deg. Fahrenheit for about 4 minutes.

3.   Spread tuna blend on biscuit parts, top each with provolone cheddar, return sandwiches to air fryer and cook them for 4 minutes, separate among plates and serve for breakfast immediately.

Enjoy the recipe!

The nutritional facts: calories 182, fat 4, fiber 7, carbs 8, protein 6

SHRIMP SANDWICHES

Prep. time: 10 minutes

The cooking time: 5 minutes

The recipe servings: 4

Fixings:

- 1 and ¼ cups cheddar, destroyed

- 6 ounces canned little shrimp, depleted 3 tablespoons mayonnaise

- 2 tablespoons green onions, cleaved 4 entire wheat bread cuts

- 2 tablespoons margarine, delicate

Guidelines:

1. In a bowl, blend shrimp in with cheddar, green onion and mayo and mix well.

2. Spread this on half of the bread cuts, top with the other bread cuts, cut into equal parts corner to corner and spread margarine on top.

3.   Place sandwiches in the air-fryer cooker and then cook at 350 Deg. Fahrenheit for about 5 minutes.

4.   Divide the shrimp sandwiches on the plates and serve them for breakfast. Enjoy the recipe!

The nutritional facts: calories 162, fat 3, fiber 7, carbs 12, protein 4

BREAKFAST PEA TORTILLA

Prep. time: 10 minutes

The cooking time: 7 minutes

The recipe servings: 8

Fixings:

½ pound child peas 4 tablespoons margarine 1 and ½ cup yogurt 8 eggs

½ cup mint, hacked

Salt and dark pepper to the taste

Guidelines:

1.   Heat up a dish that accommodates the air fryer cooker with the margarine over medium heat, include peas, mix and cook for a few minutes.

2.   Meanwhile, in a bowl, blend half of the yogurt in with salt, pepper, eggs and mint and whisk well.

3.   Pour this over the peas, hurl, present in the air fryer cooker and cook at 350 Deg. Fahrenheit for about 7 minutes.

4.   Spread the remainder of the yogurt over your tortilla, cut and serve. Enjoy the recipe!

The nutritional facts: calories 192, fat 5, fiber 4, carbs 8, protein 7

RASPBERRY ROLLS

Prep. time: 30 minutes

The cooking time: 20 minutes The recipe servings: 6

Fixings:

- 1 cup milk

- 4 tablespoons spread 3 and ¼ cups flour 2 teaspoons yeast

- ¼ cup sugar 1 egg

- For the filling:

- 8 ounces cream cheddar, delicate 12 ounces raspberries

- 1 teaspoons vanilla concentrate 5 tablespoons sugar

1   tablespoon cornstarch Zest from 1 lemon, ground

Guidelines:

1.   In a bowl, blend flour in with sugar and yeast and mix.

2.   Add milk and egg, mix until you get a batter, leave it aside to ascend for 30 minutes, move mixture to a working surface and move well.

3.   In a bowl, blend cream cheddar with sugar, vanilla and lemon pizzazz, mix well and spread over batter.

4.   In another bowl, blend raspberries in with cornstarch, mix and spread over cream cheddar blend.

5.   Roll your mixture, cut into medium pieces, place them in the air fryer cooker, shower them with cooking splash and cook them at 350 Deg. Fahrenheit for about 30 minutes.

6.   Serve your moves for breakfast. Enjoy the recipe!

The nutritional facts: calories 261, fat 5, fiber 8, carbs 9, protein 6

POTATO AND LEEK FRITTATA

Prep. time: 10 minutes

The cooking time: 18 minutes

The recipe servings: 4

Fixings:

2   gold potatoes, bubbled, stripped and cleaved 2 tablespoons margarine

2 leeks, cut

Salt and dark pepper to the taste

¼ cup entire milk 10 eggs, whisked

5 ounces fromage blanc, disintegrated

Guidelines:

1.   Heat up a container that accommodates the air fryer cooker with the margarine over medium heat, include leeks, mix and cook for 4 minutes.

2.   Add potatoes, salt, pepper, eggs, cheddar and milk, whisk well, cook for brief more, present in the air-fryer cooker and cook at 350 Deg. Fahrenheit for about 13 minutes.

3.   Slice frittata, partition among plates and serve. Enjoy the recipe!

The nutritional facts: calories 271, fat 6, fiber 8, carbs 12, protein 6

COFFEE OATMEAL

Prep. time: 10 minutes

The cooking time: 17 minutes

Recipes The recipe servings: 4

Fixings:

1 cup milk

1 cup steel cut oats 2 and ½ cups water 2 tablespoons sugar

1 teaspoon coffee powder 2 teaspoons vanilla concentrate

Guidelines:

1.   In a container that accommodates the air fryer cooker, blend oats in with water, sugar, milk and coffee powder, mix, present in the air fryer cooker and cook at 360 Deg. Fahrenheit for about 17 minutes.

2.   Add vanilla concentrate, mix, leave everything aside for 5 minutes, separate into bowls and serve for breakfast.

Enjoy the recipe!

The nutritional facts: calories 261, fat 7, fiber 6, carbs 39, protein 6

MUSHROOM OATMEAL

Prep. time: 10 minutes

The cooking time: 20 minutes

The recipe servings: 4

Fixings:

1   small yellow onion, slashed 1 cup steel cut oats

2   garlic cloves, minced 2 tablespoons margarine

½ cup water

14 ounces canned chicken stock 3 thyme springs, slashed

2 tablespoons additional virgin olive oil

½ cup gouda cheddar, ground 8 ounces mushroom, cut

Salt and dark pepper to the taste

Guidelines:

1.   Heat up a skillet that accommodates the air fryer cooker with the spread over medium heat, include onions and garlic, mix and cook for 4 minutes.

2.   Add oats, water, salt, pepper, stock and thyme, mix, present in the air fryer cooker and cook at 360 Deg. Fahrenheit for about 16 minutes.

3.   Meanwhile, heat up a skillet with the olive oil over medium heat, include mushrooms, cook them for 3 minutes, add to oatmeal and cheddar, mix, separate into bowls and serve for breakfast.

Enjoy the recipe!

The nutritional facts: calories 284, fat 8, fiber 8, carbs 20, protein 17

PECANS AND PEAR OATMEAL

Prep. Time: 5 minutes

The cooking time: 12 minutes

The recipe servings: 4

Fixings:

- 1 cup water

    1   tablespoon margarine, delicate

- ¼ cups darker sugar

- ½ teaspoon cinnamon powder 1 cup moved oats

- ½ cup pecans, slashed

    1   cups pear, stripped and slashed

½ cup raisins

Guidelines:

1.   In a heat confirmation dish that accommodates the air fryer cooker, blend milk in with sugar, spread, oats, cinnamon, raisins, pears and pecans, mix, present in your fryer and cook at 360 Deg. Fahrenheit for about 12 minutes.

2.	Divide into bowls and serve. Enjoy the recipe!

The nutritional facts: calories 230, fat 6, fiber 11, carbs 20, protein 5

CINNAMON AND CREAM CHEESE OATS

Prep. time: 10 minutes

The cooking time: 25 minutes

The recipe servings: 4

Fixings:

1 cup steel oats 3 cups milk

1 tablespoon margarine

¾ cup raisins

1	teaspoon cinnamon powder

¼ cup darker sugar

2	tablespoons white sugar

2 ounces cream cheddar, delicate

Guidelines:

1.   Heat up a skillet that accommodates the air fryer cooker with the margarine over medium heat, include oats, mix and toast them for 3 minutes.

2.   Add milk and raisins, mix, present in the air fryer cooker and cook at 350 Deg. Fahrenheit for about 20 minutes.

3.   Meanwhile, in a bowl, blend cinnamon in with dark colored sugar and mix.

4.   In a subsequent bowl, blend white sugar in with cream cheddar and whisk.

5.   Divide oats into bowls and top each with cinnamon and cream cheddar. Enjoy the recipe!

The nutritional facts: calories 152, fat 6, fiber 6, carbs 25, protein 7

FRUITS RISOTTO

Prep. time: 10 minutes

The cooking time: 12 minutes

The recipe servings: 4

Fixings:

- 1½ cups of Arborio rice

- 1½ teaspoons of the cinnamon powder 1/3 cup of darker sugar

- A touch of salt

- tablespoons spread

- apples, cored and cut 1 cup squeezed apple

- cups milk

½ cup fruits, dried

Guidelines:

1.   Heat up a container that clench hand the air fryer cooker with the margarine over medium heat, include rice, mix and cook for 4-5 minutes.

2.   Add sugar, apples, squeezed apple, milk, cinnamon and fruits, mix, present in the air fryer cooker and cook at 350 Deg. Fahrenheit for about 8 minutes.

3.   Divide into bowls and serve for breakfast. Enjoy the recipe!

The nutritional facts: calories 162, fat 12, fiber 6, carbs 23, protein 8

RICE, ALMONDS AND RAISINS PUDDING

Prep. time: 5 minutes The cooking time: 8 minutes The recipe servings: 4

Fixings:

1   cup dark colored rice

½ cup coconut chips 1 cup milk

2   cups water

½ cup maple syrup

¼ cup raisins

¼ cup almonds

A touch of cinnamon powder

Guidelines:

1.   Put the rice in a container that accommodates the air fryer cooker, include the water, heat up on the stove over medium high heat, cook until rice is delicate and channel.

2.   Add milk, coconut chips, almonds, raisins, cinnamon and maple syrup, mix well, present in the air-fryer cooker and cook at 360 deg. F for 8 minutes.

3.   Divide rice pudding in bowls and serve. Enjoy the recipe!

The nutritional facts: calories 251, fat 6, fiber 8, carbs 39, protein 12

DATES AND MILLET PUDDING

Prep. time: 10 minutes

The cooking time: 15 minutes

The recipe servings: 4

Fixings:

14 ounces milk

7 ounces water 2/3 cup millet 4 dates, pitted

HONNEY for serving

Guidelines:

1.   Put the millet in a dish that accommodates the air fryer cooker, include dates, milk and water, mix, present in the air fryer cooker and cook at 360 Deg. Fahrenheit for about 15 minutes.

2.   Divide among plates, shower HONNEY on top and serve for breakfast. Enjoy the recipe!

The nutritional facts: calories 231, fat 6, fiber 6, carbs 18, protein 6

AIR FRYER LUNCH RECIPES

LUNCH EGG ROLLS

Prep. time: 10 minutes
The cooking time: 15 minutes
The recipe servings: 4

Fixings:

½ cup mushrooms, hacked

½ cup carrots, ground

½ cup zucchini, ground 2 green onions, hacked 2 tablespoons soy sauce 8 egg move wrappers

1 egg, whisked

1 tablespoon cornstarch

Guidelines:

1. In a bowl, blend carrots in with mushrooms, zucchini, green onions, and soy sauce and mix well.

2. Arrange egg move wrappers on a working surface, partition veggie blend on each, and move well.

3. In a bowl, blend cornstarch in with the egg, whisk well and brush eggs moves with this blend.

4. Seal edges, place all moves in your preheated air fryer, and cook them at 370 Deg. Fahrenheit for about 15 minutes.

5. Arrange the recipes on a plate and serve them for lunch. Enjoy the recipe!

The nutritional facts: calories 172, fat 6, fiber 6, carbs 8, protein 7

VEGGIE TOAST

Prep. time: 10 minutes The cooking time: 15 minutes The recipe servings: 4

Fixings:

1 red chime pepper, cut into dainty strips 1 cup cremimi mushrooms, cut

1 yellow squash, cleaved 2 green onions, cut

1 tablespoon of olive oil, 4 bread cuts

2 tablespoons spread, delicate

½ cup goat cheddar, disintegrated

Guidelines:

1. In a bowl, blend red ringer pepper with mushrooms, squash, green onions and oil, hurl, move to the air fryer cooker, cook them at 350 Deg. Fahrenheit for about 10 minutes, shaking the fryer once and move them to a bowl.

2. Spread margarine on bread cuts, place them in air fryer and cook them at 350 Deg. Fahrenheit for about 5 minutes.

3. Divide veggie blend on each bread cut, top with disintegrated cheddar and serve for lunch.

Enjoy the recipe!

The nutritional facts: calories 152, fat 3, fiber 4, carbs 7, protein 2

STUFFED MUSHROOMS

Prep. time: 10 minutes

The cooking time: 20 minutes

The recipe servings: 4

Fixings:

4 big Portobello mushroom tops 1 tablespoon of olive oil

¼ cup ricotta cheddar

5 tablespoons parmesan, ground 1 cup spinach, torn

1/3 cup bread pieces

¼ teaspoon rosemary, hacked

Guidelines:

1. Rub mushrooms tops with the oil, place them in the air fryer cooker's crate and cook them at 350 Deg. Fahrenheit for about 2 minutes.

2. Meanwhile, in a bowl, blend half of the parmesan in with ricotta, spinach, rosemary and bread morsels and mix well.

3. Stuff mushrooms with this blend, sprinkle the remainder of the parmesan on top, place them in the air fryer cooker's container again and cook at 350 Deg. Fahrenheit for about 10 minutes.

4. Divide them on plates and present with a side serving of mixed greens for lunch. Enjoy the recipe!

The nutritional facts: calories 152, fat 4, fiber 7, carbs 9, protein 5

SNAPPY LUNCH PIZZAS

Prep. time: 10 minutes

The cooking time: 7 minutes

The recipe servings: 4

Fixings:

4 pitas

1 tablespoon of olive oil

¾ cup pizza sauce

4 ounces bumped mushrooms, cut

½ teaspoon basil, dried 2 green onions, slashed 2 cup mozzarella, ground

1 cup grape tomatoes, cut

Guidelines:

1. Spread pizza sauce on every pita bread, sprinkle green onions and basil, isolate mushrooms and top with cheddar.

2. Arrange pita pizzas in the air fryer cooker and cook them at 400 Deg. Fahrenheit for about 7 minutes.

3. Top every pizza with tomato cuts, separate among plates and serve. Enjoy the recipe!

The nutritional facts: calories 200, fat 4, fiber 6, carbs 7, protein 3

LUNCH GNOCCHI

Prep. time: 10 minutes

The cooking time: 17 minutes

The recipe servings: 4

Fixings:

1 yellow onion, hacked 1 tablespoon of olive oil

3 garlic cloves, minced 16 ounces gnocchi

¼ cup parmesan, ground 8 ounces spinach pesto

Guidelines:

1. Grease the air fryer cooker's dish with olive oil, include gnocchi, onion and garlic, hurl, put skillet in the air fryer cooker and cook at 400 Deg. Fahrenheit for about 10 minutes.

2. Add pesto, hurl and cook for 7 minutes more at 350 degrees F.

3. Divide among plates and serve for lunch. Enjoy the recipe!

The nutritional facts: calories 200, fat 4, fiber 4, carbs 12, protein 4

TUNA AND ZUCCHINI TORTILLAS

Prep. time: 10 minutes

The cooking time: 10 minutes

The recipe servings: 4

Fixings:

4 corn tortillas

4 tablespoons spread, delicate

6 ounces canned tuna, depleted 1 cup zucchini, destroyed

1/3 cup mayonnaise

2 tablespoons mustard

1 cup cheddar, ground

Guidelines:

1. Spread spread on tortillas, place them in the air fryer cooker's container and cook them at 400 Deg. Fahrenheit for about 3 minutes.

2. Meanwhile, in a bowl, blend tuna in with zucchini, mayo and mustard and mix.

3. Divide this blend on every tortilla, top with cheddar, move tortillas, place them in the air fryer cooker's bushel again and cook them at 400 Deg. Fahrenheit for about 4 minutes more.

4. Serve for lunch. Enjoy the recipe!

The nutritional facts: calories 162, fat 4, fiber 8, carbs 9, protein 4

SQUASH FRITTERS

Prep. time: 10 minutes

The cooking time: 7 minutes

The recipe servings: 4

Fixings:

3 ounces cream cheddar 1 egg, whisked

½ teaspoon oregano, dried

A spot of salt and dark pepper 1 yellow summer squash, ground 1/3 cup carrot, ground

2/3 cup bread morsels 2 tablespoons olive oil

Guidelines:

1. In a bowl, blend cream cheddar with salt, pepper, oregano, egg, breadcrumbs, carrot and squash and mix well.

2. Shape medium patties out of this blend and brush them with the oil.

3. Place squash patties in the air fryer cooker and cook them at 400 Deg. Fahrenheit for about 7 minutes.

4. Serve them for lunch. Enjoy the recipe!

The nutritional facts: calories 200, fat 4, fiber 7, carbs 8, protein 6

LUNCH SHRIMP CROQUETTES

Prep. time: 10 minutes

The cooking time: 8 minutes

The recipe servings: 4

Fixings:

2/3 pound shrimp, cooked, stripped, deveined and hacked 1 and ½ cups bread morsels

1 egg, whisked

2 tablespoons lemon juice 3 green onions, hacked

½ teaspoon basil, dried

Salt and dark pepper to the taste 2 tablespoons olive oil

Guidelines:

1. In a bowl, blend half of the bread pieces with egg and lemon squeeze and mix well.

2. Add green onions, basil, salt, pepper and shrimp and mix truly well.

3. In a different bowl, blend the remainder of the bread scraps with the oil and hurl well.

4. Shape balance wads of shrimp blend, dig them in bread pieces, place them in preheated air fryer and cook the for 8 minutes at 400 degrees F.

5. Serve them with a plunge for lunch. Enjoy the recipe!

The nutritional facts: calories 142, fat 4, fiber 6, carbs 9, protein 4

LUNCH SPECIAL PANCAKE

Prep. time: 10 minutes

The cooking time: 10 minutes

The recipe servings: 2

Fixings:

1 tablespoon margarine

3 eggs, whisked

½ cup flour

½ cup milk 1 cup salsa

1 cup little shrimp, stripped and deveined

Guidelines:

1. Preheat the air fryer cooker at 400 degrees F, include fryer's container, include 1 tablespoon margarine and soften it.

2. In a bowl, blend eggs in with flour and milk, whisk well and fill air fryer's container, spread, cook at 350 degrees for 12 minutes and move to a plate.

3. In a bowl, blend shrimp in with salsa, mix and serve your hotcake with this as an afterthought.

Enjoy the recipe!

The nutritional facts: calories 200, fat 6, fiber 8, carbs 12, protein 4

SCALLOPS AND DILL

Prep. time: 10 minutes

The cooking time: 5 minutes

The recipe servings: 4

Fixings:

1 pound ocean scallops, debearded 1 tablespoon lemon juice

1 teaspoon dill, slashed 2 teaspoons olive oil

Salt and dark pepper to the taste

Guidelines:

1. In the air fryer cooker, blend scallops in with dill, oil, salt, pepper and lemon squeeze, spread and cook at 360 Deg. Fahrenheit for about 5 minutes.

2. Discard unopened ones, separate scallops and dill sauce on plates and serve for lunch.

Enjoy the recipe!

The nutritional facts: calories 152, fat 4, fiber 7, carbs 19, protein 4

CHICKEN SANDWICHES

Prep. time: 10 minutes

The cooking time: 10 minutes

The recipe servings: 4

Fixings:

2 chicken bosoms, skinless, boneless and cubed 1 red onion, hacked

1 red chime pepper, cut

½ cup Italian flavoring

½ teaspoon thyme, dried 2 cups spread lettuce, torn 4 pita pockets

1 cup cherry tomatoes, split 1 tablespoon of olive oil

Guidelines:

1. In the air fryer cooker, blend chicken in with onion, ringer pepper, Italian flavoring and oil, hurl and cook at 380 Deg. Fahrenheit for about 10 minutes.

2. Transfer chicken blend to a bowl, include thyme, spread lettuce and cherry tomatoes, hurl well, stuff pita pockets with this blend and serve for lunch.

Enjoy the recipe!

The nutritional facts: calories 126, fat 4, fiber 8, carbs 14, protein 4

NEW CHICKEN MIX

Prep. time: 10 minutes

The cooking time: 22 minutes

The recipe servings: 4

Fixings:

2 chicken bosoms, skinless, boneless and cubed 8 catch mushrooms, cut

1 red chime pepper, cleaved 1 tablespoon of olive oil

½ teaspoon thyme, dried 10 ounces alfredo sauce 6 bread cuts

2 tablespoons spread, delicate

Guidelines:

1. In the air fryer cooker, blend chicken in with mushrooms, chime pepper and oil, hurl to cover well and cook at 350 Deg. Fahrenheit for about 15 minutes.

2. Transfer chicken blend to a bowl, include thyme and alfredo sauce, hurl, come back to air fryer apparatus and then cook at 350 Deg. Fahrenheit for about 4 minutes more.

3. Spread margarine on bread cuts, add it to the fryer, adulate side and cook for 4 minutes more.

4. Arrange toasted bread cuts on a platter, top each with chicken blend and serve for lunch.

Enjoy the recipe!

The nutritional facts: calories 172, fat 4, fiber 9, carbs 12, protein 4

HOT BACON SANDWICHES

Prep. time: 10 minutes

The cooking time: 7 minutes

The recipe servings: 4

Fixings:

- 1/3 cup bar-b-que sauce

- tablespoons HONNEY

- 8 bacon cuts, cooked and cut into thirds 1 red ringer pepper, cut

- 1 yellow ringer pepper, cut 3 pita pockets, divided

- 1 and ¼ cup margarine lettuce leaves, torn 2 tomatoes, cut

Guidelines:

1. In a bowl, blend bar-b-que sauce with HONNEY and whisk well.

2. Brush bacon and all chime peppers with a portion of this blend, place them in the air fryer cooker and cook at 350 Deg. Fahrenheit for about 4 minutes.

3. Shake fryer and cook them for 2 minutes more.

4. Stuff pita pockets with bacon blend, additionally stuff with tomatoes and lettuce, spread the remainder of the bar-b-que sauce and serve for lunch.

Enjoy the recipe!

The nutritional facts: calories 186, fat 6, fiber 9, carbs 14, protein 4

BUTTERMILK CHICKEN

Prep. time: 10 minutes

The cooking time: 18 minutes

The recipe servings: 4

Fixings:

1½ of pounds chicken thighs and 2 of cups buttermilk

Salt and dark pepper to the taste A touch of cayenne pepper

2 cups white flour

1 tablespoon preparing powder 1 tablespoon sweet paprika 1 tablespoon garlic powder

Guidelines:

1. In a bowl, blend chicken thighs in with buttermilk, salt, pepper and cayenne, hurl and leave aside for 6 hours.

2. In a different bowl, blend flour in with paprika, preparing powder and garlic powder and mix,

3. Drain chicken thighs, dig them in flour blend, orchestrate them in the air fryer cooker and then cook at 360 deg. F for 8 minutes.

4. The flip chicken pieces, cook it for 10 minutes more, orchestrate on a platter and serve for lunch.

Enjoy the recipe!

The nutritional facts: calories 200, fat 3, fiber 9, carbs 14, protein 4

THE CHICKEN PIE

Prep. time: 10 minutes The cooking time: 16 minutes The recipe servings: 4

Fixings:

2 chicken thighs, boneless, skinless and cubed 1 carrot, hacked

1 yellow onion, cleaved 2 potatoes, slashed

2 mushrooms, cleaved 1 teaspoon soy sauce

Salt and dark pepper to the taste 1 teaspoon Italian flavoring

½ teaspoon garlic powder

1 teaspoon Worcestershire sauce 1 tablespoon flour

1 tablespoon milk 2 puff baked good sheets

1 tablespoon spread, softened

Guidelines:

1. Heat up a container over medium high heat, include potatoes, carrots and onion, mix and cook for 2 minutes.

2. Add chicken and mushrooms, salt, soy sauce, pepper, Italian flavoring, garlic powder, Worcestershire sauce, flour and milk, mix truly well and take off heat.

3. Place 1 puff cake sheet on the base of the air fryer cooker's dish and trim edge overabundance.

4. Add chicken blend, top with the other puff cake sheet, trim overabundance also and brush pie with margarine.

5. Place in the air fryer cooker and cook at 360 Deg. Fahrenheit for about 6 minutes.

6. Leave pie to chill off, cut and serve for breakfast. Enjoy the recipe!

The nutritional facts: calories 300, fat 5, fiber 7, carbs 14, protein 7

THE MACARONI AND CHEESE

Prep. time: 10 minutes The cooking time: 30 minutes The recipe servings: 3

Fixings:

1 and ½ cups most loved macaroni Cooking splash

½ cup overwhelming cream 1 cup chicken stock

¾ cup cheddar, destroyed

½ cup mozzarella cheddar, destroyed

¼ cup parmesan, destroyed

Salt and dark pepper to the taste

Guidelines:

1. Spray a dish with cooking splash, include macaroni, overwhelming cream, stock, cheddar, mozzarella and parmesan yet in addition salt and pepper, hurl well, place skillet in the air fryer cooker's container and cook for 30 minutes.

2. Divide among plates and serve for lunch. Enjoy the recipe!

The nutritional facts: calories 341, fat 7, fiber 8, carbs 18, protein 4

THE LUNCH FAJITAS

Prep. time: 10 minutes The cooking time: 10 minutes The recipe servings: 4

Fixings:

1 teaspoon garlic powder

¼ teaspoon cumin, ground

½ teaspoon stew powder

Salt and dark pepper to the taste

¼ teaspoon coriander, ground

1 pound chicken bosoms, cut into strips 1 red chime pepper, cut

1 green chime pepper, cut 1 yellow onion, hacked 1 tablespoon lime juice Cooking splash

4 tortillas, heated up Salsa for serving

Acrid cream for serving

1 cup lettuce leaves, torn for serving

Guidelines:

1. In a bowl, blend chicken in with garlic powder, cumin, bean stew, salt, pepper, coriander, lime juice, red ringer pepper, green chime pepper and onion, hurl, leave aside for 10 minutes, move to the air fryer cooker and shower some cooking splash everywhere.

2. Toss and cook at 400 Deg. Fahrenheit for about 10 minutes.

3. Arrange tortillas on a working surface, isolate chicken blend, additionally include salsa, sharp cream and lettuce, wrap and serve for lunch.

Enjoy the recipe!

The nutritional facts: calories 317, fat 6, fiber 8, carbs 14, protein 4

LUNCH CHICKEN SALAD

Prep. time: 10 minutes The cooking time: 20 minutes The recipe servings: 4

Fixings:

2 ears of corn, hulled

1 pound chicken fingers, boneless Olive oil varying

Salt and dark pepper to the taste 1 teaspoon sweet paprika

1 tablespoon dark colored sugar

½ teaspoon garlic powder

½ ice sheet lettuce head, cut into medium strips

½ romaine lettuce head, cut into medium strips 1 cup canned dark beans, depleted

1 cup cheddar, destroyed 3 tablespoons cilantro, cleaved 4 green onions, slashed

12 cherry tomatoes, cut

¼ cup farm dressing

3 tablespoons BBQ sauce

Guidelines:

1. Put corn in the air fryer cooker, sprinkle some oil, hurl, cook at 400 Deg. Fahrenheit for about 10 minutes, move to a plate and leave aside for the time being.

2. Put chicken in the air fryer cooker's bin, include salt, pepper, darker sugar, paprika and garlic powder, hurl, sprinkle some more oil, cook at 400 Deg. Fahrenheit for about 10 minutes, flipping them midway, move tenders to a cutting board and hack them.

3. Cur bits off the cob, move corn to a bowl, include chicken, ice shelf lettuce, romaine lettuce, dark beans, cheddar, cilantro, tomatoes, onions, bar-b-que sauce and farm dressing, hurl well and serve for lunch.

Enjoy the recipe!

The nutritional facts: calories 372, fat 6, fiber 9, carbs 17, protein 6

THE FISH AND CHIPS

Prep. time: 10 minutes

The cooking time: 12 minutes

The recipe servings: 2

Fixings:

2 medium cod fillets, skinless and boneless Salt and dark pepper to the taste

¼ cup buttermilk

3 cups pot chips, cooked

Guidelines:

1. In a bowl, blend fish in with salt, pepper and buttermilk, hurl and leave aside for 5 minutes.

2. Put chips in your food processor, pulverize them and spread them on a plate.

3. Add fish and press well on all sides.

4. Transfer fish to the air fryer cooker's bin and cook at 400 Deg. Fahrenheit for about 12 minutes.

5. Serve hot for lunch. Enjoy the recipe!

The nutritional facts: calories 271, fat 7, fiber 9, carbs 14, protein 4

HARSH BROWN TOASTS

Prep. time: 10 minutes

The cooking time: 7 minutes

The recipe servings: 4

Fixings:

4 hash darker patties, solidified 1 tablespoon of olive oil

¼ cup cherry tomatoes, slashed

3 tablespoons mozzarella, destroyed 2 tablespoons parmesan, ground

1 tablespoon balsamic vinegar 1 tablespoon basil, slashed

Guidelines:

1. Put hash darker patties in the air fryer cooker, sprinkle the oil over them and cook at 400 deg. F for 7 minutes.

2. In a bowl, blend tomatoes in with mozzarella, parmesan, vinegar and basil and mix well.

3. Divide hash dark colored patties on plates, top each with tomatoes blend and serve for lunch.

Enjoy the recipe!

The nutritional facts: calories 199, fat 3, fiber 8, carbs 12, protein 4

DELECTABLE BEEF CUBES

Prep. time: 10 minutes

The cooking time: 12 minutes

The recipe servings: 4

Fixings:

1 pound sirloin, cubed

16 ounces jostled pasta sauce 1 and ½ cups bread morsels 2 tablespoons olive oil

½ teaspoon marjoram, dried

White rice, effectively cooked for serving

Guidelines:

1. In a bowl, blend meat shapes with pasta sauce and hurl well.

2. In another bowl, blend bread scraps with marjoram and oil and mix well.

3. Dip meat 3D squares right now, them in the air fryer cooker and cook at 360 Deg. Fahrenheit for about 12 minutes.

4. Divide among plates and present with white rice as an afterthought. Enjoy the recipe!

The nutritional facts: calories 271, fat 6, fiber 9, carbs 18, protein 12

PASTA SALAD

Prep. time: 10 minutes The cooking time: 12 minutes The recipe servings: 6

Fixings:

1 zucchini, cut into equal parts and generally hacked 1 orange chime pepper, generally slashed

1 green chime pepper, generally hacked 1 red onion, generally cleaved

4 ounces dark colored mushrooms, split Salt and dark pepper to the taste

1 teaspoon Italian flavoring

1 pound penne rigate, effectively cooked 1 cup cherry tomatoes, split

½ cup kalamata olive, pitted and split

¼ cup olive oil

3 tablespoons balsamic vinegar 2 tablespoons basil, hacked

Guidelines:

1. In a bowl, blend zucchini in with mushrooms, orange chime pepper, green ringer pepper, red onion, salt, pepper, Italian flavoring and oil, hurl well, move to preheated air fryer at 380 degrees F and cook them for 12 minutes.

2. Inside a large plate of mixed greens bowl, blend pasta in with cooked veggies, cherry tomatoes, olives, vinegar and basil, hurl and serve for lunch.

Enjoy the recipe!

The nutritional facts: calories 200, fat 5, fiber 8, carbs 10, protein 6

PHILADELPHIA CHICKEN LUNCH

Prep. time: 10 minutes The cooking time: 30 minutes The recipe servings: 4

Fixings:

1 teaspoon olive oil

1 yellow onion, cut

2 chicken bosoms, skinless, boneless and cut Salt and dark pepper to the taste

1 tablespoon Worcestershire sauce 14 ounces pizza mixture

1 and ½ cups cheddar, ground

½ cup jolted cheddar sauce

Guidelines:

1. Preheat the air fryer cooker at 400 degrees F, include half of the oil and onions and fry them for 8 minutes, blending once.

2. Add chicken pieces, Worcestershire sauce, salt and pepper, hurl, air fry for 8 minutes increasingly, mixing once and move everything to a bowl.

3. Roll pizza batter on a working surface and shape a square shape.

4. Spread portion of the cheddar all finished, include chicken and onion blend and top with cheddar sauce.

5. Roll your mixture and shape into a U.

6. Place your move in the air fryer cooker's container, brush with the remainder of the oil and cook at 370 degrees for 12 minutes, flipping the roll midway.

7. Slice your roll when it's warm and serve for lunch. Enjoy the recipe!

The nutritional facts: calories 300, fat 8, fiber 17, carbs 20, protein 6

SCRUMPTIOUS CHEESEBURGERS

Prep. time: 10 minutes The cooking time: 20 minutes The recipe servings: 2

Fixings:

12 ounces lean hamburger, ground 4 teaspoons ketchup

3 tablespoons yellow onion, slashed 2 teaspoons mustard

Salt and dark pepper to the taste 4 cheddar cuts

2 burger buns, divided

Guidelines:

1. In a bowl, blend hamburger in with onion, ketchup, mustard, salt and pepper, mix well and shape 4 patties out of this blend.

2. Divide cheddar on 2 patties and top with the other 2 patties.

3. Place them in preheated air fryer at 370 degrees F and fry them for 20 minutes.

4. Divide cheeseburger on 2 bun parts, top with the other 2 and serve for lunch.

Enjoy the recipe!

The nutritional facts: calories 261, fat 6, fiber 10, carbs 20, protein 6

TURKISH KOFTAS

Prep. time: 10 minutes The cooking time: 15 minutes The recipe servings: 2

Fixings:

1 leek, slashed

2 tablespoons feta cheddar, disintegrated

½ pound lean hamburger, minced 1 tablespoon cumin, ground 1 tablespoon mint, hacked

1 tablespoon parsley, slashed 1 teaspoon garlic, minced

Salt and dark pepper to the taste

Guidelines:

1. In a bowl, blend hamburger in with leek, cheddar, cumin, mint, parsley, garlic, salt and pepper, mix well, shape your koftas and spot them on sticks.

2. Add koftas to your preheated air fryer at 360 degrees F and cook them for 15 minutes.

3. Serve them with a side plate of mixed greens for lunch. Enjoy the recipe!

The nutritional facts: calories 281, fat 7, fiber 8, carbs 17, protein 6

THE CHICKEN KABOBS

Prep. time: 10 minutes The cooking time: 20 minutes The recipe servings: 2

Fixings:

3 orange chime peppers, cut into squares

¼ cup HONNEY

1/3 cup soy sauce

Salt and dark pepper to the taste Cooking splash

6 mushrooms, split

2 chicken bosoms, skinless, boneless and generally cubed

Guidelines:

1. In a bowl, blend chicken in with salt, pepper, HONNEY, state sauce and some cooking shower and hurl well.

2. Thread chicken, ringer peppers and mushrooms on sticks, place them in the air fryer cooker and cook at 338 Deg. Fahrenheit for about 20 minutes.

3. Divide among plates and serve for lunch. Enjoy the recipe!

The nutritional facts: calories 261, fat 7, fiber 9, carbs 12, protein 6

CHINESE PORK LUNCH MIX

Prep. time: 10 minutes The cooking time: 12 minutes The recipe servings: 4

Fixings:

2 eggs

2 pounds pork, cut into medium solid shapes 1 cup cornstarch

1 teaspoon sesame oil

Salt and dark pepper to the taste A spot of Chinese five zest

3 tablespoons canola oil

Sweet tomato sauce for serving

Guidelines:

1. In a bowl, blend five zest in with salt, pepper and cornstarch and mix.

2. In another bowl, blend eggs in with sesame oil and whisk well.

3. Dredge pork 3D squares in cornstarch blend, at that point dunk in eggs blend and spot them in the air fryer cooker which you've lubed with the canola oil.

4. Cook at 340 Deg. Fahrenheit for about 12 minutes, shaking the fryer once.

5. Serve pork for lunch with the sweet tomato sauce as an afterthought. Enjoy the recipe!

The nutritional facts: calories 320, fat 8, fiber 12, carbs 20, protein 5

HAMBURGER LUNCH MEATBALLS

Prep. time: 10 minutes The cooking time: 15 minutes The recipe servings: 4

Fixings:

½ pound hamburger, ground

½ pound Italian frankfurter, cleaved

½ teaspoon garlic powder

½ teaspoon onion powder

Salt and dark pepper to the taste

½ cup cheddar, ground Mashed potatoes for serving

Guidelines:

1. In a bowl, blend hamburger in with wiener, garlic powder, onion powder, salt, pepper and cheddar, mix well and shape 16 meatballs out of this blend.

2. Place meatballs in the air fryer cooker and cook them at 370 Deg. Fahrenheit for about 15 minutes.

3. Serve your meatballs with some pureed potatoes as an afterthought. Enjoy the recipe!

The nutritional facts: calories 333, fat 23, fiber 1, carbs 8, protein 20

HEAVENLY CHICKEN WINGS

Prep. time: 10 minutes

The cooking time: 45 minutes

The recipe servings: 4

Fixings:

3 pounds chicken wings

½ cup margarine

1 tablespoon old cove flavoring

¾ cup potato starch

1 teaspoon lemon juice Lemon wedges for serving

Guidelines:

1. In a bowl, blend starch in with old cove flavoring and chicken wings and hurl well.

2. Place chicken wings in the air fryer cooker's crate and cook them at 360 Deg. Fahrenheit for about 35 minutes shaking the fryer now and again.

3. Increase temperature to 400 degrees F, cook chicken wings for 10 minutes more and gap them on plates.

4. Heat up a container over medium heat, include spread and liquefy it.

5. Add lemon juice, mix well, take off heat and shower over chicken wings.

6. Serve them for lunch with lemon wedges as an afterthought. Enjoy the recipe!

The nutritional facts: calories 271, fat 6, fiber 8, carbs 18, protein 18

SIMPLE HOT DOGS

Prep. time: 10 minutes

The cooking time: 7 minutes

The recipe servings: 2

Fixings:

2 hot canine buns 2 hot mutts

1 tablespoon Dijon mustard

2 tablespoons cheddar, ground

Guidelines:

1. Put hot canines in preheated air fryer and cook them at 390 Deg. Fahrenheit for about 5 minutes.

2. Divide hot canines into hot pooch buns, spread mustard and cheddar, return everything to the air fryer cooker and cook for 2 minutes more at 390 degrees F.

3. Serve for lunch. Enjoy the recipe!

The nutritional facts: calories 211, fat 3, fiber 8, carbs 12, protein 4

JAPANESE CHICKEN MIX

Prep. time: 10 minutes The cooking time: 8 minutes The recipe servings: 2

Fixings:

2 chicken thighs, skinless and boneless 2 ginger cuts, slashed

3 garlic cloves, minced

¼ cup soy sauce

¼ cup mirin 1/8 cup purpose

½ teaspoon sesame oil 1/8 cup water

2 tablespoons sugar

1 tablespoon cornstarch blended in with 2 tablespoons water Sesame seeds for serving

Guidelines:

1. In a bowl, blend chicken thighs in with ginger, garlic, soy sauce, mirin, purpose, oil, water, sugar and cornstarch, hurl well, move to preheated air fryer and cook at 360 Deg. Fahrenheit for about 8 minutes.

2. Divide among plates, sprinkle sesame seeds on top and present with a side serving of mixed greens for lunch.

Enjoy the recipe!

The nutritional facts: calories 300, fat 7, fiber 9, carbs 17, protein 10

PROSCIUTTO SANDWICH

Prep. time: 10 minutes

The cooking time: 5 minutes

The recipe servings: 1
Fixings:

2 bread cuts

2 mozzarella cuts

2 tomato cuts

2 prosciutto cuts

2 basil leaves

1 teaspoon olive oil

A touch of salt and dark pepper

Guidelines:

1. Arrange mozzarella and prosciutto on a bread cut.

2. Seasoned with salt & pepper, place in the air fryer cooker and cook at 400 Deg. Fahrenheit for about 5 minutes.

3. Drizzle oil over prosciutto, include tomato and basil, spread with the other bread cut, cut sandwich down the middle and serve.

Enjoy the recipe!

The nutritional facts: calories 172, fat 3, fiber 7, carbs 9, protein 5

LENTILS FRITTERS

Prep. time: 10 minutes

The cooking time: 10 minutes

The recipe servings: 2

Fixings

1 cup yellow lentils, absorbed water for 1 hour and depleted 1 hot stew pepper, slashed

1 inch ginger piece, ground

½ teaspoon turmeric powder 1 teaspoon garam masala

1 teaspoon preparing powder

Salt and dark pepper to the taste 2 teaspoons olive oil

1/3 cup water

½ cup cilantro, hacked

1 and ½ cup spinach, hacked 4 garlic cloves, minced

¾ cup red onion, hacked Mint chutney for serving

Guidelines:

1. In your blender, blend lentils in with stew pepper, ginger, turmeric, garam masala, preparing powder, salt, pepper, olive oil, water, cilantro, spinach, onion and garlic, mix well and shape medium balls out of this blend.

2. Place them all in your preheated air fryer at 400 degrees F and cook for 10 minutes.

3. Serve your veggie squanders with a side plate of mixed greens for lunch. Enjoy the recipe!

The nutritional facts: calories 142, fat 2, fiber 8, carbs 12, protein 4

LUNCH POTATO SALAD

Prep. time: 10 minutes

The cooking time: 10 minutes

The recipe servings: 2

Fixings

2 pound red potatoes, split 2 tablespoons olive oil

Salt and dark pepper to the taste 2 green onions, hacked

1 red chime pepper, hacked 1/3 cup lemon juice

3 tablespoons mustard

Guidelines:

1. On the air fryer cooker's crate, blend potatoes in with half of the olive oil, salt and pepper and cook at 350 Deg. Fahrenheit for about 25 minutes shaking the fryer once.

2. In a bowl, blend onions in with ringer pepper and simmered potatoes and hurl.

3. In a little bowl, blend lemon squeeze in with the remainder of the oil and mustard and whisk truly well.

4. Add this to potato plate of mixed greens, hurl well and serve for lunch. Enjoy the recipe!

The nutritional facts: calories 211, fat 6, fiber 8, carbs 12, protein 4

CORN CASSEROLE

Prep. time: 10 minutes The cooking time: 15 minutes The recipe servings: 4

Fixings:

2 cups corn

3 tablespoons flour

1 egg

¼ cup milk

½ cup light cream

½ cup Swiss cheddar, ground 2 tablespoons margarine

Salt and dark pepper to the taste Cooking shower

Guidelines:

1. In a bowl, blend corn in with flour, egg, milk, light cream, cheddar, salt, pepper and spread and mix well.

2. Grease the air fryer cooker's dish with cooking splash, pour cream blend, spread and cook at 320 Deg. Fahrenheit for about 15 minutes.

3. Serve warm for lunch. Enjoy the recipe!

The nutritional facts: calories 281, fat 7, fiber 8, carbs 9, protein 6

BACON AND GARLIC PIZZAS

Prep. time: 10 minutes The cooking time: 10 minutes The recipe servings: 4

Fixings:

4 supper rolls, solidified 4 garlic cloves minced

½ teaspoon oregano dried

½ teaspoon garlic powder 1 cup tomato sauce

8 bacon cuts, cooked and hacked 1 and ¼ cups cheddar, ground Cooking shower

Guidelines:

1. Place supper moves on a working surface and press them to get 4 ovals.

2. Spray every oval with cooking splash, move them to the air fryer cooker and cook them at 370 Deg. Fahrenheit for about 2 minutes.

3. Spread tomato sauce on every oval, separate garlic, sprinkle oregano and garlic powder and top with bacon and cheddar.

4. Return pizzas to your heated air fryer and cook them at 370 Deg. Fahrenheit for about 8 minutes more.

5. Serve them warm for lunch. Enjoy the recipe!

The nutritional facts: calories 217, fat 5, fiber 8, carbs 12, protein 4

PREPARED SAUSAGE MIX

Prep. time: 10 minutes The cooking time: 10 minutes The recipe servings: 4

Fixings:

1 pound frankfurters, cut

1 red ringer pepper, cut into strips

½ cup yellow onion, slashed 3 tablespoons dark colored sugar 1/3 cup ketchup

2 tablespoons mustard

2 tablespoons apple juice vinegar

½ cup chicken stock

Guidelines:

1. In a bowl, blend sugar in with ketchup, mustard, stock and vinegar and whisk well.

2. In the air fryer cooker's dish, blend hotdog cuts with ringer pepper, onion and prepared blend, hurl and cook at 350 Deg. Fahrenheit for about 10 minutes.

3. Divide into bowls and serve for lunch. Enjoy the recipe!

The nutritional facts: calories 162, fat 6, fiber 9, carbs 12, protein 6

THE MEATBALLS AND TOMATO SAUCE

Prep. time: 10 minutes The cooking time: 15 minutes The recipe servings: 4

Fixings:

1 pound lean hamburger, ground 3 green onions, slashed 2 garlic cloves, minced

1 egg yolk

¼ cup bread pieces

Salt and dark pepper to the taste 1 tablespoon of olive oil

16 ounces tomato sauce 2 tablespoons mustard

Guidelines:

1. In a bowl, blend hamburger in with onion, garlic, egg yolk, bread scraps, salt and pepper, mix well and shape medium meatballs out of this blend.

2. Grease meatballs with the oil, place them in the air fryer cooker and cook them at 400 Deg. Fahrenheit for about 10 minutes.

3. In a bowl, blend tomato sauce with mustard, whisk, include over meatballs, hurl them and cook at 400 Deg. Fahrenheit for about 5 minutes more.

4. Divide meatballs and sauce on plates and serve for lunch. Enjoy the recipe!

The nutritional facts: calories 300, fat 8, fiber 9, carbs 16, protein 5

THE STUFFED MEATBALLS

Prep. time: 10 minutes The cooking time: 10 minutes The recipe servings: 4

Fixings:

- 1/3 cup bread pieces 3 tablespoons milk

- 1 tablespoon ketchup

- 1 egg

- ½ teaspoon marjoram, dried

- Salt and dark pepper to the taste 1 pound lean meat, ground

- 20 cheddar 3D squares 1 tablespoon of olive oil

Guidelines:

1. In a bowl, blend bread pieces with ketchup, milk, marjoram, salt, pepper and egg and whisk well.

2. Add hamburger, mix and shape 20 meatballs out of this blend.

3. Shape every meatball around a cheddar 3D shape, shower the oil over them and rub.

4. Place all meatballs in your preheated air fryer and cook at 390 Deg. Fahrenheit for about 10 minutes.

5. Serve them for lunch with a side plate of mixed greens. Enjoy the recipe!

The nutritional facts: calories 200, fat 5, fiber 8, carbs 12, protein 5

STEAKS AND CABBAGE

Prep. time: 10 minutes The cooking time: 10 minutes The recipe servings: 4

Fixings:

½ pound sirloin steak, cut into strips 2 teaspoons cornstarch

1 tablespoon nut oil

2 cups green cabbage, slashed 1 yellow ringer pepper, hacked 2 green onions, cleaved

2 garlic cloves, minced

Salt and dark pepper to the taste

Guidelines:

1. In a bowl, blend cabbage in with salt, pepper and nut oil, hurl, move to air fryer's bin, cook at 370 Deg. Fahrenheit for about 4 minutes and move to a bowl.

2. Add steak strips to the air fryer cooker, likewise include green onions, chime pepper, garlic, salt and pepper, hurl and cook for 5 minutes.

3. Add over cabbage, hurl, isolate among plates and serve for lunch. Enjoy the recipe!

The nutritional facts: calories 282, fat 6, fiber 8, carbs 14, protein 6

THE SUCCULENT LUNCH TURKEY BREAST

Prep. time: 10 minutes The cooking time: 47 minutes The recipe servings: 4

Fixings:

1 big turkey bosom

2 teaspoons olive oil

½ teaspoon smoked paprika 1 teaspoon thyme, dried

½ teaspoon savvy, dried

Salt and dark pepper to the taste 2 tablespoons mustard

¼ cup maple syrup

1 tablespoon margarine, delicate

Guidelines:

1. Brush turkey bosom with the olive oil, season with salt, pepper, thyme, paprika and sage, rub, place in the air fryer cooker's crate and fry at 350 Deg. Fahrenheit for about 25 minutes.

2. Flip turkey, cook for 10 minutes increasingly, flip once again and cook for an additional 10 minutes.

3. Meanwhile, heat up a skillet with the spread over medium heat, include mustard and maple syrup, mix well, cook for two or three minutes and take off heat.

4. Slice turkey bosom, isolate among plates and present with the maple coat sprinkled on top.

Enjoy the recipe!

The nutritional facts: calories 280, fat 2, fiber 7, carbs 16, protein 14

THE ITALIAN EGGPLANT SANDWICH

Prep. time: 10 minutes The cooking time: 16 minutes The recipe servings: 2

Fixings:

1 eggplant, cut

2 teaspoons parsley, dried

Salt and dark pepper to the taste

½ cup breadcrumbs

½ teaspoon Italian flavoring

½ teaspoon garlic powder

½ teaspoon onion powder 2 tablespoons milk

4 bread cuts Cooking shower

½ cup mayonnaise

¾ cup tomato sauce

2 cups mozzarella cheddar, ground

Guidelines:

1. Season eggplant cuts with salt and pepper, leave aside for 10 minutes and afterward pat dry them well.

2. In a bowl, blend parsley in with breadcrumbs, Italian flavoring, onion and garlic powder, salt and dark pepper and mix.

3. In another bowl, blend milk in with mayo and whisk well.

4. Brush eggplant cuts with mayo blend, dunk them in breadcrumbs, place them in the air fryer cooker's bushel, shower with cooking oil and cook them at 400 Deg. Fahrenheit for about 15 minutes, flipping them following 8 minutes.

5. Brush each bread cut with olive oil and organize 2 on a working surface.

6. Add mozzarella and parmesan on each, include prepared eggplant cuts, spread tomato sauce and basil and top with the other bread cuts, lubed side down.

Enjoy the recipe!

7. Divide sandwiches on plates, cut them in equal parts and serve for lunch.

The nutritional facts: calories 324, fat 16, fiber 4, carbs 39, protein 12

THE CREAMY CHICKEN STEW

Prep. time: 10 minutes The cooking time: 25 minutes The recipe servings: 4

Fixings:

1 and ½ cups canned cream of celery soup 6 chicken fingers

Salt and dark pepper to the taste 2 potatoes, slashed

1 narrows leaf

1 thyme spring, slashed 1 tablespoon milk

1 egg yolk

½ cup substantial cream

Guidelines:

1. In a bowl, blend chicken in with cream of celery, potatoes, overwhelming cream, inlet leaf, thyme, salt and pepper, hurl, immerse the air fryer cooker's skillet and cook at 320 Deg. Fahrenheit for about 25 minutes.

2. Leave your stew to chill off a piece, dispose of straight leaf, partition among plates and serve immediately.

Enjoy the recipe!

The nutritional facts: calories 300, fat 11, fiber 2, carbs 23, protein 14

THE LUNCH PORK AND POTATOES

Prep. time: 10 minutes The cooking time: 25 minutes The recipe servings: 2

Fixings:

2 pounds pork flank

Salt and dark pepper to the taste

2 red potatoes, cut into medium wedges

½ teaspoon garlic powder

½ teaspoon red pepper drops 1 teaspoon parsley, dried

A sprinkle of balsamic vinegar

Guidelines:

1. In the air fryer cooker's skillet, blend pork in with potatoes, salt, pepper, garlic powder, pepper pieces, parsley and vinegar, hurl and cook at 390 Deg. Fahrenheit for about 25 minutes.

2. Slice pork, partition it and potatoes on plates and serve for lunch.

Enjoy the recipe!

The nutritional facts: calories 400, fat 15, fiber 7, carbs 27, protein 20

TURKEY CAKES

Prep. time: 10 minutes

The cooking time: 10 minutes

The recipe servings: 4

Fixings:

6 mushrooms, cleaved

1 teaspoon of garlic powder and 1 teaspoon of onion powder

Salt and dark pepper to the taste

1 and ¼ pounds turkey meat, ground Cooking shower

Tomato sauce for serving

Guidelines:

1. In your blender, blend mushrooms in with salt and pepper, beat well and move to a bowl.

2. Add turkey, onion powder, garlic powder, salt and pepper, mix and shape cakes out of this blend.

3. Spray them with cooking splash, move them to the air fryer cooker and cook at 320 Deg. Fahrenheit for about 10 minutes.

4. Serve them with tomato sauce as an afterthought and a delicious side serving of mixed greens.

Enjoy the recipe!

The nutritional facts: calories 202, fat 6, fiber 3, carbs 17, protein 10

CHEDDAR RAVIOLI AND MARINARA SAUCE

Prep. time: 10 minutes

The cooking time: 8 minutes

The recipe servings: 6

Fixings:

20 ounces cheddar ravioli 10 ounces marinara sauce 1 tablespoon of olive oil

1 cup buttermilk

2 cups bread pieces

¼ cup parmesan, ground

Guidelines:

1. Put buttermilk in a bowl and breadcrumbs in another bowl.

2. Dip ravioli in buttermilk, at that point in breadcrumbs and spot them in the air fryer cooker on a preparing sheet.

3. Drizzle olive oil over them, cook at 400 Deg. Fahrenheit for about 5 minutes, isolate them on plates, sprinkle parmesan on top and serve for lunch

Enjoy the recipe!

The nutritional facts: calories 270, fat 12, fiber 6, carbs 30, protein 15

HAMBURGER STEW

Prep. time: 10 minutes

The cooking time: 20 minutes

The recipe servings: 4

Fixings:

2 pounds hamburger meat, cut into medium lumps 2 carrots, hacked

4 potatoes, slashed

Salt and dark pepper to the taste 1 quart veggie stock

½ teaspoon smoked paprika A bunch thyme, slashed

Guidelines:

1. In a dish that accommodates the air fryer cooker, blend hamburger in with carrots, potatoes, stock, salt, pepper, paprika and thyme, mix, place in air fryer's bin and cook at 375 Deg. Fahrenheit for about 20 minutes.

2. Divide into bowls and serve immediately for lunch.

Enjoy the recipe!

The nutritional facts: calories 260, fat 5, fiber 8, carbs 20, protein 22

MEATBALLS SANDWICH

Prep. time: 10 minutes

The cooking time: 22 minutes

The recipe servings: 4

Fixings:

3 loaves, cut more than partially through 14 ounces hamburger, ground

7 ounces tomato sauce 1 little onion, hacked 1 egg, whisked

1 tablespoon bread pieces

2 tablespoons cheddar, ground 1 tablespoon oregano, hacked

1 tablespoon of olive oil

Salt and dark pepper to the taste 1 teaspoon thyme, dried

1 teaspoon basil, dried

Guidelines:

1. In a bowl, consolidate meat with salt, pepper, onion, breadcrumbs, egg, cheddar, oregano, thyme and basil, mix, shape medium meatballs and add them to the air fryer cooker after you've lubed it with the oil.

2. Cook them at 375 Deg. Fahrenheit for about 12 minutes, flipping them midway.

3. Add tomato sauce, cook meatballs for 10 minutes more and orchestrate them on cut rolls.

4. Serve them immediately.

Enjoy the recipe!

The nutritional facts: calories 380, fat 5, fiber 6, carbs 34, protein 20

THE BACON PUDDING

Prep. time: 10 minutes

The cooking time: 30 minutes

The recipe servings: 4

Fixings:

4 bacon strips, cooked and cleaved 1 tablespoon margarine, delicate

2 cups corn

1 yellow onion, cleaved

¼ cup celery, cleaved

½ cup red ringer pepper, cleaved 1 teaspoon thyme, slashed

2 teaspoons garlic, minced

Salt and dark pepper to the taste

½ cup substantial cream 1 and ½ cups milk 3 eggs, whisked

3 cups bread, cubed

4 tablespoons parmesan, ground Cooking shower

Guidelines:

1. Grease the air fryer cooker's container with coking shower.

2. In a bowl, blend bacon in with margarine, corn, onion, ringer pepper, celery, thyme, garlic, salt, pepper, milk, substantial cream, eggs and bread shapes, hurl, fill lubed container and sprinkle cheddar everywhere

3. Add this to your preheated air fryer at 320 degrees and cook for 30 minutes.

4. Divide among plates and serve warm for a snappy lunch.

Enjoy the recipe!

The nutritional facts: calories 276, fat 10, fiber 2, carbs 20, protein 10

UNCOMMON LUNCH SEAFOOD STEW

Prep. time: 10 minutes

The cooking time: 20 minutes

The recipe servings: 4

Fixings:

5ounces white rice 2 ounces peas

1 red ringer pepper, hacked 14 ounces white wine

3 ounces water

2 ounces squid pieces 7 ounces mussels

3 ounces ocean bass filet, skinless, boneless and hacked 6 scallops

3.5 ounces mollusks 4 shrimp

4 crayfish

Salt and dark pepper to the taste 1 tablespoon of olive oil

Guidelines:

1. In the air fryer cooker's dish, blend ocean bass in with shrimp, mussels, scallops, crayfish, shellfishes and squid.

2. Add the oil, salt and pepper and hurl to cover.

3. In a bowl, blend peas salt, pepper, chime pepper and rice and mix.

4. Add this over seafood, additionally include cry and water, place container in the air fryer cooker and cook at 400 Deg. Fahrenheit for about 20 minutes, mixing midway.

5. Divide into bowls and serve for lunch.

Enjoy the recipe!

The nutritional facts: calories 300, fat 12, fiber 2, carbs 23, protein 25

AIR FRIED THAI SALAD

Prep. time: 10 minutes

The cooking time: 5 minutes

The recipe servings: 4

Fixings:

1 cup carrots, ground

1 cup red cabbage, destroyed

A spot of salt and dark pepper A bunch cilantro, slashed

1 small cucumber, slashed Juice from 1 lime

2 teaspoons red curry glue

12 major shrimp, cooked, stripped and deveined

Guidelines:

1. In a skillet that accommodates your, blend cabbage in with carrots, cucumber and shrimp, hurl, present in the air fryer cooker and cook at 360 Deg. Fahrenheit for about 5 minutes.

2. Add salt, pepper, cilantro, lime juice and red curry glue, hurl once more, partition among plates and serve immediately.

Enjoy the recipe!

The nutritional facts: calories 172, fat 5, fiber 7, carbs 8, protein 5

SWEET POTATO LUNCH CASSEROLE

Prep. time: 10 minutes The cooking time: 50 minutes The recipe servings: 6

Fixings:

3 major sweet potatoes, pricked with a fork 1 cup chicken stock

Salt and dark pepper to the taste A spot of cayenne pepper

¼ teaspoon nutmeg, ground 1/3 cup coconut cream

Guidelines:

1. Place sweet potatoes in the air fryer cooker, cook them at 350 Deg. Fahrenheit for about 40 minutes, chill them off, strip, generally hack and move to a container that accommodates the air fryer cooker.

2. Add stock, salt, pepper, cayenne and coconut cream, hurl, present in the air fryer cooker and cook at 360 deg. F for 10 minutes more.

3. Divide meal into bowls and serve. Enjoy the recipe!

The nutritional facts: calories 245, fat 4, fiber 5, carbs 10, protein 6

ZUCCHINI CASEROLE

Prep. time: 10 minutes The cooking time: 16 minutes The recipe servings: 8

Fixings:

1 cup veggie stock

1 tablespoons olive oil

2 sweet potatoes, stripped and cut into medium wedges 8 zucchinis, cut into medium wedges

2 yellow onions, slashed 1 cup coconut milk

Salt and dark pepper to the taste 1 tablespoon soy sauce

¼ teaspoon thyme, dried

¼ teaspoon rosemary, dried 4 tablespoons dill, slashed

½ teaspoon basil, slashed

Guidelines:

1. Heat a skillet that accommodates the air fryer cooker with the oil over medium heat, include onion, mix and cook for 2 minutes.

2. Add zucchinis, thyme, rosemary, basil, potato, salt, pepper, stock, milk, soy sauce and dill, mix, present in the air fryer cooker, cook at 360 Deg. Fahrenheit for about 14 minutes, isolate among plates and serve immediately.

Enjoy the recipe!

The nutritional facts: calories 133, fat 3, fiber 4, carbs 10, protein 5

COCONUT AND CHICKEN CASEROLE

Prep. time: 10 minutes The cooking time: 25 minutes The recipe servings: 4

Fixings:

4 lime leaves, torn 1 cup veggie stock

1 lemongrass stalk, hacked 1 inch piece, ground

1 pound chicken bosom, skinless, boneless and cut into dainty strips 8 ounces mushrooms, hacked

4 Thai chilies, hacked 4 tablespoons fish sauce 6 ounces coconut milk

¼ cup lime juice

¼ cup cilantro, hacked

Salt and dark pepper to the taste

Guidelines:

1. Put stock into a dish that accommodates the air fryer cooker, bring to a stew over medium heat, include lemongrass, ginger and lime leaves, mix and cook for 10 minutes.

2. Strain soup, come back to container, include chicken, mushrooms, milk, chilies, fish sauce, lime juice, cilantro, salt and pepper, mix, present in the air fryer cooker and cook at 360 Deg. Fahrenheit for about 15 minutes.

3. Divide into bowls and serve. Enjoy the recipe!

The nutritional facts: calories 150, fat 4, fiber 4, carbs 6, protein 7

TURKEY BUGGERS

Prep. time: 10 minutes

The cooking time: 8 minutes

The recipe servings: 4

Fixings:

1 pound turkey meat, ground 1 shallot, minced

A shower of olive oil

1 little jalapeno pepper, minced 2 teaspoons lime juice

Pizzazz from 1 lime, ground

Salt and dark pepper to the taste 1 teaspoon cumin, ground

1 teaspoon sweet paprika Guacamole for serving
Guidelines:

1. In a bowl, blend turkey meat in with salt, pepper, cumin, paprika, shallot, jalapeno, lime squeeze and pizzazz, mix well, shape burgers from this blend, sprinkle the oil over them, present in preheated air fryer and cook them at 370 Deg. Fahrenheit for about 8 minutes on each side.

2. Divide among plates and present with guacamole on top.

Enjoy the recipe!

The nutritional facts: calories 200, fat 12, fiber 0, carbs 0, protein 12

SALMON AND ASPARAGUS

Prep. time: 10 minutes The cooking time: 23 minutes The recipe servings: 4

Fixings:

1 pound asparagus, cut 1 tablespoon of olive oil

A spot of sweet paprika

Salt and dark pepper to the taste A spot of garlic powder

A spot of cayenne pepper

1 red ringer pepper, cut into equal parts 4 ounces smoked salmon

Guidelines:

1. Put asparagus lances and chime pepper on a lined preparing sheet that accommodates the air fryer cooker, include salt, pepper, garlic powder, paprika, olive oil, cayenne pepper, hurl to cover, present in the fryer, cook at 390 Deg. Fahrenheit for about 8 minutes, flip and cook for 8 minutes more.

2. Add salmon, cook for 5 minutes, more, isolate everything on plates and serve.

Enjoy the recipe!

The nutritional facts: calories 90, fat 1, fiber 1, carbs 1.2, protein 4

SIMPLE CHICKEN LUNCH

Prep. time: 10 minutes The cooking time: 20 minutes The recipe servings: 6

Fixings:

1 bundle kale, hacked

Salt and dark pepper to the taste

¼ cup chicken stock

1 cup chicken, destroyed 3 carrots, slashed

1 cup shiitake mushrooms, generally cut

Guidelines:

1. In a blender, blend stock in with kale, heartbeat a couple of times and fill a container that accommodates the air fryer cooker.

2. Add chicken, mushrooms, carrots, salt and pepper to the taste, hurl, present in the air fryer cooker and cook at 350 Deg. Fahrenheit for about 18 minutes.

Enjoy the recipe!

The nutritional facts: calories 180, fat 7, fiber 2, carbs 10, protein 5

CHICKEN AND CORN CASSEROLE

Prep. time: 10 minutes The cooking time: 30 minutes The recipe servings: 6

Fixings:

1 cup clean chicken stock 2 teaspoons garlic powder

Salt and dark pepper to the taste 6 ounces canned coconut milk

1 and ½ cups green lentils

2 pounds chicken bosoms, skinless, boneless and cubed 1/3 cup cilantro, cleaved

3 cups corn

3 bunches spinach

3 green onions, cleaved

Guidelines:

1. In a container that accommodates the air fryer cooker, blend stock in with coconut milk, salt, pepper, garlic powder, chicken and lentils.

2. Add corn, green onions, cilantro and spinach, mix well, present in the air fryer cooker and cook at 350 deg. F for 30 minutes.

Enjoy the recipe!

The nutritional facts: calories 345, fat 12, fiber 10, carbs 20, protein 44

CHICKEN AND ZUCCHINI LUNCH MIX

Prep. time: 10 minutes The cooking time: 20 minutes The recipe servings: 4

Fixings:

4 zucchinis, cut with a spiralizer

1 pound chicken bosoms, skinless, boneless and cubed 2 garlic cloves, minced

1 teaspoon olive oil

Salt and dark pepper to the taste 2 cups cherry tomatoes, divided

½ cup almonds, slashed

For the pesto:

2 cups basil

2 cups kale, slashed

1 tablespoon lemon juice 1 garlic clove

¾ cup pine nuts

½ cup olive oil A spot of salt

Guidelines:

1. In your food processor, blend basil in with kale, lemon juice, garlic, pine nuts, oil and a spot of salt, beat truly well and leave aside.

2. Heat up a dish that accommodates the air fryer cooker with the oil over medium heat, include garlic, mix and cook for 1 moment.

3. Add chicken, salt, pepper, mix, almonds, zucchini noodles, garlic, cherry tomatoes and the pesto you've made toward the start, mix delicately, present in preheated air fryer and cook at 360 Deg. Fahrenheit for about 17 minutes.

4. Divide among plates and serve for lunch.

Enjoy the recipe!

The nutritional facts: calories 344, fat 8, fiber 7, carbs 12, protein 16

CHICKEN, BEANS, CORN AND THE QUINOA CASSEROLE

Prep. time: 10 minutes The cooking time: 30 minutes The recipe servings: 8

Fixings:

1 cup quinoa, effectively cooked

3 cups chicken bosom, cooked and destroyed 14 ounces canned dark beans

12 ounces corn

½ cup cilantro, hacked 6 kale leaves, slashed

½ cup green onions, cleaved 1 cup clean tomato sauce

1 cup clean salsa

2 teaspoons bean stew powder

2 teaspoons cumin, ground

3 cups mozzarella cheddar, destroyed 1 tablespoon garlic powder Cooking splash

2 jalapeno peppers, cleaved

Guidelines:

1. Spray a preparing dish that accommodates the air fryer cooker with cooking shower, include quinoa, chicken, dark beans, corn, cilantro, kale, green onions, tomato sauce, salsa, stew powder, cumin, garlic powder, jalapenos and mozzarella, hurl, present in your fryer and cook at 350 Deg. Fahrenheit for about 17 minutes.

2. Slice and serve warm for lunch.

Enjoy the recipe!

The nutritional facts: calories 365, fat 12, fiber 6, carbs 22, protein 26

AIR FRYER SIDE DISH RECIPES

POTATO WEDGES

Prep. time: 10 minutes The cooking time: 25 minutes The recipe servings: 4

Fixings:

2 potatoes, cut into wedges 1 tablespoon of olive oil

Salt and dark pepper to the taste 3 tablespoons acrid cream

2 tablespoons sweet bean stew sauce

Guidelines:

1. In a bowl, blend potato wedges with oil, salt and pepper, hurl well, add to air fryer's container and cook at 360 Deg. Fahrenheit for about 25 minutes, flipping them once.

2. Divide potato wedges on plates, sprinkle acrid cream and stew sauce all finished and serve them as a side dish.

Enjoy the recipe!

The nutritional facts: calories 171, fat 8, fiber 9, carbs 18, protein 7

MUSHROOM SIDE DISH

Prep. time: 10 minutes The cooking time: 8 minutes The recipe servings: 4

Fixings:

10 catch mushrooms, stems evacuated 1 tablespoon Italian flavoring

Salt and dark pepper to the taste

2 tablespoons cheddar, ground 1 tablespoon of olive oil

2 tablespoons mozzarella, ground 1 tablespoon dill, slashed

Guidelines:

1. In a bowl, blend mushrooms in with Italian flavoring, salt, pepper, oil and dill and rub well.

2. Arrange mushrooms in the air fryer cooker's container, sprinkle mozzarella and cheddar in each and cook them at 360 Deg. Fahrenheit for about 8 minutes.

3. Divide them on plates and serve them as a side dish. Enjoy the recipe!

The nutritional facts: calories 241, fat 7, fiber 8, carbs 14, protein 6

SWEET POTATO FRIES

Prep. time: 10 minutes The cooking time: 20 minutes The recipe servings: 2

Fixings:

2 sweet potatoes, stripped and cut into medium fries Salt and dark pepper to the taste

2 tablespoons olive oil

½ teaspoon curry powder

¼ teaspoon coriander, ground

¼ cup ketchup

2 tablespoons mayonnaise

½ teaspoon cumin, ground A touch of ginger powder

A touch of cinnamon powder

Guidelines:

1. In the air fryer cooker's crate, blend sweet potato fries with salt, pepper, coriander, curry powder and oil, hurl well and cook at 370 Deg. Fahrenheit for about 20 minutes, flipping them once.

2. Meanwhile, in a bowl, blend ketchup in with mayo, cumin, ginger and cinnamon and whisk well.

3. Divide fries on plates, sprinkle ketchup blend over them and fill in as a side dish.

Enjoy the recipe!

The nutritional facts: calories 200, fat 5, fiber 8, carbs 9, protein 7

CORN WITH LIME AND CHEESE

Prep. time: 10 minutes The cooking time: 15 minutes The recipe servings: 2

Fixings:

2 corns on the cob, husks evacuated A sprinkle of olive oil

½ cup feta cheddar, ground 2 teaspoons sweet paprika Juice from 2 limes

Guidelines:

1. Rub corn with oil and paprika, place in the air fryer cooker and cook at 400 Deg. Fahrenheit for about 15 minutes, flipping once.

2. Divide corn on plates, sprinkle cheddar on top, shower lime squeeze and fill in as a side dish.

Enjoy the recipe!

The nutritional facts: calories 200, fat 5, fiber 2, carbs 6, protein 6

HASSELBACK POTATOES

Prep. time: 10 minutes The cooking time: 20 minutes The recipe servings: 2

Fixings:

2 potatoes, stripped and daintily cut practically as far as possible on a level plane 2 tablespoons olive oil

1 teaspoon garlic, minced

Salt and dark pepper to the taste

½ teaspoon oregano, dried

½ teaspoon basil, dried

½ teaspoon sweet paprika

Guidelines:

1. In a bowl, blend oil in with garlic, salt, pepper, oregano, basil and paprika and whisk truly well.

2. Rub potatoes with this blend, place them in the air fryer cooker's bin and fry them at 360 Deg. Fahrenheit for about 20 minutes.

3. Divide them on plates and fill in as a side dish. Enjoy the recipe!

The nutritional facts: calories 172, fat 6, fiber 6, carbs 9, protein 6

BRUSSELS SPROUTS SIDE DISH

Prep. time: 10 minutes The cooking time: 15 minutes The recipe servings: 4

Fixings:

1 pound Brussels grows, cut and divided Salt and dark pepper to the taste

6 teaspoons olive oil

½ teaspoon thyme, slashed

½ cup mayonnaise

2 tablespoons simmered garlic, squashed

Guidelines:

1. In the air fryer cooker, blend Brussels grows with salt, pepper and oil, hurl well and cook them at 390 Deg. Fahrenheit for about 15 minutes.

2. Meanwhile, in a bowl, blend thyme in with mayo and garlic and whisk well.

3. Divide Brussels grows on plates, shower garlic sauce all finished and fill in as a side dish.

Enjoy the recipe!

The nutritional facts: calories 172, fat 6, fiber 8, carbs 12, protein 6

CREAMY AIR FRIED POTATO SIDE DISH

Prep. time: 10 minutes

The cooking time: 1 hour and 20 minutes

The recipe servings: 2

Fixings:

1 big potato

2 bacon strips, cooked and cleaved 1 teaspoon olive oil

1/3 cup cheddar, destroyed

1 tablespoon green onions, cleaved Salt and dark pepper to the taste

1 tablespoon margarine

2 tablespoons substantial cream

Guidelines:

1. Rub potato with oil, season with salt and pepper, place in preheated air fryer and cook at 400 Deg. Fahrenheit for about 30 minutes.

2. Flip potato, cook for 30 minutes more, move to a cutting board, chill it off, cut into equal parts longwise and scoop mash in a bowl.

3. Add bacon, cheddar, margarine, overwhelming cream, green onions, salt and pepper, mix well and stuff potato skins with this blend.

4. Return potatoes to the air fryer cooker and cook them at 400 Deg. Fahrenheit for about 20 minutes.

5. Divide among plates and fill in as a side dish. Enjoy the recipe!

The nutritional facts: calories 172, fat 5, fiber 7, carbs 9, protein 4

GREEN BEANS SIDE DISH

Prep. time: 10 minutes The cooking time: 25 minutes The recipe servings: 4

Fixings:

1 and ½ pounds green beans, cut and steamed for 2 minutes Salt and dark pepper to the taste

½ pound shallots, cleaved

¼ cup almonds, toasted 2 tablespoons olive oil

Guidelines:

1. In the air fryer cooker's bin, blend green beans in with salt, pepper, shallots, almonds and oil, hurl well and cook at 400 Deg. Fahrenheit for about 25 minutes.

2. Divide among plates and fill in as a side dish. Enjoy the recipe!

The nutritional facts: calories 152, fat 3, fiber 6, carbs 7, protein 4

BROILED PUMPKIN

Prep. time: 10 minutes The cooking time: 12 minutes The recipe servings: 4

Fixings:

1 and ½ pound pumpkin, deseeded, cut and generally hacked 3 garlic cloves, minced

1 tablespoon of olive oil A touch of ocean salt

A touch of darker sugar

A touch of nutmeg, ground A spot of cinnamon powder

Guidelines:

1. In the air fryer cooker's bushel, blend pumpkin in with garlic, oil, salt, dark colored sugar, cinnamon and nutmeg, hurl well, spread and cook at 370 Deg. Fahrenheit for about 12 minutes.

2. Divide among plates and fill in as a side dish. Enjoy the recipe!

The nutritional facts: calories 200, fat 5, fiber 4, carbs 7, protein 4

PARMESAN MUSHROOMS

Prep. time: 10 minutes The cooking time: 15 minutes The recipe servings: 3

Fixings:

9 catch mushroom tops

3 cream saltine cuts, disintegrated 1 egg white

2 tablespoons parmesan, ground 1 teaspoon Italian flavoring

A spot of salt and dark pepper 1 tablespoon spread, liquefied

Guidelines:

1. In a bowl, blend saltines in with egg white, parmesan, Italian flavoring, spread, salt and pepper, mix well and stuff mushrooms with this blend.

2. Arrange mushrooms in the air fryer cooker's container and cook them at 360 Deg. Fahrenheit for about 15 minutes.

3. Divide among plates and fill in as a side dish. Enjoy the recipe!

The nutritional facts: calories 124, fat 4, fiber 4, carbs 7, protein 3

GARLIC POTATOES

Prep. time: 10 minutes The cooking time: 20 minutes The recipe servings: 6

Fixings:

2 tablespoons parsley, slashed 5 garlic cloves, minced

½ teaspoon basil, dried

½ teaspoon oregano, dried

2 pounds red potatoes, divided 1 teaspoon thyme, dried

2 tablespoons olive oil

Salt and dark pepper to the taste 2 tablespoons margarine

1/3 cup parmesan, ground

Guidelines:

1. In a bowl, blend potato parts with parsley, garlic, basil, oregano, thyme, salt, pepper, oil and spread, hurl truly well and move to the air fryer cooker's bushel.

2. Cover and cook at 400 Deg. Fahrenheit for about 20 minutes, flipping them once.

3. Sprinkle parmesan on top, separate potatoes on plates and fill in as a side dish.

Enjoy the recipe!

The nutritional facts: calories 162, fat 5, fiber 5, carbs 7, protein 5

EGGPLANT SIDE DISH

Prep. time: 10 minutes The cooking time: 10 minutes The recipe servings: 4

Fixings:

8 child eggplants, scooped in the inside and mash saved Salt and dark pepper to the taste

A touch of oregano, dried

1 green chime pepper, slashed 1 tablespoon tomato glue

1 pack coriander, slashed

½ teaspoon garlic powder 1 tablespoon of olive oil

1 yellow onion, hacked 1 tomato slashed

Guidelines:

1. Heat up a dish with the oil over medium heat, include onion, mix and cook for 1 moment.

2. Add salt, pepper, eggplant mash, oregano, green chime pepper, tomato glue, garlic force, coriander and tomato, mix, cook for 1-2 minutes more, bring off heat and chill off.

3. Stuff eggplants with this blend, place them in the air fryer cooker's bin and cook at 360 Deg. Fahrenheit for about 8 minutes.

4. Divide eggplants on plates and serve them as a side dish. Enjoy the recipe!

The nutritional facts: calories 200, fat 3, fiber 7, carbs 12, protein 4

MUSHROOMS AND SOUR CREAM

Prep. time: 10 minutes The cooking time: 10 minutes The recipe servings: 6

Fixings:

2 bacon strips, cleaved 1 yellow onion, slashed

1 green ringer pepper, cleaved 24 mushrooms, stems expelled 1 carrot, ground

½ cup acrid cream

1 cup cheddar, ground Salt and dark pepper to the taste

Guidelines:

1. Heat up a container over medium high heat, include bacon, onion, ringer pepper and carrot, mix and cook for 1 moment.

2. Add salt, pepper and acrid cream, mix cook for brief more, bring off heat and chill off.

3. Stuff mushrooms with this blend, sprinkle cheddar on top and cook at 360 Deg. Fahrenheit for about 8 minutes.

4. Divide among plates and fill in as a side dish. Enjoy the recipe!

The nutritional facts: calories 211, fat 4, fiber 7, carbs 8, protein 3

EGGPLANT FRIES

Prep. time: 10 minutes The cooking time: 5 minutes The recipe servings: 4

Fixings:

Cooking shower

1 eggplant, stripped and cut into medium fries 2 tablespoons milk

1 egg, whisked

2 cups panko bread scraps

½ cup Italian cheddar, destroyed

A touch of salt and dark pepper to the taste

Guidelines:

1. In a bowl, blend egg in with milk, salt and pepper and whisk well.

2. In another bowl, blend panko with cheddar and mix.

3. Dip eggplant fries in egg blend, at that point coat in panko blend, place them in the air fryer cooker lubed with cooking splash and cook at 400 Deg. Fahrenheit for about 5 minutes.

4. Divide among plates and fill in as a side dish. Enjoy the recipe!

The nutritional facts: calories 162, fat 5, fiber 5, carbs 7, protein 6

FRIED TOMATOES DISH

Prep. time: 10 minutes The cooking time: 5 minutes The recipe servings: 4

Fixings:

2 green tomatoes, cut

Salt and dark pepper to the taste

½ cup flour

1 cup buttermilk

1 cup panko bread pieces

½ tablespoon Creole flavoring Cooking splash

Guidelines:

1. Season tomato cuts with salt and pepper.

2. Put flour in a bowl, buttermilk in another and panko pieces and Creole flavoring in a third one.

3. Dredge tomato cuts in flour, at that point in buttermilk and panko bread pieces, place them in the air fryer cooker's bin lubed with cooking shower and cook them at 400 Deg. Fahrenheit for about 5 minutes.

4. Divide among plates and fill in as a side dish. Enjoy the recipe!

The nutritional facts: calories 124, fat 5, fiber 7, carbs 9, protein 4

CAULIFLOWER CAKES

Prep. time: 10 minutes The cooking time: 10 minutes The recipe servings: 6

Fixings:

3 and ½ cups cauliflower rice 2 eggs

¼ cup white flour

½ cup parmesan, ground

Salt and dark pepper to the taste Cooking splash

Guidelines:

1.   In a bowl, blend cauliflower rice with salt and pepper, mix and press abundant water.

2.   Transfer cauliflower to another bowl, include eggs, salt, pepper, flour, and parmesan, mix truly well and shape your cakes.

3.   Grease the air fryer cooker with a cooking splash, heat it up at 400 degrees, include cauliflower cakes, and cook them for 10 minutes, flipping them midway.

4.   Divide cakes between plates and fill in as a side dish. Enjoy the recipe!

The nutritional facts: calories 125, fat 2, fiber 6, carbs 8, protein 3

CREAMY BRUSSELS SPROUTS

Prep. time: 10 minutes The cooking time: 25 minutes The recipe servings: 8

Fixings:

3 pounds Brussels grows, split A shower of olive oil

1 pound bacon, hacked

Salt and dark pepper to the taste 4 tablespoons spread.

3 shallots, hacked

1   cup milk

2   cups overwhelming cream

¼ teaspoon nutmeg, ground

3   tablespoons arranged horseradish

Guidelines:

1.   Preheated the air fryer at 370 degrees F, include oil, bacon, salt and pepper and Brussels sprouts and hurl.

2.	Add spread, shallots, overwhelming cream, milk, nutmeg and horseradish, hurl again and cook for 25 minutes.

3.	Divide among plates and fill in as a side dish. Enjoy the recipe!

The nutritional facts: calories 214, fat 5, fiber 8, carbs 12, protein 5

CHADDAR BISCUITS

Prep. time: 10 minutes The cooking time: 20 minutes The recipe servings: 8

Fixings:

2 and 1/3 cup self-rising flour

½ cup butter+ 1 tablespoon, dissolved 2 tablespoons sugar

½ cup cheddar, ground 1 and 1/3 cup buttermilk

1 cup flour

Guidelines:

1.	In a bowl, blend self-rising flour with ½ cup spread, sugar, cheddar and buttermilk, and mix until you get a mixture.

2.	Spread 1 cup flour on a working surface, move mixture, level it, cut 8 circles with a cookie shaper and coat them with flour.

3.   Line, the air fryer cooker's bin with tin foil, include rolls, brush them with liquefied margarine and cook them at 380 Deg. Fahrenheit for about 20 minutes.

4.   Divide among plates and fill in as a side. Enjoy the recipe!

The nutritional facts: calories 221, fat 3, fiber 8, carbs 12, protein 4

ZUCCHINI FRIES

Prep. time: 10 minutes The cooking time: 12 minutes The recipe servings: 4

Fixings:

1 zucchini, cut into medium sticks A shower of olive oil

Salt and dark pepper to the taste 2 eggs, whisked

1 cup bread scraps

½ cup flour

Guidelines:

1.   Put flour in a bowl and blend in with salt and pepper and mix.

2.   Put breadcrumbs in another bowl.

3.   In a third bowl blend eggs in with a touch of salt and pepper.

4.   Dredge zucchini fries in flour, at that point in eggs and in bread morsels toward the end.

5.   Grease the air fryer cooker with some olive oil, heat up at 400 degrees F, include zucchini fries and then cook the recipes for 12 minutes.

6.   Serve them as a side dish. Enjoy the recipe!

The nutritional facts: calories 172, fat 3, fiber 3, carbs 7, protein 3

HERBED TOMATOES

Prep. time: 10 minutes The cooking time: 15 minutes The recipe servings: 4

Fixings:

4 major tomatoes, divided and inner parts scooped out Salt and dark pepper to the taste

½ teaspoon thyme, slashed

Guidelines:

1.   In the air fryer cooker, blend tomatoes in with salt, pepper, oil, garlic and thyme, hurl and cook at 390 deg. F for another 15 minutes.

2.   Divide among plates and serve them as a side dish. Enjoy the recipe!

The nutritional facts: calories 112, fat 1, fiber 3, carbs 4, protein 4

THE ROASTED PEPPERS

Prep. time: 10 minutes The cooking time: 20 minutes The recipe servings: 4

Fixings:

1 tablespoon sweet paprika 1 tablespoon of olive oil

4 red chime peppers, cut into medium strips

4 green chime peppers, cut into medium strips 4 yellow ringer peppers, cut into medium strips 1 yellow onion, hacked

Salt and dark pepper to the taste

Guidelines:

1.   In the air fryer cooker, blend red chime peppers with green and yellow ones.

2.   Add paprika, oil, onion, salt and pepper, hurl and cook at 350 Deg. Fahrenheit for about 20 minutes.

3.   Divide among plates and fill in as a side dish. Enjoy the recipe!

The nutritional facts: calories 142, fat 4, fiber 4, carbs 7, protein 4

CREAMY ENDIVES

Prep. time: 10 minutes The cooking time: 10 minutes The recipe servings: 6

Fixings:

6 endives, cut and divided 1 teaspoon garlic powder

½ cup Greek yogurt

½ teaspoon curry powder

Salt and dark pepper to the taste 3 tablespoons lemon juice

Guidelines:

1.   In a bowl, blend endives in with garlic powder, yogurt, curry powder, salt, pepper and lemon juice, hurl, leave aside for 10 minutes and move to your preheated air fryer at 350 degrees F.

2.   Cook endives for 10 minutes, partition them on plates and fill in as a side dish.

Enjoy the recipe!

The nutritional facts: calories 100, fat 2, fiber 2, carbs 7, protein 4

DELIGHTFUL ROASTED CARROTS

Prep. time: 10 minutes The cooking time: 20 minutes The recipe servings: 4

Fixings:

1 pound child carrots 2 teaspoons olive oil

1 teaspoon herbs de Provence 4 tablespoons squeezed orange

Guidelines:

1.	In the air fryer cooker's crate, blend carrots in with herbs de Provence, oil and squeezed orange, hurl and cook at 320 Deg. Fahrenheit for about 20 minutes.

2.	Divide among plates and fill in as a side dish. Enjoy the recipe!

The nutritional facts: calories 112, fat 2, fiber 3, carbs 4, protein 3

VERMOUTH MUSHROOMS

Prep. time: 10 minutes The cooking time: 25 minutes The recipe servings: 4

Fixings:

1 tablespoon of olive oil

1	pounds white mushrooms

2 tablespoons white vermouth 2 teaspoons herbs de Provence 2 garlic cloves, minced

Guidelines:

1.   In the air fryer cooker, blend oil in with mushrooms, herbs de Provence and garlic, hurl and cook at 350 deg. F for about 20 minutes.

2.   Add vermouth, hurl and cook for 5 minutes more.

3.   Divide among plates and fill in as a side dish. Enjoy the recipe!

The nutritional facts: calories 121, fat 2, fiber 5, carbs 7, protein 4

THE ROASTED PARSNIPS

Prep. time: 10 minutes The cooking time: 40 minutes The recipe servings: 6

Fixings:

2 pounds parsnips, stripped and cut into medium pieces 2 tablespoons maple syrup

1 tablespoon parsley pieces, dried 1 tablespoon of olive oil

Guidelines:

1.   Preheat the air fryer cooker at 360 degrees F, include oil and heat it up also.

2.   Add parsnips, parsley drops and maple syrup, hurl and cook them for 40 minutes.

3.   Divide among plates and fill in as a side dish. Enjoy the recipe!

The nutritional facts: calories 124, fat 3, fiber 3, carbs 7, protein 4

GRAIN RISOTTO

Prep. time: 10 minutes The cooking time: 30 minutes The recipe servings: 8

Fixings:

- 5 cups veggie stock

- tablespoons olive oil

- yellow onions, slashed 2 garlic cloves, minced

- ¾ pound grain

- ounces mushrooms, cut 2 ounces skim milk

- 1 teaspoon thyme, dried

- teaspoon tarragon, dried

- Salt and dark pepper to the taste

- pounds sweet potato, stripped and slashed

Guidelines:

1.   Put stock in a pot, include grain, mix, heat to the point of boiling over medium heat and cook for 15 minutes.

2.   Heat up the air fryer cooker at 350 degrees F, include oil and heat it up.

3.   Add grain, onions, garlic, mushrooms, milk, salt, pepper, tarragon and sweet potato, mix and cook for 15 minutes more.

4.   Divide among plates and fill in as a side dish. Enjoy the recipe!

The nutritional facts: calories 124, fat 4, fiber 4, carbs 6, protein 4

THE GLAZED BEETS

Prep. time: 10 minutes The cooking time: 40 minutes The recipe servings: 8

Fixings:

3 pounds little beets, cut 4 tablespoons maple syrup

1   tablespoon duck fat

Guidelines:

·

1.   Heat up the air fryer cooker at 360 degrees F, include duck fat and heat it up.

2.   Add beets and maple syrup, hurl and cook for 40 minutes.

3.   Divide among plates and fill in as a side dish. Enjoy the recipe!

The nutritional facts: calories 121, fat 3, fiber 2, carbs 3, protein 4

THE BEER RISOTTO

Prep. time: 10 minutes The cooking time: 30 minutes The recipe servings: 4

Fixings:

2 tablespoons olive oil

2 yellow onions, slashed 1 cup mushrooms, cut 1 teaspoon basil, dried

1   teaspoon oregano, dried 1 and ½ cups rice

2   cups lager

2 cups chicken stock 1 tablespoon margarine

½ cup parmesan, ground

Guidelines:

1.   In a dish that accommodates the air fryer cooker, blend oil in with onions, mushrooms, basil and oregano and mix.

2.   Add rice, lager, spread, stock and margarine, mix once more, place in the air fryer cooker's bushel and cook at 350 Deg. Fahrenheit for about 30 minutes.

3.   Divide among plates and present with ground parmesan on top as a side dish. Enjoy the recipe!

The nutritional facts: calories 142, fat 4, fiber 4, carbs 6, protein 4

CAULIFLOWER RICE

Prep. time: 10 minutes The cooking time: 40 minutes The recipe servings: 8

Fixings:

1 tablespoon nut oil 1 tablespoon sesame oil 4 tablespoons soy sauce 3 garlic cloves, minced

1 tablespoon ginger, ground Juice from ½ lemon

1 cauliflower head, riced

9 ounces water chestnuts, depleted

¾ cup peas

15 ounces mushrooms, slashed 1 egg, whisked

Guidelines:

1.   In the air fryer cooker, blend cauliflower rice with nut oil, sesame oil, soy sauce, garlic, ginger and lemon juice, mix, spread and cook at 350 Deg. Fahrenheit for about 20 minutes.

2.	Add chestnuts, peas, mushrooms and egg, hurl and cook at 360 Deg. Fahrenheit for about 20 minutes more.

3.	Divide among plates and serve for breakfast. Enjoy the recipe!

The nutritional facts: calories 142, fat 3, fiber 2, carbs 6, protein 4

CARROTS AND RHUBARB

Prep. time: 10 minutes The cooking time: 40 minutes The recipe servings: 4

Fixings:

1 pound infant carrots 2 teaspoons pecan oil

1 pound rhubarb, generally slashed

1 orange, stripped, cut into medium fragments and pizzazz ground

½ cup pecans, divided

½ teaspoon stevia

Guidelines:

1.	Put the oil in the air fryer cooker, include carrots, hurl and fry them at 380 Deg. Fahrenheit for about 20 minutes.

2.	Add rhubarb, orange pizzazz, stevia and pecans, hurl and cook for 20 minutes more.

3.   Add orange fragments, hurl and fill in as a side dish. Enjoy the recipe!

The nutritional facts: calories 172, fat 2, fiber 3, carbs 4, protein 4

BROILED EGGPLANT

Prep. time: 10 minutes The cooking time: 20 minutes The recipe servings: 6

Fixings:

1 and ½ pounds eggplant, cubed 1 tablespoon of olive oil

1 teaspoon of the garlic powder & 1 teaspoon of onion powder plus 1 teaspoon sumac

2   teaspoons za'atar Juice from ½ lemon 2 inlet leaves

Guidelines:

1.   In the air fryer cooker, blend eggplant 3D squares with oil, garlic powder, onion powder, sumac, za'atar, lemon squeeze and sound leaves, hurl and cook at 370 Deg. Fahrenheit for about 20 minutes.

2.   Divide among plates and fill in as a side dish. Enjoy the recipe!

The nutritional facts: calories 172, fat 4, fiber 7, carbs 12, protein 3

DELIGHTFUL AIR FRIED BROCCOLI

Prep. time: 10 minutes The cooking time: 20 minutes The recipe servings:4

Fixings:

1 tablespoon duck fat

1 broccoli head, florets isolated 3 garlic cloves, minced

Juice from ½ lemon

1 tablespoon sesame seeds

Guidelines:

1.   Heat up the air fryer cooker at 350 degrees F, include duck fat and heat also.

2.   Add broccoli, garlic, lemon juice and sesame seeds, hurl and cook for 20 minutes.

3.   Divide among plates and fill in as a side dish. Enjoy the recipe!

The nutritional facts: calories 132, fat 3, fiber 3, carbs 6, protein 4

ONION RINGS SIDE DISH

Prep. time: 10 minutes The cooking time: 10 minutes The recipe servings: 3

Fixings:

1 onion cut into medium cuts and rings isolated 1 and ¼ cups white flour

A spot of salt 1 egg

1 cup milk

1   teaspoon heating powder

¾ cup bread scraps

Guidelines:

1.   In a bowl, blend flour in with salt and heating powder, mix, dig onion rings right now place them on a different plate.

2.   Add milk and egg to flour blend and whisk well.

3.   Dip onion rings right now, them in breadcrumbs, put them in the air fryer cooker's bushel and cook it at 360 deg. F for 10 minutes.

4.   Divide among plates and fill in as a side dish for a steak.

Enjoy the recipe!

The nutritional facts: calories 140, fat 8, fiber 20, carbs 12, protein 3

RICE AND SAUSAGE SIDE DISH

Prep. time: 10 minutes The cooking time: 20 minutes The recipe servings: 4

Fixings:

2   cups white rice, effectively bubbled 1 tablespoon spread

Salt and dark pepper to the taste 4 garlic cloves, minced

1   pork hotdog, slashed

2   tablespoons carrot, hacked

3   tablespoons cheddar, ground

2 tablespoons mozzarella cheddar, destroyed

Guidelines:

1.   Heat up the air fryer cooker at 350 degrees F, include spread, soften it, add garlic, mix and dark colored for 2 minutes.

2.   Add hotdog, salt, pepper, carrots and rice, mix and cook at 350 Deg. Fahrenheit for about 10 minutes.

3.   Add cheddar and mozzarella, hurl, separate among plates and fill in as a side dish.

Enjoy the recipe!

The nutritional facts: calories 240, fat 12, fiber 5, carbs 20, protein 13

POTATOES PATTIES

Prep. time: 10 minutes The cooking time: 8 minutes The recipe servings: 4

Fixings:

- 4 potatoes, cubed, bubbled and squashed 1 cup parmesan, ground

- Salt and dark pepper to the taste A touch of nutmeg

- egg yolks

- tablespoons white flour

- tablespoons chives, cleaved

For the breading:

¼ cup white flour

3   tablespoons vegetable oil 2 eggs, whisked

¼ cup bread scraps

Guidelines:

1.   In a bowl, blend pureed potatoes with egg yolks, salt, pepper, nutmeg, parmesan, chives and 2 tablespoons flour, mix well, shape medium cakes and spot them on a plate.

2.   In another bowl, blend vegetable oil in with bread morsels and mix,.

3.   Put whisked eggs in a third bowl and ¼ cup flour in a forward one.

4.   Dip cakes in flour, at that point in eggs and in breadcrumbs toward the end, place them in the air fryer cooker's crate, cook them at 390 Deg. Fahrenheit for about 8 minutes, separate among plates and fill in as a side dish.

Enjoy the recipe!

The nutritional facts: calories 140, fat 3, fiber 4, carbs 17, protein 4

STRAIGHTFORWARD POTATO CHIPS

Prep. time: 30 minutes The cooking time: 30 minutes The recipe servings: 4

Fixings:

4   potatoes, scoured, stripped into slim chips, absorbed water for 30 minutes, depleted and pat dried

Salt the taste

1   tablespoon of olive oil

2   teaspoons rosemary, cleaved

Guidelines:

1.   In a bowl, blend potato chips with salt and oil hurl to cover, place them in the air fryer cooker's bushel and cook at 330 Deg. Fahrenheit for about 30 minutes.

2.   Divide among plates, sprinkle rosemary all finished and fill in as a side dish.

Enjoy the recipe!

The nutritional facts: calories 200, fat 4, fiber 4, carbs 14, protein 5

AVOCADO FRIES

Prep. time: 10 minutes The cooking time: 10 minutes The recipe servings: 4

Fixings:

1 avocado, hollowed, stripped, cut and cut into medium fries Salt and dark pepper to the taste

½ cup panko bread pieces 1 tablespoon lemon juice

1 egg, whisked

1 tablespoon of olive oil

Guidelines:

1.   In a bowl, blend panko with salt and pepper and mix.

2.   In another bowl, blend egg in with a spot of salt and whisk.

3.   In a third bowl, blend avocado fries in with lemon squeeze and oil and hurl.

4.   Dip fries in egg, at that point in panko, place them in the air fryer cooker's crate and cook at 390 Deg. Fahrenheit for about 10 minutes, shaking midway.

5.   Divide among plates and fill in as a side dish.

Enjoy the recipe!

The nutritional facts: calories 130, fat 11, fiber 3, carbs 16, protein 4

VEGGIE FRIES

Prep. time: 10 minutes The cooking time: 30 minutes The recipe servings: 4

Fixings:

- 4 parsnips, cut into medium sticks

- sweet potatoes cut into medium sticks 4 blended carrots cut into medium sticks Salt and dark pepper to the taste

- tablespoons rosemary, hacked 2 tablespoons olive oil

- 1 tablespoon flour

- ½ teaspoon garlic powder

Guidelines:

1.   Put veggie fries in a bowl, include oil, garlic powder, salt, pepper, flour and rosemary and hurl to cover.

2.   Put sweet potatoes in your preheated air fryer, cook them for 10 minutes at 350 degrees F and move them to a platter.

3.   Put parsnip fries in the air fryer cooker, cook for 5 minutes and move over potato fries.

4.   Put carrot fries in the air fryer cooker, cook for 15 minutes at 350 degrees F and move to the platter with different fries.

5.   Divide veggie fries on plates and serve them as a side dish.

Enjoy the recipe!

The nutritional facts: calories 100, fat 0, fiber 4, carbs 7, protein 4

AIR FRIED CREAMY CABBAGE

Prep. time: 10 miinutes

The cooking time: 20 moment

The recipe servings: 4

Fixings:

1 green cabbage head, hacked 1 yellow onion, cleaved

Salt and dark pepper to the taste 4 bacon cuts, hacked

1   cup whipped cream

2   tablespoons cornstarch

Guidelines:

1.   Put cabbage, bacon and onion in the air fryer cooker.

2.   In a bowl, blend cornstarch in with cream, salt and pepper, mix and include over cabbage.

3.   Toss, cook at 400 Deg. Fahrenheit for about 20 minutes, isolate among plates and fill in as a side dish.

Enjoy the recipe!

The nutritional facts: calories 208, fat 10, fiber 3, carbs 16, protein 5

THE TORTILLA CHIPS

Prep. time: 10 miinutes

The cooking time: 6 minutes

The recipe servings: 4

Fixings:

8 tortillas corn, cut it into triangles Salt and dark pepper to the taste 1 tablespoon of olive oil

A touch of garlic powder A spot of sweet paprika

Guidelines:

1.   In a bowl, blend tortilla chips with oil, include salt, pepper, garlic powder and paprika, hurl well, place them in the air fryer cooker's crate and cook them at 400 Deg. Fahrenheit for about 6 minutes.

2.   Serve them as a side for a fish dish.

Enjoy the recipe!

The nutritional facts: calories 53, fat 1, fiber 1, carbs 6, protein 4

ZUCCHINI CROQUETTES

Prep. time: 10 minutes The cooking time: 10 minutes The recipe servings: 4

Fixings:

1 carrot, ground

1   zucchini, ground

2   slices of bread, disintegrated 1 egg

Salt and dark pepper to the taste

½ teaspoon sweet paprika 1 teaspoon garlic, minced

2 tablespoons parmesan cheddar, ground 1 tablespoon corn flour

Guidelines:

1.   Put zucchini in a bowl, include salt, leave aside for 10 minutes, crush abundance water and move them to another bowl.

2.   Add carrots, salt, pepper, paprika, garlic, flour, parmesan, egg and bread scraps, mix well, shape 8 croquettes, place them in the air fryer cooker and cook at 360 Deg. Fahrenheit for about 10 minutes.

3.   Divide among plates and fill in as a side dish

Enjoy the recipe!

The nutritional facts: calories 100, fat 3, fiber 1, carbs 7, protein 4

CREAMY POTATOES

Prep. time: 10 minutes The cooking time: 20 minutes The recipe servings: 4

Fixings:

1 a ½ pounds potatoes, stripped and cubed 2 tablespoons olive oil

Salt and dark pepper to the taste 1 tablespoon hot paprika

1 cup Greek yogurt

Guidelines:

1.   Put potatoes in a bowl, add water to cover, leave aside for 10 minutes, channel, pat dry them, move to another bowl, include salt, pepper, paprika and half of the oil and hurl them well.

2.   Put potatoes in the air fryer cooker's container and cook at 360 Deg. Fahrenheit for about 20 minutes.

3.   In a bowl, blend yogurt in with salt, pepper and the remainder of the oil and whisk.

4.   Divide potatoes on plates, shower yogurt dressing all finished, hurl them and fill in as a side dish.

Enjoy the recipe!

The nutritional facts: calories 170, fat 3, fiber 5, carbs 20, protein 5

MUSHROOM CAKES

The cooking time: 8 minutes

Prep. time: 10 minutes

The recipe servings: 8

Fixings:

4 ounces mushrooms, cleaved 1 yellow onion, slashed

Salt and dark pepper to the taste

½ teaspoon nutmeg, ground 2 tablespoons olive oil

1 tablespoon margarine

1 and ½ tablespoon flour

1 tablespoon bread scraps 14 ounces milk

Guidelines:

1.   Heat up a container with the margarine over medium high heat, include onion and mushrooms, mix, cook for 3 minutes, include flour, mix well again and take off heat.

2.   Add milk step by step, salt, pepper and nutmeg, mix and leave aside to chill off totally.

3.	In a bowl, blend oil in with bread pieces and whisk.

4.	Take spoonfuls of the mushroom filling, add to breadcrumbs blend, coat well, shape patties out of this blend, place them in the air fryer cooker's container and cook at 400 Deg. Fahrenheit for about 8 minutes.

5.	Divide among plates and fill in as a side for a steak

Enjoy the recipe!

The nutritional facts: calories 192, fat 2, fiber 1, carbs 16, protein 6

CREAMY ROASTED PEPPERS SIDE

Prep. time: 10 minutes

The cooking time: 10 minutes

The recipe servings: 4

Fixings:

1 tablespoon lemon juice 1 red chime pepper

1 green ringer pepper 1 yellow chime pepper

1	lettuce head, cut into strips 1 ounce rocket leaves

Salt and dark pepper to the taste 3 tablespoons Greek yogurt

2   tablespoons olive oil

Guidelines:

1.   Place ringer peppers in the air fryer cooker's container, cook at 400 Deg. Fahrenheit for about 10 minutes, move to a bowl, leave aside for 10 minutes, strip them, dispose of seeds, cut them in strips, move to a bigger bowl, include rocket leaves and lettuce strips and hurl.

2.   In a bowl, blend oil in with lemon juice, yogurt, salt and pepper and whisk well.

3.   Add this over ringer peppers blend, prepare to cover, partition among plates and fill in as a side serving of mixed greens.

Enjoy the recipe!

The nutritional facts: calories 170, fat 1, fiber 1, carbs 2, protein 6

GREEK VEGGIES SIDE DISH MUSHROOM CAKES

Prep. time: 10 minutes

The cooking time: 45 minutes

The recipe servings: 4

Fixings:

1 eggplant, cut

1   zucchini, cut

2   red ringer peppers, cleaved 2 garlic cloves, minced

3   tablespoons olive oil 1 cove leaf

1 thyme spring, slashed 2 onions, cleaved

4 tomatoes, cut into quarters

Salt and dark pepper to the taste

Guidelines:

1.   In the air fryer cooker's skillet, blend eggplant cuts with zucchini ones, ringer peppers, garlic, oil, cove leaf, thyme, onions, tomatoes, salt and pepper, hurl and cook them at 300 Deg. Fahrenheit for about 35 minutes.

2.   Divide among plates and fill in as a side dish.

Enjoy the recipe!

The nutritional facts: calories 200, fat 1, fiber 3, carbs 7, protein 6

YELLOW SQUASH AND ZUCCHINIS SIDE DISH

Prep. time: 10 minutes

The cooking time: 35 minutes

The recipe servings: 4

Fixings:

6 teaspoons olive oil

1 pound zucchinis, cut

½ pound carrots, cubed

1 yellow squash, split, deseeded and cut into pieces Salt and white pepper to the taste

1 tablespoon tarragon, cleaved

Guidelines:

1.   In the air fryer cooker's crate, blend zucchinis in with carrots, squash, salt, pepper and oil, hurl well and cook at 400 Deg. Fahrenheit for about 25 minutes.

2.   Divide them on plates and fill in as a side dish with tarragon sprinkled on top.

Enjoy the recipe!

The nutritional facts: calories 160, fat 2, fiber 1, carbs 5, protein 5

ENHANCED CAULIFLOWER SIDE DISH

Prep. time: 10 minutes

The cooking time: 10 minutes

The recipe servings: 4

Fixings:

Salt and dark pepper to the taste

¼ teaspoon turmeric powder

1   and ½ teaspoon red bean stew powder 1 tablespoon ginger, ground

2   teaspoons lemon juice 3 tablespoons white flour 2 tablespoons water Cooking shower

½ teaspoon corn flour

Guidelines:

1.   In a bowl, blend stew powder with turmeric powder, ginger glue, salt, pepper, lemon juice, white flour, corn flour and water, mix, include cauliflower, hurl well and move them to the air fryer cooker's crate.

2.   Coat them with cooking splash, cook them at 400 Deg. Fahrenheit for about 10 minutes, isolate among plates and fill in as a side dish.

Enjoy the recipe!

The nutritional facts: calories 70, fat 1, fiber 2, carbs 12, protein 3

COCONUT CREAM POTATOES

Prep. time: 10 minutes

The cooking time: 20 minutes

The recipe servings: 4

Fixings:

Salt and dark pepper to the taste

1   tablespoon cheddar, ground 1 tablespoon flour

2   potatoes, cut

4 ounces coconut cream

Guidelines:

1.   Place potato cuts in the air fryer cooker's bushel and cook at 360 Deg. Fahrenheit for about 10 minutes.

2.   Meanwhile, in a bowl, blend eggs in with coconut cream, salt, pepper and flour.

3.   Arrange potatoes in the air fryer cooker's dish, include coconut cream blend over them, sprinkle cheddar, come back to air fryer's container and cook at 400 Deg. Fahrenheit for about 10 minutes more.

4.   Divide among plates and fill in as a side dish.

Enjoy the recipe!

The nutritional facts: calories 170, fat 4, fiber 1, carbs 15, protein 17

CAJUM ONION WEDGES

Prep. time: 10 minutes

The cooking time: 15 minutes

The recipe servings: 4

Fixings:

Salt and dark pepper to the taste 2 eggs

¼ cup milk 1/3 cup panko

A shower of olive oil

1 and ½ teaspoon paprika 1 teaspoon garlic powder

½ teaspoon Cajun flavoring

Guidelines:

1.   In a bowl, blend panko with Cajun flavoring and oil and mix.

2.   In another bowl, blend egg in with milk, salt and pepper and mix.

3.   Sprinkle onion wedges with paprika and garlic powder, plunge them in egg blend, at that point in bread pieces blend, place in the air fryer cooker's bushel, cook at 360 Deg. Fahrenheit for about about 10 minutes, flip and then cook for 5 minutes more.

4.   Divide among plates and fill in as a side dish.

Enjoy the recipe!

The nutritional facts: calories 200, fat 2, fiber 2, carbs 14, protein 7

WILD RICE PILAF

Prep. time: 10 minutes The cooking time: 25 minutes The recipe servings: 12

Fixings:

1 shallot, slashed

1 teaspoon garlic, minced A sprinkle of olive oil

1 cup farro

¾ cup wild rice

4 cups chicken stock

Salt and dark pepper to the taste 1 tablespoon parsley, slashed

½ cup hazelnuts, toasted and slashed

¾ cup fruits, dried Chopped chives for serving

Guidelines:

1.   In a dish that accommodates the air fryer cooker, blend shallot in with garlic, oil, faro, wild rice, stock, salt, pepper, parsley, hazelnuts and fruits, mix, place in the air fryer cooker's bushel and cook at 350 Deg. Fahrenheit for about 25 minutes.

2.   Divide among plates and fill in as a side dish. Enjoy the recipe!

The nutritional facts: calories 142, fat 4, fiber 4, carbs 16, protein 4

PUMPKIN RI CE

Prep. time: 5 minutes The cooking time: 30 minutes The recipe servings: 4

Fixings:

2 tablespoons olive oil

1 little yellow onion, hacked 2 garlic cloves, minced

12 ounces white rice 4 cups chicken stock

6 ounces pumpkin puree

½ teaspoon nutmeg

1 teaspoon thyme, hacked

½ teaspoon ginger, ground

½ teaspoon cinnamon powder

½ teaspoon allspice

4 ounces overwhelming cream

Guidelines:

1.   In a dish that accommodates the air fryer cooker, blend oil in with onion, garlic, rice, stock, pumpkin puree, nutmeg, thyme, ginger, cinnamon, allspice and cream, mix well, place in the air fryer cooker's crate and cook at 360 Deg. Fahrenheit for about 30 minutes.

2.   Divide among plates and fill in as a side dish.

Enjoy the recipe!

The nutritional facts: calories 261, fat 6, fiber 7, carbs 29, protein 4

HUED VEGGIES RICE

Prep. time: 10 minutes

The cooking time: 25 minutes

The recipe servings: 4

Fixings:

2 cups basmati rice

1   cup blended carrots, peas, corn and green beans 2 cups water

½ teaspoon green bean stew, minced

½ teaspoon ginger, ground 3 garlic cloves, minced

2   tablespoons margarine

1   teaspoon cinnamon powder 1 tablespoon cumin seeds

2   bay leaves

3   whole cloves

5 dark peppercorns

2 entire cardamoms

1 tablespoon sugar Salt to the taste

Guidelines:

1.   Put the water in a heat verification dish that accommodates the air fryer cooker, include rice, blended veggies, green stew, ground ginger, garlic cloves, cinnamon, cloves, margarine, cumin seeds, sound leaves, cardamoms, dark peppercorns, salt and sugar, mix, put in the air fryer cooker's container and cook at 370 Deg. Fahrenheit for about 25 minutes.

2.   Divide among plates and fill in as a side dish.

Enjoy the recipe!

The nutritional facts: calories 283, fat 4, fiber 8, carbs 34, protein 14

POTATO CASSEROLE

Prep. time: 15 minutes

The cooking time: 40 minutes

The recipe servings: 4

Fixings:

3 pounds sweet potatoes, cleaned

¼ cup milk

½ teaspoon nutmeg, ground 2 tablespoons white flour

¼ teaspoon allspice, ground Salt to the taste

For the garnish:

½ cup almond flour

½ cup pecans, drenched, depleted and ground

¼ cup walnuts, drenched, depleted and ground

¼ cup coconut, destroyed 1 tablespoon chia seeds

¼ cup sugar

1   teaspoon cinnamon powder 5 tablespoons margarine

Guidelines:

1.   Place potatoes in the air fryer cooker's bin, prick them with a fork and cook at 360 Deg. Fahrenheit for about 30 minutes.

2.   Meanwhile, in a bowl, blend almond flour with walnuts, pecans, ¼ cup coconut, ¼ cup sugar, chia seeds, 1 teaspoon cinnamon and the margarine and mix everything.

3.   Transfer potatoes to a cutting board, cool them, strip and spot them in a preparing dish that accommodates the air fryer cooker.

4.   Add milk, flour, salt, nutmeg and allspice and mix

5.   Add disintegrate blend you've made before on top, place dish in the air fryer cooker's bushel and cook at 400 Deg. Fahrenheit for about 8 minutes.

6.   Divide among plates and fill in as a side dish.

Enjoy the recipe!

The nutritional facts: calories 162, fat 4, fiber 8, carbs 18, protein 4

LEMONY ARTICHOKES

Prep. time: 10 minutes

The cooking time: 15 minutes

The recipe servings: 4

Fixings:

2   medium artichokes, cut and split Cooking shower

2 tablespoons lemon juice

Salt and dark pepper to the taste

Guidelines:

1.   Grease the air fryer cooker with cooking splash, include artichokes, shower lemon squeeze and sprinkle salt and dark pepper and cook them at 380 Deg. Fahrenheit for about 15 minutes.

2.   Divide them on plates and fill in as a side dish.

Enjoy the recipe!

The nutritional facts: calories 121, fat 3, fiber 6, carbs 9, protein 4

CAULIFLOWER AND BROCCOLI DELIGHT

Prep. time: 10 minutes

The cooking time: 7 minutes

The recipe servings: 4

Fixings:

2 cauliflower heads, florets isolated and steamed 1 broccoli head, florets isolated and steamed Zest from 1 orange, ground

Juice from 1 orange

A touch of hot pepper chips 4 anchovies

1 tablespoon tricks, hacked Salt and dark pepper to the taste 4 tablespoons olive oil

Guidelines:

1.   In a bowl, blend orange pizzazz in with squeezed orange, pepper drops, anchovies, escapades salt, pepper and olive oil and whisk well.

2.   Add broccoli and cauliflower, hurl well, move them to the air fryer cooker's container and cook at 400 Deg. Fahrenheit for about 7 minutes.

3.   Divide among plates and fill in as a side dish with a portion of the orange vinaigrette sprinkled on top.

Enjoy the recipe!

The nutritional facts: calories 300, fat 4, fiber 7, carbs 28, protein 4

GARLIC BEET WEDGES

Prep. time: 10 minutes

The cooking time: 15 minutes

The recipe servings: 4

Fixings:

4 beets, washed, stripped and cut into enormous wedges 1 tablespoon of olive oil

Salt and dark to the taste 2 garlic cloves, minced

1 teaspoon lemon juice

Guidelines:

1.   In a bowl, blend beets in with oil, salt, pepper, garlic and lemon juice, hurl well, move to the air fryer cooker's bin and cook them at 400 Deg. Fahrenheit for about 15 minutes.

2.   Divide beets wedges on plates and fill in as a side dish.

Enjoy the recipe!

The nutritional facts: calories 182, fat 6, fiber 3, carbs 8, protein 2

FRIED RED CABBAGE

Prep. time: 10 minutes

The cooking time: 15 minutes

The recipe servings: 4

Fixings:

4 garlic cloves, minced

½ cup yellow onion, hacked 1 tablespoon of olive oil

6 cups red cabbage, hacked 1 cup veggie stock

1 tablespoon apple juice vinegar 1 cup fruit purée

Salt and dark pepper to the taste

Guidelines:

1.   In a heat evidence dish that accommodates the air fryer cooker, blend cabbage in with onion, garlic, oil, stock, vinegar, fruit purée, salt and pepper, hurl truly well, place dish in the air fryer cooker's container and cook at 380 Deg. Fahrenheit for about 15 minutes.

2.   Divide among plates and fill in as a side dish.

Enjoy the recipe!

The nutritional facts: calories 172, fat 7, fiber 7, carbs 14, protein 5

ARTICHOKES AND TARRAGON SAUCE

Prep. time: 10 minutes

The cooking time: 18 minutes

The recipe servings: 4

Fixings:

4 artichokes, cut

2 tablespoons tarragon, slashed 2 tablespoons chicken stock

Lemon pizzazz from 2 lemons, ground 2 tablespoons lemon juice

1 celery stalk, hacked

½ cup olive oil Salt to the taste

Guidelines:

1.   In your food processor, blend tarragon, chicken stock, lemon get-up-and-go, lemon juice, celery, salt and olive oil and heartbeat well indeed.

2.   In a bowl, blend artichokes in with tarragon and lemon sauce, hurl well, move them to the air fryer cooker's bushel and cook at 380 Deg. Fahrenheit for about 18 minutes.

3. Divide artichokes on plates, shower the remainder of the sauce all finished and fill in as a side dish.

Enjoy the recipe!

The nutritional facts: calories 215, fat 3, fiber 8, carbs 28, protein 6

BRUSSELS SPROUTS AND POMEGRANATE SEEDS SIDE DISH

Prep. time: 5 minutes The cooking time: 10 minutes The recipe servings: 4

Fixings:

1 pound Brussels grows, cut and divided Salt and dark pepper to the taste

1   cup pomegranate seeds

¼ cup pine nuts, toasted 1 tablespoons olive oil

2   tablespoons veggie stock

Guidelines:

1. In a heat verification dish that accommodates the air fryer cooker, blend Brussels grows with salt, pepper, pomegranate seeds, pine nuts, oil and stock, mix, place in the air fryer cooker's container and cook at 390 deg. F for another 10 minutes.

2. Divide among plates and fill in as a side dish.

Enjoy the recipe!

The nutritional facts: calories 152, fat 4, fiber 7, carbs 12, protein 3

FIRM BRUSSELS SPROUTS AND POTATOES

Prep. time: 10 minutes The cooking time: 8 minutes The recipe servings: 4

Fixings:

1 and ½ pounds Brussels grows, washed and cut 1 cup new potatoes, hacked

1 and ½ tablespoons bread pieces Salt and dark pepper to the taste 1 and ½ tablespoons margarine

Guidelines:

1. Put Brussels sprouts and potatoes in the air fryer cooker's container, include bread scraps, salt, pepper and margarine, hurl well and cook at 400 Deg. Fahrenheit for about 8 minutes.

2. Divide among plates and fill in as a side dish.

Enjoy the recipe!

The nutritional facts: calories 152, fat 3, fiber 7, carbs 17, protein 4

258

AIR FRYER SNACK AND APPETIZER RECIPES

COCONUT CHICKEN BITES

Prep. time: 10 minutes The cooking time: 13 minutes The recipe servings: 4

Fixings:

- teaspoons garlic powder 2 eggs

- Salt and dark pepper to the taste

- ¾ cup panko bread scraps

- ¾ cup coconut, destroyed Cooking splash

- 8 chicken strips

Guidelines:

1. In a bowl, blend eggs in with salt, pepper and garlic powder and whisk well.

2. In another bowl, blend coconut in with panko and mix well.

3. Dip chicken strips in eggs blend and afterward coat in coconut one well.

4.   Spray chicken chomps with cooking shower, place them in the air fryer cooker's bushel and cook them at 350 deg. F for about 10 minutes.

5.   Arrange them on a platter and fill in as a tidbit.

Enjoy the recipe!

The nutritional facts: calories 252, fat 4, fiber 2, carbs 14, protein 24

CAULIFLOWER SNACKS

Prep. time: 10 minutes

The cooking time: 15 minutes

The recipe servings: 4

Fixings:

4 cups of cauliflower florets and 1 cup of panko bread scraps

¼ cup margarine, liquefied

¼ cup wild ox sauce Mayonnaise for serving

Guidelines:

1.   In a bowl, blend wild ox sauce with margarine and whisk well.

2.   Dip cauliflower florets right now coat them in panko bread pieces.

3.   Place them in the air fryer cooker's container and cook at 350 Deg. Fahrenheit for about 15 minutes.

4.   Arrange them on a platter and present with mayo as an afterthought.

Enjoy the recipe!

The nutritional facts: calories 241, fat 4, fiber 7, carbs 8, protein 4

BANANA SNACKS

Prep. time: 10 minutes

The cooking time: 5 minutes

The recipe servings: 8

Fixings:

16 heating cups outside layer

¼ cup nutty spread

¾ cup chocolate chips

1 banana, stripped and cut into 16 pieces 1 tablespoon vegetable oil

Guidelines:

1.   Put chocolate contributes a little pot, heat up over low heat, mix until it melts and take off heat.

2.   In a bowl, blend nutty spread in with coconut oil and whisk well.

3.   Spoon 1 teaspoon chocolate blend in a cup, include 1 banana cut and top with 1 teaspoon spread blend

4.   Repeat with the remainder of the cups, place them all into a dish that accommodates the air fryer cooker, cook at 320 Deg. Fahrenheit for about 5 minutes, move to a cooler and keep there until you serve them as a bite.

Enjoy the recipe!

The nutritional facts: calories 70, fat 4, fiber 1, carbs 10, protein 1

POTATO SPREAD

Prep. time: 10 minutes

The cooking time: 10 minutes

The recipe servings: 10

Fixings:

19 ounces canned garbanzo beans, depleted 1 cup sweet potatoes, stripped and hacked

¼ cup tahini

2 tablespoons lemon juice 1 tablespoon of olive oil

5 garlic cloves, minced

½ teaspoon cumin, ground 2 tablespoons water

A touch of salt and white pepper

Guidelines:

1.   Put potatoes in the air fryer cooker's bushel, cook them at 360 Deg. Fahrenheit for about 15 minutes, chill them off, strip, put them in your food processor and heartbeat well. crate,

2.   Add sesame glue, garlic, beans, lemon juice, cumin, water and oil and heartbeat truly well.

3.   Add salt and pepper, beat once more, partition into bowls and serve.

Enjoy the recipe!

The nutritional facts: calories 200, fat 3, fiber 10, carbs 20, protein 11

MEXICAN APPLE SNACKS

Prep. time: 10 minutes

The cooking time: 5 minutes

The recipe servings: 4

Fixings:

3 major apples, cored, stripped and cubed 2 teaspoons lemon juice

¼ cup walnuts, hacked

½ cup dull chocolate chips

½ cup clean caramel sauce

Guidelines:

1.   In a bowl, blend apples in with lemon squeeze, mix and move to a dish that accommodates the air fryer cooker.

2.   Add chocolate chips, walnuts, sprinkle the caramel sauce, hurl, present in the air fryer cooker and cook at 320 Deg. Fahrenheit for about 5 minutes.

3.   Toss delicately, isolate into little dishes and serve immediately as a bite.

Enjoy the recipe!

The nutritional facts: calories 200, fat 4, fiber 3, carbs 20, protein 3

SHRIMP MUFFINS

Prep. time: 10 minutes

The cooking time: 26 minutes

The recipe servings: 6

Fixings:

1 spaghetti squash, stripped and split 2 tablespoons mayonnaise

1 cup mozzarella, destroyed

8 ounces shrimp, stripped, cooked and hacked 1 and ½ cups panko

1   teaspoon parsley chips 1 garlic clove, minced

Salt and dark pepper to the taste Cooking splash

Guidelines:

1.   Put squash parts in the air fryer cooker, cook at 350 Deg. Fahrenheit for about 16 minutes, leave aside to chill off and scratch tissue into a bowl.

2.   Add salt, pepper, parsley chips, panko, shrimp, mayo and mozzarella and mix well.

3.   Spray a biscuit plate that accommodates the air fryer cooker with cooking splash and gap squash and shrimp blend in each cup.

4.   Introduce in the fryer and cook at 360 Deg. Fahrenheit for about 10 minutes.

5.   Arrange biscuits on a platter and fill in as a bite.

Enjoy the recipe!

The nutritional facts: calories 60, fat 2, fiber 0.4, carbs 4, protein 4

ZUCCHINI CAKES

Prep. time: 10 minutes

The cooking time: 12 minutes

The recipe servings: 12

Fixings:

Cooking splash

½ cup dill, cleaved 1 egg

½ cup entire wheat flour

Salt and dark pepper to the taste 1 yellow onion, cleaved

2   garlic cloves, minced 3 zucchinis, ground

Guidelines:

1.   In a bowl, blend zucchinis in with garlic, onion, flour, salt, pepper, egg and dill, mix well, shape little patties out of this blend, splash them with cooking shower, place them in the air fryer cooker's bin and cook at 370 Deg. Fahrenheit for about 6 minutes on each side.

2.   Serve them as a bite immediately.

Enjoy the recipe!

The nutritional facts: calories 60, fat 1, fiber 2, carbs 6, protein 2

CAULIFLOWER BARS

Prep. time: 10 minutes

The cooking time: 25 minutes

The recipe servings: 12

Fixings:

1 major cauliflower head, florets isolated

½ cup mozzarella, destroyed

¼ cup egg whites

1   teaspoon Italian flavoring

Salt and dark pepper to the taste

Guidelines:

1.   Put cauliflower florets in your food processor, beat well, spread on a lined preparing sheet that accommodates the air fryer cooker, present in the fryer and cook at 360 Deg. Fahrenheit for about 10 minutes.

2.   Transfer cauliflower to a bowl, include salt, pepper, cheddar, egg whites and Italian flavoring, mix truly well, spread this into a square shape container that accommodates the air fryer cooker, press well, present in the fryer and cook at 360 Deg. Fahrenheit for about 15 minutes more.

3.   Cut into 12 bars, organize them on a platter and fill in as a bite

Enjoy the recipe!

The nutritional facts: calories 50, fat 1, fiber 2, carbs 3, protein 3

PESTO CRACKERS

Prep. time: 10 minutes

The cooking time: 17 minutes

The recipe servings: 6

Fixings:

½ teaspoon preparing powder

Salt and dark pepper to the taste 1 and ¼ cups flour

¼ teaspoon basil, dried 1 garlic clove, minced

2   tablespoons basil pesto 3 tablespoons spread

Guidelines:

1.   In a bowl, blend salt, pepper, preparing powder, flour, garlic, cayenne, basil, pesto and spread and mix until you acquire a batter.

2.   Spread this mixture on a lined heating sheet that accommodates the air fryer cooker, present in the fryer at 325 degrees F and prepare for 17 minutes.

3.   Leave aside to chill off, cut saltines and serve them as a tidbit.

Enjoy the recipe!

The nutritional facts: calories 200, fat 20, fiber 1, carbs 4, protein 7

PUMPKIN MUFFINS

Prep. time: 10 minutes

The cooking time: 15 minutes

The recipe servings: 18

Fixings:

¼ cup margarine

¾ cup pumpkin puree

2   tablespoons flaxseed meal

¼ cup flour

½ cup sugar

½ teaspoon nutmeg, ground 1 teaspoon cinnamon powder

½ teaspoon heating soft drink 1 egg

½ teaspoon heating powder

Guidelines:

1.   In a bowl, blend margarine in with pumpkin puree and egg and mix well.

2.   Add flaxseed meal, flour, sugar, heating pop, preparing powder, nutmeg and cinnamon and mix well.

3.   Spoon this into a biscuit skillet that accommodates your fryer present in the fryer at 350 degrees F and prepare for 15 minutes.

4.   Serve biscuits cold as a tidbit.

Enjoy the recipe!

The nutritional facts: calories 50, fat 3, fiber 1, carbs 2, protein 2

ZUCCHINI CHIPS

Prep. time: 10 minutes

The cooking time: 60 minutes

The recipe servings: 6

Fixings:

3   zucchinis, daintily cut

Salt and dark pepper to the taste 2 tablespoons olive oil

2 tablespoons balsamic vinegar

Guidelines:

1.   In a bowl, blend oil in with vinegar, salt and pepper and whisk well.

2.   Add zucchini cuts, hurl to cover well, present in the air fryer cooker and cook at 200 Deg. Fahrenheit for about 60 minutes.

3.   Serve zucchini chips cold as a bite.

Enjoy the recipe!

The nutritional facts: calories 40, fat 3, fiber 7, carbs 3, protein 7

MEAT JERKY SNACKS

Prep. time: 2 hours

The cooking time: 1 hour and 30 minutes

The recipe servings: 6

Fixings:

2 cups soy sauce

½ cup Worcestershire sauce

2 tablespoons dark peppercorns 2 tablespoons dark pepper

2 pounds meat round, cut

Guidelines:

1.   In a bowl, blend soy sauce with dark peppercorns, dark pepper and Worcestershire sauce and whisk well.

2.   Add meat cuts, hurl to cover and leave aside in the ice chest for 6 hours.

3.   Introduce meat adjusts in the air fryer cooker and cook them at 370 Deg. Fahrenheit for about 1 hour and 30 minutes.

4.   Transfer to a bowl and serve cold.

Enjoy the recipe!

The nutritional facts: calories 300, fat 12, fiber 4, carbs 3, protein 8

HONEY PARTY WINGS

Prep. time: 1 hour and 10 minutes

The cooking time: 12 minutes

The recipe servings: 8

Fixings:

16 chicken wings, divided 2 tablespoons soy sauce 2 tablespoons HONNEY

Salt and dark pepper to the taste 2 tablespoons lime juice

Guidelines:

1.   In a bowl, blend chicken wings in with soy sauce, HONNEY, salt, pepper and lime juice, hurl well and keep in the cooler for 60 minutes.

2.   Transfer chicken wings to the air fryer cooker and cook them at 360 Deg. Fahrenheit for about 12 minutes, flipping them midway.

3.   Arrange them on a platter and fill in as a starter. Enjoy the recipe!

The nutritional facts: calories 211, fat 4, fiber 7, carbs 14, protein 3

SALMON PARTY PATTIES

Prep. time: 10 minutes

The cooking time: 22 minutes

The recipe servings: 4

Fixings:

3 major potatoes, bubbled, depleted and squashed 1 major salmon filet, skinless, boneless

2 tablespoons parsley, cleaved 2 tablespoon dill, slashed

Salt and dark pepper to the taste 1 egg

2 tablespoons bread scraps Cooking shower

Guidelines:

1.   Place salmon in the air fryer cooker's bin and cook for 10 minutes at 360 degrees F.

2.   Transfer salmon to a cutting board, chill it off, drop it and put it in a bowl.

3.   Add pureed potatoes, salt, pepper, dill, parsley, egg and bread morsels, mix well and shape 8 patties out of this blend.

4.   Place salmon patties in the air fryer cooker's container, spry them with cooking oil, cook at 360 deg. F for about 12 minutes, flipping them midway, move them to a platter and fill in as a starter.

Enjoy the recipe!

The nutritional facts: calories 231, fat 3, fiber 7, carbs 14, protein 4

BANANA CHIPS

Prep. time: 10 minutes

The cooking time: 15 minutes

The recipe servings: 4

Fixings:

4 bananas, stripped and cut A spot of salt

½ teaspoon turmeric powder

½ teaspoon chaat masala 1 teaspoon olive oil

Guidelines:

1.   In a bowl, blend banana cuts with salt, turmeric, chaat masala and oil, hurl and leave aside for 10 minutes.

2.   Transfer banana cuts to your preheated air fryer at 360 degrees F and cook them for 15 minutes flipping them once.

3.   Serve as a bite. Enjoy the recipe!

The nutritional facts: calories 121, fat 1, fiber 2, carbs 3, protein 3

SPRING ROLLS

Prep. time: 10 minutes

The cooking time: 25 minutes

The recipe servings: 8

Fixings:

2 cups green cabbage, destroyed 2 yellow onions, hacked

1 carrot, ground

½ stew pepper, minced

1 tablespoon ginger, ground 3 garlic cloves, minced

1   teaspoon sugar

Salt and dark pepper to the taste 1 teaspoon soy sauce

2   tablespoons olive oil 10 spring move sheets

2 tablespoons corn flour 2 tablespoons water

Guidelines:

1.   Heat up a dish with the oil over medium heat, include cabbage, onions, carrots, stew pepper, ginger, garlic, sugar, salt, pepper and soy sauce, mix well, cook for 2-3 minutes, bring off heat and chill off.

2.   Cut spring move sheets in squares, separate cabbage blend on each and move them.

3.   In a bowl, blend corn flour with water, mix well and seal spring moves with this blend.

4.   Place spring abounds in the air fryer cooker's bin and cook them at 360 Deg. Fahrenheit for about 10 minutes.

5.   Flip roll and cook them for 10 minutes more.

6.   Arrange on a platter and serve them as a hors d'oeuvre. Enjoy the recipe!

The nutritional facts: calories 214, fat 4, fiber 4, carbs 12, protein 4

FIRM RADDISH CHIPS

Prep. time: 10 minutes

The cooking time: 10 minutes

The recipe servings: 4

Fixings:

Cooking splash

15 radishes, cut

Salt and dark pepper to the taste 1 tablespoon chives, hacked

Guidelines:

1.   Arrange radish cuts in the air fryer cooker's crate, splash them with cooking oil, season with salt and dark pepper to the taste, cook them at 350 Deg. Fahrenheit for about 10 minutes, flipping them midway, move to bowls and present with chives sprinkled on top.

Enjoy the recipe!

The nutritional facts: calories 80, fat 1, fiber 1, carbs 1, protein 1

CRAB STICKS

Prep. time: 10 minutes

The cooking time: 12 minutes

The recipe servings: 4

Fixings:

10 crabsticks, split 2 teaspoons sesame oil

2 teaspoons Cajun flavoring

Guidelines:

1.   Put crab sticks in a bowl, include sesame oil and Cajun flavoring, hurl, move them to the air fryer cooker's bushel and cook at 350 Deg. Fahrenheit for about 12 minutes.

Orchestrate on a platter and fill in as a starter.

Enjoy the recipe!

The nutritional facts: calories 110, fat 0, fiber 1, carbs 4, protein 2

AIR FRIED DILL PICKLES

Prep. time: 10 minutes

The cooking time: 5 minutes

The recipe servings: 4

Fixings:

16 ounces jostled dill pickles, cut into wedges and pat dried

½ cup white flour 1 egg

¼ cup milk

½ teaspoon garlic powder

½ teaspoon sweet paprika Cooking splash

¼ cup farm sauce

Guidelines:

1.   In a bowl, consolidate milk with egg and whisk well.

2.   In a subsequent bowl, blend flour in with salt, garlic powder and paprika and mix also

3.	Dip pickles in flour, at that point in egg blend and again in flour and spot them in the air fryer cooker.

4.	Grease them with cooking splash, cook pickle wedges at 400 Deg. Fahrenheit for about 5 minutes, move to a bowl and present with farm sauce as an afterthought.

Enjoy the recipe!

The nutritional facts: calories 109, fat 2, fiber 2, carbs 10, protein 4

CHICKPEAS SNACK

Prep. time: 10 minutes

The cooking time: 10 minutes

The recipe servings: 4

Fixings:

15 ounces canned chickpeas, depleted

½ teaspoon cumin, ground 1 tablespoon of olive oil

1 teaspoon smoked paprika

Salt and dark pepper to the taste

Guidelines:

1.   In a bowl, blend chickpeas in with oil, cumin, paprika, salt and pepper, hurl to cover, place them in your fryer's bin and cook at 390 Deg. Fahrenheit for about 10 minutes.

2.   Divide into bowls and fill in as a tidbit.

Enjoy the recipe!

The nutritional facts: calories 140, fat 1, fiber 6, carbs 20, protein 6

FRANKFURTER BALLS

Prep. time: 10 minutes

The cooking time: 15 minutes

The recipe servings: 4

Fixings:

4 ounces frankfurter meat, ground Salt and dark pepper to the taste 1 teaspoon sage

½ teaspoon garlic, minced 1 little onion, slashed

3 tablespoons breadcrumbs

Guidelines:

1.   In a bowl, blend hotdog in with salt, pepper, sage, garlic, onion and breadcrumbs, mix well and shape little balls out of this blend.

2.   Put them in the air fryer cooker's container, cook at 360 Deg. Fahrenheit for about 15 minutes, isolate into bowls and fill in as a tidbit.

Enjoy the recipe!

The nutritional facts: calories 130, fat 7, fiber 1, carbs 13, protein 4

CHICKEN DIP

Prep. time: 10 minutes

The cooking time: 25 minutes

The recipe servings: 10

Fixings:

3 tablespoons margarine, softened 1 cup yogurt

12 ounces cream cheddar

2 cups chicken meat, cooked and destroyed 2 teaspoons curry powder

4 scallions, slashed

6 ounces Monterey jack cheddar, ground 1/3 cup raisins

¼ cup cilantro, slashed

½ cup almonds, cut

Salt and dark pepper to the taste

½ cup chutney

Guidelines:

1. In a bowl blend cream cheddar with yogurt and whisk utilizing your blender.

2. Add curry powder, scallions, chicken meat, raisins, cheddar, cilantro, salt and pepper and mix everything.

3. Spread this into a preparing dish that clench hand the air fryer cooker, sprinkle almonds on top, place in the air fryer cooker, heat at 300 degrees for 25 minutes, partition into bowls, top with chutney and fill in as a tidbit.

Enjoy the recipe!

The nutritional facts: calories 240, fat 10, fiber 2, carbs 24, protein 12

SWEET POPCORN

Prep. time: 5 minutes The cooking time: 10 minutes The recipe servings: 4

Fixings:

2 tablespoons corn portions 2 and ½ tablespoons margarine 2 ounces dark colored sugar

Guidelines:

1.   Put corn portions in the air fryer cooker's container, cook at 400 Deg. Fahrenheit for about 6 minutes, move them to a plate, spread and leave aside for the present.

2.   Heat up a container over low heat, include margarine, liquefy it, include sugar and mix until it breaks down.

3.   Add popcorn, hurl to cover, take off heat and spread on the plate once more.

4.   Cool down, separate into bowls and fill in as a bite.

Enjoy the recipe!

The nutritional facts: calories 70, fat 0.2, fiber 0, carbs 1, protein 1

APPLE CHIPS

Prep. time: 10 minutes

The cooking time: 10 minutes

The recipe servings: 2

Fixings:

1 apple, cored and cut A touch of salt

½ teaspoon cinnamon powder 1 tablespoon white sugar

Guidelines:

1.   In a bowl, blend apple cuts with salt, sugar and cinnamon, hurl, move to the air fryer cooker's crate, cook for 10 minutes at 390 degrees F flipping once.

2.   Divide apple contributes bowls and fill in as a bite.

Enjoy the recipe!

The nutritional facts: calories 70, fat 0, fiber 4, carbs 3, protein 1

BREAD STICKS

Prep. time: 10 minutes

The cooking time: 10 minutes

The recipe servings: 2

Fixings:

4 bread cuts, each cut into 4 sticks 2 eggs

¼ cup milk

1 teaspoon cinnamon powder 1 tablespoon HONNEY

¼ cup darker sugar A spot of nutmeg

Guidelines:

1.   In a bowl, blend eggs in with milk, darker sugar, cinnamon, nutmeg and HONNEY and whisk well.

2.   Dip bread sticks right now, them in the air fryer cooker's container and cook at 360 Deg. Fahrenheit for about 10 minutes.

3.   Divide bread sticks into bowls and fill in as a tidbit.

Enjoy the recipe!

The nutritional facts: calories 140, fat 1, fiber 4, carbs 8, protein 4

FRESH SHRIMP

Prep. time: 10 minutes

The cooking time: 5 minutes

The recipe servings: 4

Fixings:

12 major shrimp, deveined and stripped 2 egg whites

1 cup coconut, destroyed

1 cup panko bread morsels 1 cup white flour

Salt and dark pepper to the taste

Guidelines:

1.   In a bowl, blend panko with coconut and mix.

2.   Put flour, salt and pepper in a subsequent bowl and whisk egg whites in a third one.

3.   Dip shrimp in flour, egg whites blend and coconut, place them all in the air fryer cooker's crate, cook at 350 Deg. Fahrenheit for about 10 minutes flipping midway.

4.   Arrange on a platter and fill in as a tidbit.

Enjoy the recipe!

The nutritional facts: calories 140, fat 4, fiber 0, carbs 3, protein 4

CAJUM SHRIMP APPATIZERS

Prep. time: 10 minutes

The cooking time: 5 minutes

The recipe servings: 2

Fixings:

20 tiger shrimp, stripped and deveined Salt and dark pepper to the taste

½ teaspoon old straight flavoring 1 tablespoon of olive oil

¼ teaspoon smoked paprika

Guidelines:

1.   In a bowl, blend shrimp in with oil, salt, pepper, old straight flavoring and paprika and hurl to cover.

2.   Place shrimp in the air fryer cooker's bin and cook at 390 Deg. Fahrenheit for about 5 minutes.

3.   Arrange them on a platter and fill in as a tidbit.

Enjoy the recipe!

The nutritional facts: calories 162, fat 6, fiber 4, carbs 8, protein 14

FRESH FISH STICKS

Prep. time: 10 minutes

The cooking time: 12 minutes

The recipe servings: 2

Fixings:

4 ounces bread scraps 4 tablespoons olive oil 1 egg, whisked

4 white fish fillets, boneless, skinless and cut into medium sticks Salt and dark pepper to the taste

Guidelines:

1.   In a bowl, blend bread pieces with oil and mix well.

2.   Put egg in a subsequent bowl, include salt and pepper and whisk well.

3.   Dip fish stick in egg and them in bread morsel blend, place them in the air fryer cooker's container and cook at 360 Deg. Fahrenheit for about 12 minutes.

4.   Arrange fish sticks on a platter and fill in as a canapé.

Enjoy the recipe!

The nutritional facts: calories 160, fat 3, fiber 5, carbs 12, protein 3

FISH NUGGETS

Prep. time: 10 minutes

The cooking time: 12 minutes

The recipe servings: 4

Fixings:

28 ounces fish fillets, skinless and cut into medium pieces Salt and dark pepper to the taste

5 tablespoons flour

1 egg, whisked

5 tablespoons water

3 ounces panko bread pieces 1 tablespoon garlic powder

1 tablespoon smoked paprika

4 tablespoons hand crafted mayonnaise Lemon juice from ½ lemon

1   teaspoon dill, dried Cooking splash

Guidelines:

1. In a bowl, blend flour in with water and mix well.

2. Add egg, salt and grinded pepper then whisk well.

3. In a subsequent bowl, blend panko with garlic powder and paprika and mix well.

4. Dip fish pieces in flour and egg blend and afterward in panko blend, place them in the air fryer cooker's crate, shower them with cooking oil and cook at 400 Deg. Fahrenheit for about 12 minutes.

5. Meanwhile, in a bowl blend mayo in with dill and lemon squeeze and whisk well.

6. Arrange fish pieces on a platter and present with dill mayo as an afterthought.

Enjoy the recipe!

The nutritional facts: calories 332, fat 12, fiber 6, carbs 17, protein 15

SHRIMP AND CHESTNUT ROLLS

Prep. time: 10 minutes

The cooking time: 15 minutes

The recipe servings: 4

Fixings:

½ pound previously cooked shrimp, hacked 8 ounces water chestnuts, cleaved

½ pounds shiitake mushrooms, cleaved 2 cups cabbage, hacked

1 teaspoon ginger, ground 3 scallions, cleaved

Salt and dark pepper to the taste 1 tablespoon water

1 egg yolk

6 spring move wrappers

Guidelines:

1.   Heat up a container with the oil over medium high heat, include cabbage, shrimp, chestnuts, mushrooms, garlic, ginger, scallions, salt and pepper, mix and cook for 2 minutes.

2.   In a bowl, blend egg in with water and mix well.

3.   Arrange move wrappers on a working surface, isolate shrimp and veggie blend on them, seal edges with egg wash, place them all in the air fryer cooker's bin, cook at 360 Deg. Fahrenheit for about 15 minutes, move to a platter and fill in as a hors d'oeuvre.

Enjoy the recipe!

The nutritional facts: calories 140, fat 3, fiber 1, carbs 12, protein 3

SEAFOODS APPETIZER

Prep. time: 10 minutes

The cooking time: 25 minutes

The recipe servings: 4

Fixings:

½ cup yellow onion, slashed

1 cup green ringer pepper, cleaved 1 cup celery, hacked

1 cup infant shrimp, stripped and deveined 1 cup crabmeat, chipped

1 cup natively constructed mayonnaise

1 teaspoon Worcestershire sauce Salt and dark pepper to the taste 2 tablespoons bread morsels

1 tablespoon margarine

1 teaspoon sweet paprika

Guidelines:

1.   In a bowl, blend shrimp in with crab meat, chime pepper, onion, mayo, celery, salt and pepper and mix.

2.   Add Worcestershire sauce, mix again and empty everything into a preparing dish that accommodates the air fryer cooker.

3.   Sprinkle bread pieces and include margarine, present in the air fryer cooker and cook at 320 Deg. Fahrenheit for about 25 minutes, shaking midway.

4.   Divide into bowl and present with paprika sprinkled on top as a hors d'oeuvre.

Enjoy the recipe!

The nutritional facts: calories 200, fat 1, fiber 2, carbs 5, protein 1

SALMON MEATBALLS

Prep. time: 10 minutes

The cooking time: 12 minutes

The recipe servings: 4

Fixings:

3 tablespoons cilantro, minced

1 pound salmon, skinless and hacked 1 little yellow onion, slashed

1 egg white

Salt and dark pepper to the taste 2 garlic cloves, minced

½ teaspoon paprika

¼ cup panko

½ teaspoon oregano, ground Cooking splash

Guidelines:

1.   In your food processor, blend salmon in with onion, cilantro, egg white, garlic cloves, salt, pepper, paprika and oregano and mix well.

2.   Add panko, mix again and shape meatballs from this blend utilizing your palms.

3.   Place them in the air fryer cooker's bushel, shower them with cooking splash and cook at 320 deg. F for about 12 minutes shaking the fryer midway.

4.   Arrange the meatballs on a plate and serve them as a hors d'oeuvre.

Enjoy the recipe!

The nutritional facts: calories 289, fat 12, fiber 3, carbs 22, protein 23

SIMPLE CHICKEN WINGS

Prep. time: 10 minutes

The cooking time: 1 hours

The recipe servings: 2

Fixings:

16 pieces chicken wings

Salt and dark pepper to the taste

¼ cup spread

¾ cup potato starch

¼ cup HONNEY

4 tablespoons garlic, minced

Guidelines:

1.   In a bowl, blend chicken wings in with salt, pepper and potato starch, hurl well, move to the air fryer cooker's bushel, cook them at 380 Deg. Fahrenheit for about 25 minutes and at 400 Deg. Fahrenheit for about 5 minutes more.

2.   Meanwhile, heat up a dish with the spread over medium high heat, soften it, include garlic, mix, cook for 5 minutes and afterward blend in with salt, pepper and HONNEY.

3.   Whisk well, cook over medium heat for 20 minutes and take off heat.

4.   Arrange chicken wings on a platter, shower HONNEY sauce all finished and fill in as a hors d'oeuvre.

Enjoy the recipe!

The nutritional facts: calories 244, fat 7, fiber 3, carbs 19, protein 8

CHICKEN BREAST ROLLS

Prep. time: 10 minutes

The cooking time: 22 minutes

The recipe servings: 4

Fixings:

2 cups infant spinach

4 chicken bosoms, boneless and skinless 1 cup sun-dried tomatoes, slashed

Salt and dark pepper to the taste

1 and ½ tablespoons Italian flavoring 4 mozzarella cuts

A sprinkle of olive oil

Guidelines:

1.   Flatten chicken bosoms utilizing a meat tenderizer, isolate tomatoes, mozzarella and spinach, season with salt, pepper, and Italian flavoring, roll, and seal them.

2.   Place them in the air fryer cooker's bin, shower some oil over them and cook at 375 Deg. Fahrenheit for about 17 minutes, flipping once.

3.   Arrange chicken moves on a platter and serve them as a starter.

Enjoy the recipe!

The nutritional facts: calories 300, fat 1, fiber 4, carbs 7, protein 10

FRESH CHICKEN BREAST STICKS

Prep. time: 10 minutes

The cooking time: 16 minutes

The recipe servings: 4

Fixings:

¾ cup white flour

1 pound chicken bosom, skinless, boneless and cut into medium sticks 1 teaspoon sweet paprika

1   cup panko bread morsels 1 egg, whisked

Salt and dark pepper to the taste

½ tablespoon of olive oil Zest from 1 lemon, ground

Guidelines:

1.   In a bowl, blend paprika in with the flour, salt, pepper, and lemon pizzazz and mix.

2.   Put the whisked egg in another bowl and the panko breadcrumbs in a third one.

3.   Dredge chicken pieces in flour, egg, and panko and place them in your lined air fryer's crate, sprinkle the oil over them, cook at 400 Deg. Fahrenheit for about 8 minutes, flip and cook for 8 additional minutes.

4.   Arrange them on a platter and fill in as a tidbit.

Enjoy the recipe!

The nutritional facts: calories 254, fat 4, fiber 7, carbs 20, protein 22

HAMBURGER ROLLS

Prep. time: 10 minutes

The cooking time:14 minutes

The recipe servings: 4

Fixings:

2 pounds hamburger steak, opened and smoothed with a meat tenderizer Salt and dark pepper to the taste

1 cup infant spinach

3 ounces red ringer pepper, cooked and slashed 6 cuts provolone cheddar

3 tablespoons pesto

Guidelines:

1.   Arrange straightened hamburger steak on a cutting board, spread pesto all finished, include cheddar in a solitary layer, include ringer peppers, spinach, salt, and pepper to the taste.

2.   Roll your steak, secure with toothpicks, season again with salt and pepper, place move in the air fryer cooker's bin, and cook at 400 Deg. Fahrenheit for about 14 minutes, pivoting roll midway.

3.   Leave aside to chill off, cut into 2 inches littler rolls, organize on a platter and serve them as a tidbit.

Enjoy the recipe!

The nutritional facts: calories 230, fat 1, fiber 3, carbs 12, protein 10

EMPANADAS

Prep. time: 10 minutes

The cooking time: 25 minutes

The recipe servings: 4

Fixings:

1 bundle empanada shells 1 tablespoon of olive oil

1 pound hamburger meat, ground 1 yellow onion, slashed

Salt and dark pepper to the taste 2 garlic cloves, minced

½ teaspoon cumin, ground

¼ cup tomato salsa

1 egg yolk raced with 1 tablespoon water 1 green ringer pepper, cleaved

Guidelines:

1.   Heat up a skillet with the oil over medium-high heat, include hamburger and dark-colored all sides.

2.   Add onion, garlic, salt, pepper, ringer pepper, and tomato salsa, mix and cook for 15 minutes.

3.   Divide cooked meat in empanada shells, brush them with egg wash and seal.

4.   Place them in the air fryer cooker's steamer container and cook at 350 Deg. Fahrenheit for about 10 minutes.

5.   Arrange on a platter and fill in as a canapé.

Enjoy the recipe!

The nutritional facts: calories 274, fat 17, fiber 14, carbs 20, protein 7

GREEK LAMB MEATBALLS

Prep. time: 10 minutes

The cooking time: 8 minutes

The recipe servings: 10

Fixings:

4 ounces lamb meat, minced Salt and dark pepper to the taste

1 cut of bread, toasted and disintegrated 2 tablespoons feta cheddar, disintegrated

½ tablespoon lemon strip, ground 1 tablespoon oregano, slashed

Guidelines:

1.   In a bowl, join meat with bread morsels, salt, pepper, feta, oregano, and lemon strip, mix well, shape 10 meatballs, and spot them in your air fryer.

2.   Cook the recipes at 400 deg. F for about 8 minutes, organize them on a platter, and fill in as a tidbit.

Enjoy the recipe!

The nutritional facts: calories 234, fat 12, fiber 2, carbs 20, protein 30

MEAT PARTY ROLLS

Prep. time: 10 minutes The cooking time: 15 minutes The recipe servings: 4

Fixings:

14 ounces meat stock 7 ounces white wine 4 hamburger cutlets

Salt and dark pepper to the taste 8 sage leaves

4 ham cuts

1 tablespoon spread, liquefied

Guidelines:

1.   Heat up a container with the stock over medium-high heat, include wine, cook until it diminishes, take off heat and partition into little dishes

2.   Season cutlets with salt and pepper spread with sage and roll each in ham cuts.

3.   Brush moves with spread, place them in the air fryer cooker's crate, and cook at 400 Deg. Fahrenheit for about 15 minutes.

4.   Arrange moves on a platter and serve them with the sauce as an afterthought.

Enjoy the recipe!

The nutritional facts: calories 260, fat 12, fiber 1, carbs 22, protein 21

PORK ROLLS

Prep. time: 10 minutes

The cooking time: 40 minutes

The recipe servings: 4

Fixings:

 15 ounces pork filet

½ teaspoon bean stew powder

1 teaspoon cinnamon powder 1 garlic clove, minced

Salt and dark pepper to the taste 2 tablespoons olive oil

1 and ½ teaspoon cumin, ground 1 red onion, hacked

3 tablespoons parsley, hacked

Guidelines:

1.   In a bowl, blend cinnamon in with garlic, salt, pepper, stew powder, oil, onion, parsley, and cumin and mix well

2.   Put pork filet on a cutting board, straighten it utilizing a meat tenderizer. What's more, utilize a meat tenderizer to straighten it.

3.   Spread onion blend on pork, roll tight, cut into medium moves, place them in your preheated air fryer at 360 degrees F and cook them for 35 minutes.

4.   Arrange them on a platter and fill in as an hors d'oeuvre

Enjoy the recipe!

The nutritional facts: calories 304, fat 12, fiber 1, carbs 15, protein 23

MEAT PATTIES

Prep. time: 10 minutes

The cooking time: 8 minutes

The recipe servings: 4

Fixings:

14 ounces meat, minced

2   tablespoons ham, cut into strips 1 leek, hacked

3   tablespoons bread pieces

Salt and dark pepper to the taste

½ teaspoon nutmeg, ground

Guidelines:

1.   In a bowl, blend meat in with leek, salt, pepper, ham, breadcrumbs and nutmeg, mix well and shape little patties out of this blend.

2.   Place them in the air fryer cooker's bushel, cook at 400 Deg. Fahrenheit for about 8 minutes, orchestrate on a platter and fill in as a hors d'oeuvre.

Enjoy the recipe!

The nutritional facts: calories 260, fat 12, fiber 3, carbs 12, protein 21

BROILED BELL PEPPER ROLLS

Prep. time: 10 minutes

The cooking time: 10 minutes

The recipe servings: 8

Fixings:

1   yellow chime pepper, split 1 orange ringer pepper, divided

Salt and dark pepper to the taste 4 ounces feta cheddar, disintegrated 1 green onion, hacked

2   tablespoons oregano, hacked

Guidelines:

1.   In a bowl, blend cheddar in with onion, oregano, salt and pepper and whisk well.

2.   Place ringer pepper parts in the air fryer cooker's bin, cook at 400 Deg. Fahrenheit for about 10 minutes, move to a cutting board, chill off and strip.

3.   Divide cheddar blend on each ringer pepper half, roll, secure with toothpicks, mastermind on a platter and fill in as a starter.

Enjoy the recipe!

The nutritional facts: calories 170, fat 1, fiber 2, carbs 8, protein 5

STUFFED PEPPERS

Prep. time: 10 minutes

The cooking time: 8 minutes

The recipe servings: 8

Fixings:

8 little ringer peppers, finishes cut off and seeds expelled 1 tablespoon of olive oil

Salt and dark pepper to the taste

3.5   ounces goat cheddar, cut into 8 pieces

Guidelines:

1.   In a bowl, blend cheddar in with oil with salt and pepper and hurl to cover.

2.   Stuff each pepper with goat cheddar, place them in the air fryer cooker's container, cook at 400 Deg. Fahrenheit for about 8 minutes, orchestrate on a platter and fill in as a canapé.

Enjoy the recipe!

The nutritional facts: calories 120, fat 1, fiber 1, carbs 12, protein 8

HERBED TOMATOES APPETIZER

Prep. time: 10 minutes

The cooking time: 20 minutes

The recipe servings: 2

Fixings:

2 tomatoes, split Cooking shower

Salt and dark pepper to the taste 1 teaspoon parsley, dried

1 teaspoon basil, dried

1 teaspoon oregano, dried 1 teaspoon rosemary, dried

Guidelines:

1.   Spray tomato parts with cooking oil, season with salt, pepper, parsley, basil, oregano and rosemary over them.

2.   Place them in the air fryer cooker's bushel and cook at 320 Deg. Fahrenheit for about 20 minutes.

3.   Arrange them on a platter and fill in as a hors d'oeuvre.

Enjoy the recipe!

The nutritional facts: calories 100, fat 1, fiber 1, carbs 4, protein 1

OLIVES BALLS

Prep. time: 10 minutes

The cooking time: 4 minutes

The recipe servings: 6

Fixings:

8 dark olives, pitted and minced Salt and dark pepper to the taste

2 tablespoons sun dried tomato pesto 14 pepperoni cuts, hacked

4 ounces cream cheddar

1 tablespoons basil, hacked

Guidelines:

1.   In a bowl, blend cream cheddar with salt, pepper, basil, pepperoni, pesto and dark olives, mix well and shape little balls out of this blend.

2.   Place them in the air fryer cooker's crate, cook at 350 Deg. Fahrenheit for about 4 minutes, orchestrate on a platter and fill in as a tidbit.

Enjoy the recipe!

The nutritional facts: calories 100, fat 1, fiber 0, carbs 8, protein 3

JALAPENO BALLS

Prep. time: 10 minutes

The cooking time: 4 minutes

The recipe servings: 3

Fixings:

3 bacon cuts, cooked and disintegrated 3 ounces cream cheddar

¼ teaspoon onion powder

Salt and dark pepper to the taste 1 jalapeno pepper, slashed

½ teaspoon parsley, dried

¼ teaspoon garlic powder

Guidelines:

1.   In a bowl, blend cream cheddar with jalapeno pepper, onion and garlic powder, parsley, bacon salt and pepper and mix well.

2.   Shape little balls out of this blend, place them in the air fryer cooker's container, cook at 350 Deg. Fahrenheit for about 4 minutes, mastermind on a platter and fill in as a starter.

Enjoy the recipe!

The nutritional facts: calories 172, fat 4, fiber 1, carbs 12, protein 5

WRAPPED SHRIMP

Prep. time: 10 minutes

The cooking time: 8 minutes

The recipe servings: 16

Fixings:

2 tablespoons olive oil

10 ounces previously cooked shrimp, stripped and deveined 1 tablespoons mint, slashed

1/3 cup blackberries, ground 11 prosciutto cut

1/3 cup red wine

Guidelines:

1.   Wrap each shrimp in a prosciutto cuts, shower the oil over them, rub well, place in your preheated air fryer at 390 degrees F and fry them for 8 minutes.

2.   Meanwhile, heat up a container with ground blackberries over medium heat, include mint and wine, mix, cook for 3 minutes and take off heat.

3. Arrange shrimp on a platter, shower blackberries sauce over them and fill in as a tidbit.

Enjoy the recipe!

The nutritional facts: calories 224, fat 12, fiber 2, carbs 12, protein 14

BROCCOLI PATTIES

Prep. time: 10 minutes

The cooking time: 10 minutes

The recipe servings: 12

Fixings:

4 cups broccoli florets

1   and ½ cup almond flour 1 teaspoon paprika

Salt and dark pepper to the taste 2 eggs

¼ cup olive oil

2   cups cheddar, ground 1 teaspoon garlic powder

½ teaspoon apple juice vinegar

½ teaspoon preparing pop

Guidelines:

1.   Put broccoli florets in your food processor, include salt and pepper, mix well and move to a bowl.

2.   Add almond flour, salt, pepper, paprika, garlic powder, preparing pop, cheddar, oil, eggs and vinegar, mix well and shape 12 patties out of this blend.

3.   Place them in your preheated air fryer's crate and cook at 350 Deg. Fahrenheit for about 10 minutes.

4.   Arrange patties on a platter and fill in as a tidbit.

Enjoy the recipe!

The nutritional facts: calories 203, fat 12, fiber 2, carbs 14, protein 2

DISTINCTIVE STUFFED PEPPERS

Prep. time: 10 minutes

The cooking time: 20 minutes

The recipe servings: 6

Fixings:

1 pound smaller than expected ringer peppers, split Salt and dark pepper to the taste 1 teaspoon garlic powder

1 teaspoon sweet paprika

½ teaspoon oregano, dried

¼ teaspoon red pepper pieces 1 pound hamburger meat, ground

1 and ½ cups cheddar, destroyed 1 tablespoons bean stew powder

1 teaspoon cumin, ground Sour cream for serving

Guidelines:

1.   In a bowl, blend bean stew powder with paprika, salt, pepper, cumin, oregano, pepper drops and garlic powder and mix.

2.   Heat up a dish over medium heat, include meat, mix and dark colored for 10 minutes.

3.   Add stew powder blend, mix, take off heat and stuff pepper parts with this blend.

4.   Sprinkle cheddar all finished, place peppers in the air fryer cooker's bushel and cook them at 350 Deg. Fahrenheit for about 6 minutes.

5.   Arrange peppers on a platter and serve them with sharp cream as an afterthought.

Enjoy the recipe!

The nutritional facts: calories 170, fat 22, fiber 3, carbs 6, protein 27

GOOEY ZUCCHINI SNACK

Prep. time: 10 minutes

The cooking time: 8 minutes

The recipe servings: 4

Fixings:

1 cup mozzarella, destroyed

¼ cup tomato sauce 1 zucchini, cut

Salt and dark pepper to the taste A touch of cumin

Cooking splash

Guidelines:

1.   Arrange zucchini cuts in the air fryer cooker's bushel, splash them with cooking oil, spread tomato sauce all finished, them, season with salt, pepper, cumin, sprinkle mozzarella toward the end and cook them at 320 Deg. Fahrenheit for about 8 minutes.

2.   Arrange them on a platter and fill in as a tidbit.

Enjoy the recipe!

The nutritional facts: calories 150, fat 4, fiber 2, carbs 12, protein 4

SPINACH BALLS

Prep. time: 10 minutes

The cooking time: 7 minutes

The recipe servings: 30

Fixings:

4 tablespoons margarine, dissolved 2 eggs

1 cup flour

16 ounces spinach

1/3 cup feta cheddar, disintegrated

¼ teaspoon nutmeg, ground 1/3 cup parmesan, ground

Salt and dark pepper to the taste 1 tablespoon onion powder

3 tablespoons whipping cream 1 teaspoon garlic powder

Guidelines:

1.   In your blender, blend spinach in with margarine, eggs, flour, feta cheddar, parmesan, nutmeg, whipping cream, salt, pepper, onion and garlic pepper, mix well indeed and keep in the cooler for 10 minutes.

2.   Shape 30 spinach balls, place them in the air fryer cooker's bushel and cook at 300 Deg. Fahrenheit for about 7 minutes.

3.   Serve as a gathering hors d'oeuvre.

Enjoy the recipe!

The nutritional facts: calories 60, fat 5, fiber 1, carbs 1, protein 2

MUSHROOMS APPETIZER

Prep. time: 10 minutes

The cooking time: 10 minutes

The recipe servings: 4

Fixings:

¼ cup mayonnaise

1 teaspoon garlic powder

1 little yellow onion, slashed 24 ounces white mushroom tops Salt and dark pepper to the taste 1 teaspoon curry powder

4 ounces cream cheddar, delicate

¼ cup harsh cream

½ cup Mexican cheddar, destroyed

1 cup shrimp, cooked, stripped, deveined and slashed

Guidelines:

1.   In a bowl, blend mayo in with garlic powder, onion, curry powder, cream cheddar, acrid cream, Mexican cheddar, shrimp, salt and pepper to the taste and whisk well.

2.   Stuff mushrooms with this blend, place them in the air fryer cooker's crate and cook at 300 Deg. Fahrenheit for about 10 minutes.

3.   Arrange on a platter and fill in as a hors d'oeuvre.

Enjoy the recipe!

The nutritional facts: calories 200, fat 20, fiber 3, carbs 16, protein 14

GOOEY PARTY WINGS

Prep. time: 10 minutes

The cooking time: 12 minutes

The recipe servings: 6

Fixings:

6 pound chicken wings, split Salt and dark pepper to the taste

½ teaspoon Italian flavoring 2 tablespoons spread

½ cup parmesan cheddar, ground

A touch of red pepper pieces, squashed 1 teaspoon garlic powder

1   egg

Guidelines:

1.   Arrange chicken wings in the air fryer cooker's crate and cook at 390 degrees F and cook for 9 minutes.

2.   Meanwhile, in your blender, blend margarine in with cheddar, egg, salt, pepper, pepper chips, garlic powder and Italian flavoring and mix well indeed.

3.   Take chicken wings out, pour cheddar sauce over them, hurl to cover well and cook in the air fryer cooker's bin at 390 Deg. Fahrenheit for about 3 minutes.

4.   Serve them as a tidbit.

Enjoy the recipe!

The nutritional facts: calories 204, fat 8, fiber 1, carbs 18, protein 14

CHEDDAR STICKS

Prep. time: 1 hour and 10 minutes

The cooking time: 8 minutes

The recipe servings: 16

Fixings:

2   eggs, whisked

Salt and dark pepper to the taste

8 mozzarella cheddar strings, cut into equal parts 1 cup parmesan, ground

1 tablespoon Italian flavoring Cooking shower

. 1 garlic clove, minced

Guidelines:

1.   In a bowl, blend parmesan in with salt, pepper, Italian flavoring and garlic and mix well.

2.   Put whisked eggs in another bowl.

3.   Dip mozzarella sticks in egg blend, at that point in cheddar blend.

4.   Dip them again in egg and in parmesan blend and save them in the cooler for 60 minutes.

5.   Spray cheddar sticks with cooking oil, place them in the air fryer cooker's container and cook at 390 Deg. Fahrenheit for about 8 minutes flipping them midway.

6.   Arrange them on a platter and fill in as a starter.

Enjoy the recipe!

The nutritional facts: calories 140, fat 5, fiber 1, carbs 3, protein 4

SWEET BACON SNACK

Prep. time: 10 minutes The cooking time: 30 minutes The recipe servings: 16

Fixings:

½ teaspoon cinnamon powder 16 bacon cuts

1 tablespoon avocado oil 3 ounces dim chocolate 1 teaspoon maple extricate

Guidelines:

1.   Arrange bacon cuts in the air fryer cooker's container, sprinkle cinnamon blend over them and cook them at 300 Deg. Fahrenheit for about 30 minutes.

2.   Heat up a pot with the oil over medium heat, include chocolate and mix until it softens.

3.   Add maple separate, mix, take off heat and leave aside to chill off a piece.

4.   Take bacon strips out of the oven, leave them to chill off, dunk each in chocolate blend, place them on a material paper and leave them to chill off totally.

5.   Serve cold as a tidbit.

Enjoy the recipe!

The nutritional facts: calories 200, fat 4, fiber 5, carbs 12, protein 3

CHICKEN ROLLS

Prep. time: 2 hours and 10 minutes

The cooking time: 10 minutes

The recipe servings: 12

Fixings:

4 ounces blue cheddar, disintegrated

2 cups chicken, cooked and slashed Salt and dark pepper to the taste

2 green onions, slashed

2 celery stalks, finely slashed

½ cup tomato sauce 12 egg move wrappers Cooking shower

Guidelines:

1.   In a bowl, blend chicken meat in with blue cheddar, salt, pepper, green onions, celery and tomato sauce, mix well and keep in the ice chest for 2 hours.

2.   Place egg wrappers on a working surface, separate chicken blend on them, roll and seal edges.

3.   Place moves in the air fryer cooker's bushel, splash them with cooking oil and cook at 350 Deg. Fahrenheit for about 10 minutes, flipping them midway.

Enjoy the recipe!

The nutritional facts: calories 220, fat 7, fiber 2, carbs 14, protein 10

DELICIOUS KALE AND CELERY CRACKERS

Prep. time: 10 minutes The cooking time: 20 minutes The recipe servings: 6

Fixings:

2 cups flax seed, ground

2 cups flax seed, splashed medium-term and depleted 4 packs kale, slashed

1   bunch basil, hacked

½ pack celery, hacked 4 garlic cloves, minced 1/3 cup olive oil

Guidelines:

1.   In your food processor blend ground flaxseed with celery, kale, basil and garlic and mix well.

2.   Add oil and drenched flaxseed and mix once more, spread in the air fryer cooker's dish, cut into medium saltines and cook them at 380 Deg. Fahrenheit for about 20 minutes.

3.   Divide into bowls and fill in as a tidbit.

Enjoy the recipe!

The nutritional facts: calories 143, fat 1, fiber 2, carbs 8, protein 4

EGG WHITE CHIPS

Prep. time: 5 minutes The cooking time: 8 minutes The recipe servings: 2

Fixings:

½ tablespoon water

2   tablespoons parmesan, destroyed 4 eggs whites

Salt and dark pepper to the taste

Guidelines:

1.   In a bowl, blend egg whites with salt, pepper and water and whisk well.

2.   Spoon this into a biscuit dish that accommodates the air fryer cooker, sprinkle cheddar on top, present in the air fryer cooker and cook at 350 Deg. Fahrenheit for about 8 minutes.

3.   Arrange egg white chips on a platter and fill in as a bite.

Enjoy the recipe!

The nutritional facts: calories 180, fat 2, fiber 1, carbs 12, protein 7

TUNA CAKES

Prep. time: 10 minutes The cooking time: 10 minutes The recipe servings: 12

Fixings:

15 ounces canned tuna, channel and chipped 3 eggs

½ teaspoon dill, dried

1 teaspoon parsley, dried

½ cup red onion, hacked 1 teaspoon garlic powder

Salt and dark pepper to the taste Cooking splash

Guidelines:

1.   In a bowl, blend tuna in with salt, pepper, dill, parsley, onion, garlic powder and eggs, mix well and shape medium cakes out of this blend.

2.   Place tuna cakes in the air fryer cooker's bin, splash them with cooking oil and cook at 350 Deg. Fahrenheit for about 10 minutes, flipping them midway.

3.   Arrange them on a platter and fill in as a canapé.

Enjoy the recipe!

The nutritional facts: calories 140, fat 2, fiber 1, carbs 8, protein 6

CALAMARI AND SHRIMP SNACK

Prep. time: 10 minutes The cooking time: 20 minutes The recipe servings: 1

Fixings:

- 8 ounces calamari, cut into medium rings 7 ounces shrimp, stripped and deveined

- 1 eggs

- tablespoons white flour 1 tablespoon of olive oil

- tablespoons avocado, slashed 1 teaspoon tomato glue

- tablespoon mayonnaise

- A sprinkle of Worcestershire sauce 1 teaspoon lemon juice

- Salt and dark pepper to the taste

- ½ teaspoon turmeric powder

Guidelines:

1.   In a bowl, whisk egg with oil, include calamari rings and shrimp and hurl to cover.

2.   In another bowl, blend flour in with salt, pepper and turmeric and mix.

3.   Dredge calamari and shrimp right now, them in the air fryer cooker's container and cook at 350 Deg. Fahrenheit for about 9 minutes, flipping them once.

4.   Meanwhile, in a bowl, blend avocado in with mayo and tomato glue and pound utilizing a fork.

5.   Add Worcestershire sauce, lemon squeeze, salt and pepper and mix well.

6.   Arrange calamari and shrimp on a platter and present with the sauce as an afterthought.

Enjoy the recipe!

The nutritional facts: calories 288, fat 23, fiber 3, carbs 10, protein 15

AIR FRYER FISH AND SEAFOOD RECIPES

TASTY AIR FRIED COD

Prep. time: 10 minutes The cooking time: 12 minutes The recipe servings: 4

Fixings:

2   cod fish, 7 ounces each A shower of sesame oil

Salt and dark pepper to the taste 1 cup water

1 teaspoon dull soy sauce

3 tablespoons olive oil 4 ginger cuts

3 spring onions, hacked

2 tablespoons coriander, hacked

Guidelines:

1.   Season fish with salt, pepper, shower sesame oil, rub well and leave aside for 10 minutes.

2.   Add fish to the air fryer cooker and cook at 356 Deg. Fahrenheit for about 12 minutes.

3.   Meanwhile, heat up a pot with the water over medium heat, include dull and light soy sauce and sugar, mix, bring to a stew and take off heat.

4.   Heat up a skillet with the olive oil over medium heat, include ginger and green onions, mix, cook for a couple of moments and take off heat.

5.   Divide fish on plates, top with ginger and green onions, shower soy sauce blend, sprinkle coriander and serve immediately.

Enjoy the recipe!

The nutritional facts: calories 300, fat 17, fiber 8, carbs 20, protein 22

SCRUMPTIOUS CATFISH

Prep. time: 10 minutes The cooking time: 20 minutes The recipe servings: 4

Fixings:

4 feline fish fillets

Salt and dark pepper to the taste A touch of sweet paprika

1 tablespoon parsley, cleaved 1 tablespoon lemon juice

1   tablespoon of olive oil

Guidelines:

1.   Season catfish fillets with salt, pepper, paprika, shower oil, rub well, place in the air fryer cooker's bushel and cook at 400 Deg. Fahrenheit for about 20 minutes, flipping the fish following 10 minutes.

2.   Divide fish on plates, shower lemon squeeze all finished, sprinkle parsley and serve.

Enjoy the recipe!

The nutritional facts: calories 253, fat 6, fiber 12, carbs 26, protein 22

COD FILLETS WITH FENNEL AND GRAPES SALAD

Prep. time: 10 minutes The cooking time: 15 minutes The recipe servings: 2

Fixings:

2   black cod fillets, boneless 1 tablespoon of olive oil

Salt and dark pepper to the taste 1 fennel bulb, meagerly cut

1 cup grapes, divided

½ cup walnuts

Guidelines:

1.   Drizzle portion of the oil over fish fillets, season with salt and pepper, rub well, place fillets in the air fryer cooker's container, cook for 10 minutes at 400 degrees F and move to a plate.

2.	In a bowl, blend walnuts in with grapes, fennel, the remainder of the oil, salt and pepper, hurl to cover, add to a skillet that accommodates the air fryer cooker and cook at 400 Deg. Fahrenheit for about 5 minutes.

3.	Divide cod on plates, include fennel and grapes blend the side and serve.

Enjoy the recipe!

The nutritional facts: calories 300, fat 4, fiber 2, carbs 32, protein 22

TABASCO SHRIMP

Prep. time: 10 minutes

The cooking time: 10 minutes

The recipe servings: 4

Fixings:

1	pound shrimp, stripped and deveined 1 teaspoon red pepper drops

2	tablespoon of olive oil

1 teaspoon Tabasco sauce 2 tablespoons water

1 teaspoon oregano, dried

Salt and dark pepper to the taste

½ teaspoon parsley, dried

½ teaspoon smoked paprika

Guidelines:

1.   In a bowl, blend oil in with water, Tabasco sauce, pepper drops, oregano, parsley, salt, pepper, paprika and shrimp and hurl well to cover.

2.   Transfer shrimp to your preheated air fryer at 370 degrees F and cook for 10 minutes shaking the fryer once.

3.   Divide shrimp on plates and present with a side serving of mixed greens.

Enjoy the recipe!

The nutritional facts: calories 200, fat 5, fiber 6, carbs 13, protein 8

BUTTERED SHRIMP SKEWERS

Prep. time: 10 minutes

The cooking time: 6 minutes

The recipe servings: 2

Fixings:

8 shrimps, stripped and deveined 4 garlic cloves, minced

Salt and dark pepper to the taste 8 green chime pepper cuts

1   tablespoon rosemary, cleaved 1 tablespoon margarine, softened

Guidelines:

1.   In a bowl, blend shrimp in with garlic, spread, salt, pepper, rosemary and ringer pepper cuts, hurl to cover and leave aside for 10 minutes.

2.   Arrange 2 shrimp and 2 ringer pepper cuts on a stick and rehash with the remainder of the shrimp and chime pepper pieces.

3.   Place them all in the air fryer cooker's crate and cook at 360 Deg. Fahrenheit for about 6 minutes.

4.   Divide among plates and serve immediately.

Enjoy the recipe!

The nutritional facts: calories 140, fat 1, fiber 12, carbs 15, protein 7

ASIAN SALMON

Prep. time: 1 hour The cooking time: 15 minutes The recipe servings: 2

Fixings:

2   medium salmon fillets

6 tablespoons light soy sauce 3 teaspoons mirin

1 teaspoon water

6 tablespoons HONNEY

Guidelines:

1.   In a bowl, blend soy sauce with HONNEY, water and mirin, whisk well, include salmon, rub well and leave aside in the ice chest for 60 minutes.

2.   Transfer salmon to the air fryer cooker and cook at 360 Deg. Fahrenheit for about 15 minutes, flipping them following 7 minutes.

3.   Meanwhile, put the soy marinade in a container, heat up over medium heat, whisk well, cook for 2 minutes and take off heat.

4.   Divide salmon on plates, shower marinade all finished and serve.

Enjoy the recipe!

The nutritional facts: calories 300, fat 12, fiber 8, carbs 13, protein 24

C OD STEAKS WITH PLUM SAUCE

Prep. time: 10 minutes The cooking time: 20 minutes The recipe servings: 2

Fixings:

2 major cod steaks

Salt and dark pepper to the taste

½ teaspoon garlic powder

½ teaspoon ginger powder

¼ teaspoon turmeric powder 1 tablespoon plum sauce Cooking splash

Guidelines:

1.	Season cod steaks with salt and pepper, splash them with cooking oil, include garlic powder, ginger powder and turmeric powder and rub well.

2.	Place cod steaks in the air fryer cooker and cook at 360 Deg. Fahrenheit for about 15 minutes, flipping them following 7 minutes.

3.	Heat up a dish over medium heat, include plum sauce, mix and cook for 2 minutes.

4.	Divide cod steaks on plates, shower plum sauce all finished and serve.

Enjoy the recipe!

The nutritional facts: calories 250, fat 7, fiber 1, carbs 14, protein 12

ENHANCED AIR FRIED SALMON

Prep. time: 1 hour The cooking time: 8 minutes The recipe servings: 2

Fixings:

2 salmon fillets

2   tablespoons lemon juice

Salt and dark pepper to the taste

½ teaspoon garlic powder 1/3 cup water

1/3 cup soy sauce

3   scallions, cleaved 1/3 cup darker sugar

2 tablespoons olive oil

Guidelines:

1.   In a bowl, blend sugar in with water, soy sauce, garlic powder, salt, pepper, oil and lemon juice, whisk well, include salmon fillets, hurl to cover and leave aside in the cooler for 60 minutes.

2.   Transfer salmon fillets to the fryer's bin and cook at 360 Deg. Fahrenheit for about 8 minutes flipping them midway.

3.   Divide salmon on plates, sprinkle scallions on top and serve immediately.

Enjoy the recipe!

The nutritional facts: calories 300, fat 12, fiber 10, carbs 23, protein 20

SALMON WITH CAPPERS AND MASH

Prep. time: 10 minutes

The cooking time: 20 minutes

The recipe servings: 4

Fixings:

4 salmon fillets, skinless and boneless 1 tablespoon escapades, depleted

Salt and dark pepper to the taste Juice from 1 lemon

2 teaspoons olive oil

For the potato squash:

2 tablespoons of the olive-oil & 1 tablespoon dill, dried

1 pound potatoes, cleaved

½ cup milk

Guidelines:

1.   Put potatoes in a pot, add water to cover, include some salt, heat to the point of boiling over medium high heat, cook for 15 minutes, channel, move to a bowl, squash with a potato masher, include 2 tablespoons oil, dill, salt, pepper and milk, whisk well and leave aside for the time being.

2.   Season salmon with salt and pepper, sprinkle 2 teaspoons oil over them, rub, move to the air fryer cooker's bin, include escapades top, cook at 360 degrees F and cook for 8 minutes.

3.   Divide salmon and escapades on plates, include pureed potatoes the side, sprinkle lemon squeeze all finished and serve.

Enjoy the recipe!

The nutritional facts: calories 300, fat 17, fiber 8, carbs 12, protein 18

LEMONY SABA FISH

Prep. time: 10 minutes

The cooking time: 8 minutes

The recipe servings: 1

Fixings:

4 Saba fish filet, boneless

Salt and dark pepper to the taste 3 red bean stew pepper, cleaved

2 tablespoons lemon juice 2 tablespoon of olive oil

2 tablespoon garlic, minced

Guidelines:

1.   Season fish fillets with salt and pepper and put in a bowl.

2.   Add lemon juice, oil, stew and garlic hurl to cover, move fish to the air fryer cooker and cook at 360 Deg. Fahrenheit for about 8 minutes, flipping midway.

3.   Divide among plates and present with certain fries.

Enjoy the recipe!

The nutritional facts: calories 300, fat 4, fiber 8, carbs 15, protein 15

ASIAN HALIBUT

Prep. time: 10 minutes

The cooking time: 10 minutes

The recipe servings: 3

Fixings:

1   pound halibut steaks 2/3 cup soy sauce

¼ cup sugar

1   tablespoons lime juice

½ cup mirin

¼ teaspoon red pepper chips, squashed

¼ cup squeezed orange

¼ teaspoon ginger, ground 1 garlic clove, minced

Guidelines:

1.   Put soy sauce in a dish, heat up over medium heat, include mirin, sugar, lime and squeezed orange, pepper pieces, ginger and garlic, mix well, heat to the point of boiling and take off heat.

2.   Transfer portion of the marinade to a bowl, include halibut, hurl to cover and leave aside in the refrigerator for 30 minutes.

3.   Transfer halibut to the air fryer cooker and cook at 390 Deg. Fahrenheit for about 10 minutes, flipping once.

4.   Divide halibut steaks on plates, shower the remainder of the marinade all finished and serve hot.

Enjoy the recipe!

The nutritional facts: calories 286, fat 5, fiber 12, carbs 14, protein 23

COD AND VINAIGRETTE

Prep. time: 10 minutes

The cooking time: 15 minutes

The recipe servings: 4

Fixings:

4 cod fillets, skinless and boneless 12 cherry tomatoes, split

8 dark olives, pitted and generally cleaved 2 tablespoons lemon juice

Salt and dark pepper to the taste 2 tablespoons olive oil

Cooking shower

1 bundle basil, slashed

Guidelines:

1.   Season cod with salt and pepper to the taste, place in the air fryer cooker's container and cook at 360 Deg. Fahrenheit for about 10 minutes, flipping following 5 minutes.

2. Meanwhile, heat up a skillet with the oil over medium heat, include tomatoes, olives and lemon juice, mix, bring to a stew, include basil, salt and pepper, mix well and take off heat.

3. Divide fish on plates and present with the vinaigrette sprinkled on top.

Enjoy the recipe!

The nutritional facts: calories 300, fat 5, fiber 8, carbs 12, protein 8

SHRIMP AND CRAB MIX

Prep. time: 10 minutes

The cooking time: 25 minutes

The recipe servings: 4

Fixings:

½ cup yellow onion, slashed

1 cup green ringer pepper, hacked 1 cup celery, cleaved

1 pound shrimp, stripped and deveined 1 cup crabmeat, chipped

1 cup mayonnaise

1 teaspoon Worcestershire sauce Salt and dark pepper to the taste 2 tablespoons breadcrumbs

1 tablespoon margarine, dissolved 1 teaspoon sweet paprika

Guidelines:

1.   In a bowl, blend shrimp in with crab meat, ringer pepper, onion, mayo, celery, salt, pepper and Worcestershire sauce, hurl well and move to a dish that accommodates the air fryer cooker.

2.   Sprinkle bread pieces and paprika, include softened margarine, place in the air fryer cooker and cook at 320 Deg. Fahrenheit for about 25 minutes, shaking midway.

3.   Divide among plates and serve immediately.

Enjoy the recipe!

The nutritional facts: calories 200, fat 13, fiber 9, carbs 17, protein 19

SEAFOOD CASEROLE

Prep. time: 10 minutes

The cooking time: 40 minutes

The recipe servings: 6

Fixings:

6 tablespoons spread

2 ounces mushrooms, hacked

1   small green chime pepper, slashed 1 celery stalk, cleaved

2   garlic cloves, minced

1 little yellow onion, hacked Salt and dark pepper to the taste 4 tablespoons flour

½ cup white wine 1 and ½ cups milk

½ cup overwhelming cream 4 ocean scallops, cut

4 ounces haddock, skinless, boneless and cut into little pieces 4 ounces lobster meat, effectively cooked and cut into little pieces

½ teaspoon of mustard powder & 1 tablespoon of lemon juice 1/3 cup bread morsels

Salt and dark pepper to the taste

3 tablespoons cheddar, ground A bunch parsley, slashed

1 teaspoon sweet paprika

Guidelines:

1.   Heat up a skillet with 4 tablespoons margarine over medium high heat, include chime pepper, mushrooms, celery, garlic, onion and wine, mix and cook for 10 minutes

2.   Add flour, cream and milk, mix well and cook for 6 minutes.

3.   Add lemon juice, salt, pepper, mustard powder, scallops, lobster meat and haddock, mix well, take off heat and move to a skillet that accommodates the air fryer cooker.

4.   In a bowl, blend the remainder of the margarine in with bread morsels, paprika and

Enjoy the recipe!

cheddar and sprinkle over seafood blend.

5.   Transfer container to the air fryer cooker and cook at 360 Deg. Fahrenheit for about 16 minutes.

6.   Divide among plates and present with parsley sprinkled on top.

The nutritional facts: calories 270, fat 32, fiber 14, carbs 15, protein 23

TROUT FILET AND ORANGES SAUCE

Prep. time: 10 minutes

The cooking time: 10 minutes

The recipe servings: 4

Fixings:

4 trout fillets, skinless and boneless 4 spring onions, cleaved

1 tablespoon of olive oil

1 tablespoon ginger, minced

Salt and dark pepper to the taste Juice and get-up-and-go from 1 orange

Guidelines:

1.   Season trout fillets with salt, pepper, rub them with the olive oil, place in a dish that accommodates the air fryer cooker, include ginger, green onions, orange pizzazz and juice, hurl well, place in the air fryer cooker and cook at 360 Deg. Fahrenheit for about 10 minutes.

2.   Divide fish and sauce on plates and serve immediately.

Enjoy the recipe!

The nutritional facts: calories 239, fat 10, fiber 7, carbs 18, protein 23

COD FILLETS AND PEAS

Prep. time: 10 minutes

The cooking time: 10 minutes

The recipe servings: 4

Fixings:

- 4 cod fillets, boneless

- tablespoons parsley, hacked 2 cups peas

- tablespoons wine

- ½ teaspoon oregano, dried

- ½ teaspoon sweet paprika 2 garlic cloves, minced Salt and pepper to the taste

Guidelines:

1. In your food processor blend garlic in with parsley, salt, pepper, oregano, paprika and wine and mix well.

2. Rub fish with half of this blend, place in the air fryer cooker and cook at 360 Deg. Fahrenheit for about 10 minutes.

3. Meanwhile, put peas in a pot, add water to cover, include salt, heat to the point of boiling over medium high heat, cook for 10 minutes, channel and partition among plates.

4. Also partition fish on plates, spread the remainder of the herb dressing all finished and serve.

Enjoy the recipe!

The nutritional facts: calories 261, fat 8, fiber 12, carbs 20, protein 22

THYME AND PARSLEY SALMON

Prep. time: 10 minutes

The cooking time: 15 minutes

The recipe servings: 4

Fixings:

4 salmon fillets, boneless Juice from 1 lemon

1 yellow onion, hacked 3 tomatoes, cut

4 thyme springs

4 parsley springs

3 tablespoons of additional virgin olive-oil Salt and dark pepper to the taste

Guidelines:

1.   Drizzle 1 tablespoon oil in a container that accommodates the air fryer cooker,, include a layer of tomatoes, salt and pepper, sprinkle 1 more tablespoon oil, include fish, season them with salt and pepper, shower the remainder of the oil, include thyme and parsley springs, onions, lemon squeeze, salt and then pepper, also place in the air fryer cooker's crate and cook at 360 Deg. Fahrenheit for about 12 minutes shaking once.

2.   Divide everything on plates and serve immediately.

Enjoy the recipe!

The nutritional facts: calories 242, fat 9, fiber 12, carbs 20, protein 31

TROUT AND BUTTER SAUSE

Prep. time: 10 minutes

The cooking time: 10 minutes

The recipe servings: 4

Fixings:

4 trout fillets, boneless

Salt and dark pepper to the taste 3 teaspoons lemon pizzazz, ground

3 tablespoons chives, hacked 6 tablespoons margarine

2 tablespoons of the olive oil & 2 teaspoons of lemon juice

Guidelines:

1. Season trout with salt and pepper, shower the olive oil, rub, move to the air fryer cooker and cook at 360 Deg. Fahrenheit for about 10 minutes, flipping once.

2.   Meanwhile, heat up a dish with the margarine over medium heat, include salt, pepper, chives, lemon squeeze and pizzazz, whisk well, cook for 1-2 minutes and take off heat

3.   Divide fish fillets on plates, sprinkle spread sauce all finished and serve.

Enjoy the recipe!

The nutritional facts: calories 300, fat 12, fiber 9, carbs 27, protein 24

REAMY SALMON

Prep. time: 10 minutes

The cooking time: 10 minutes

The recipe servings: 4

Fixings:

4 salmon fillets, boneless 1 tablespoons olive oil

Salt and dark pepper to the taste 1/3 cup cheddar, ground

1 and ½ teaspoon mustard

½ cup coconut cream

Guidelines:

1. Season salmon with salt and pepper, shower the oil and rub well.

2. In a bowl, blend coconut cream with cheddar, mustard, salt and pepper and mix well.

3. Transfer salmon to a skillet that accommodates the air fryer cooker, include coconut cream blend, present in the air fryer cooker and cook at 320 Deg. Fahrenheit for about 10 minutes.

4. Divide among plates and serve.

Enjoy the recipe!

The nutritional facts: calories 200, fat 6, fiber 14, carbs 17, protein 20

SALMON AND AVOCADO SALSA

Prep. time: 30 minutes

The cooking time: 10 minutes

The recipe servings: 4

Fixings:

4 salmon fillets

1 tablespoon of olive oil

Salt and dark pepper to the taste 1 teaspoon cumin, ground

1 teaspoon sweet paprika

½ teaspoon bean stew powder 1 teaspoon garlic powder

For the salsa:

1 little red onion, slashed

1   avocado, hollowed, stripped and slashed 2 tablespoons cilantro, cleaved

Juice from 2 limes

Salt and dark pepper to the taste

Guidelines:

1.   In a bowl, blend salt, pepper, bean stew powder, onion powder, paprika and cumin, mix, rub salmon with this blend, sprinkle the oil, rub once more, move to the air fryer cooker and cook at 350 Deg. Fahrenheit for about 5 minutes on each side.

2.   Meanwhile, in a bowl, blend avocado in with red onion, salt, pepper, cilantro and lime squeeze and mix.

3.   Divide fillets on plates, top with avocado salsa and serve.

Enjoy the recipe!

The nutritional facts: calories 300, fat 14, fiber 4, carbs 18, protein 16

ITALIAN BARRAMUNDI FILLETS AND TOMATO SALSA

Prep. time: 10 minutes

The cooking time: 8 minutes

The recipe servings: 4

Fixings:

2   barramundi fillets, boneless

1   tablespoon of olive oil+ 2 teaspoons 2 teaspoons Italian flavoring

¼ cup green olives, hollowed and slashed

¼ cup cherry tomatoes, cleaved

¼ cup dark olives, cleaved 1 tablespoon lemon pizzazz

2   tablespoons lemon pizzazz

Salt and dark pepper to the taste 2 tablespoons parsley, cleaved

Guidelines:

1.   Rub fish with salt, pepper, Italian flavoring and 2 teaspoons olive oil, move to the air fryer cooker and cook at 360 Deg. Fahrenheit for about 8 minutes, flipping them midway.

2.   In a bowl, blend tomatoes in with dark olives, green olives, salt, pepper, lemon pizzazz and lemon juice, parsley and 1 tablespoon of olive oil and hurl well

3.   Divide fish on plates, include tomato salsa top and serve.

Enjoy the recipe!

The nutritional facts: calories 270, fat 4, fiber 2, carbs 18, protein 27

CREAMY SHRIMP AND VEGGIES

Prep. time: 10 minutes

The cooking time: 30 minutes

The recipe servings: 4

Fixings:

8 ounces mushrooms, slashed

1   asparagus bundle, cut into medium pieces 1 pound shrimp, stripped and deveined

Salt and dark pepper to the taste 1 spaghetti squash, cut into equal parts 2 tablespoons olive oil

2   teaspoons Italian flavoring 1 yellow onion, cleaved

1 teaspoon red pepper pieces, squashed

¼ cup margarine, dissolved

1 cup parmesan cheddar, ground 2 garlic cloves, minced

1 cup substantial cream

Guidelines:

1.   Place squash parts in you air fryer's bin, cook at 390 Deg. Fahrenheit for about 17 minutes, move to a cutting board, scoop inner parts and move to a bowl.

2.   Put water in a pot, include some salt, heat to the point of boiling over medium heat, include asparagus, steam for several minutes, move to a bowl loaded up with ice water, channel and leave aside also.

3.   Heat up a skillet that accommodates the air fryer cooker with the oil over medium heat, include onions and mushrooms, mix and cook for 7 minutes.

4.   Add pepper drops, Italian flavoring, salt, pepper, squash, asparagus, shrimp, softened spread, cream, parmesan and garlic, hurl and cook in the air fryer cooker at 360 Deg. Fahrenheit for about 6 minutes.

5.   Divide everything on plates and serve.

Enjoy the recipe!

The nutritional facts: calories 325, fat 6, fiber 5, carbs 14, protein 13

TUNA AND CHIMICHURI SAUSE

Prep. time: 10 minutes

The cooking time: 8 minutes

The recipe servings: 4

Fixings:

½ cup cilantro, slashed

1/3 cup olive oil+ 2 tablespoons 1 little red onion, slashed

3 tablespoon balsamic vinegar 2 tablespoons parsley, slashed 2 tablespoons basil, cleaved

1 jalapeno pepper, slashed 1 pound sushi tuna steak

Salt and dark pepper to the taste 1 teaspoon red pepper drops

1   teaspoon thyme, slashed 3 garlic cloves, minced

2   avocados, hollowed, stripped and cut 6 ounces infant arugula

Guidelines:

1.   In a bowl, blend 1/3 cup oil with jalapeno, vinegar, onion, cilantro, basil, garlic, parsley, pepper drops, thyme, salt and pepper, whisk well and leave aside for the time being.

2.   Season tuna with salt and pepper, rub with the remainder of the oil, place in the air fryer cooker and cook at 360 Deg. Fahrenheit for about 3 minutes on each side.

3.   Mix arugula with half of the chimichuri blend you've made and hurl to cover.

4.   Divide arugula on plates, cut tuna and furthermore separate among plates, top with the remainder of the chimichuri and serve.

Enjoy the recipe!

The nutritional facts: calories 276, fat 3, fiber 1, carbs 14, protein 20

SQUID AND GUACAMOLE

Prep. time: 10 minutes

The cooking time: 6 minutes

The recipe servings: 2

Fixings:

2 medium squids, appendages isolated and tubes scored the long way 1 tablespoon of olive oil

Juice from 1 lime

Salt and dark pepper to the taste

For the guacamole:

2 avocados, hollowed, stripped and cleaved 1 tablespoon coriander, slashed

2 red chilies, cleaved 1 tomato, slashed

1 red onion, slashed Juice from 2 limes

Guidelines:

1. Season squid and squid arms with salt, pepper, shower the olive oil all finished, put in the air fryer cooker's container and cook at 360 Deg. Fahrenheit for about 3 minutes on each side.

2. Transfer squid to a bowl, sprinkle lime squeeze all finished and hurl.

3. Meanwhile, put avocado in a bowl, squash with a fork, include coriander, chilies, tomato, onion and juice from 2 limes and hurl.

4. Divide squid on plates, top with guacamole and serve.

Enjoy the recipe!

The nutritional facts: calories 500, fat 43, fiber 6, carbs 7, protein 20

SHRIMP AND CAULIFLOWER

Prep. time: 10 minutes

The cooking time: 12 minutes

The recipe servings: 2

Fixings:

1 tablespoon margarine Cooking splash

1 cauliflower head, riced

1 pound shrimp, stripped and deveined

¼ cup substantial cream

8 ounces mushrooms, generally slashed A touch of red pepper pieces

Salt and dark pepper to the taste 2 garlic cloves, minced

4 bacon cuts, cooked and disintegrated

½ cup hamburger stock

1   tablespoon parsley, finely slashed 1 tablespoon chives, hacked

Guidelines:

1.   Season shrimp with salt and pepper, shower with cooking oil, place in the air fryer cooker and cook at 360 Deg. Fahrenheit for about 7 minutes.

2.   Meanwhile, heat up a container with the margarine over medium heat, include mushrooms, mix and cook for 3-4 minutes.

3.   Add garlic, cauliflower rice, pepper pieces, stock, cream, chives, parsley, salt and pepper, mix, cook for a couple of moments and take off heat.

4.   Divide shrimp on plates, include cauliflower blend the side, sprinkle bacon on top and serve.

Enjoy the recipe!

The nutritional facts: calories 245, fat 7, fiber 4, carbs 6, protein 20

THE STUFFED SALMON

Prep. time: 10 minutes

The cooking time: 20 minutes

The recipe servings: 2

Fixings:

2 salmon fillets, skinless and boneless 1 tablespoon of olive oil

5 ounces tiger shrimp, stripped, deveined and hacked 6 mushrooms, slashed

3 green onions, hacked 2 cups spinach, torn

¼ cup macadamia nuts, toasted and hacked Salt and dark pepper to the taste

Guidelines:

1.   Heat up a dish with half of the oil over medium high heat, include mushrooms, onions, salt and pepper, mix and cook for 4 minutes.

2.   Add macadamia nuts, spinach and shrimp, mix, cook for 3 minutes and take off heat.

3.   Make a cut the long way in every salmon filet, season with salt and pepper, separate spinach and shrimp blend into entry points and rub with the remainder of the olive oil.

4.   Place in the air fryer cooker's container and cook at 360 degrees F and cook for 10 minutes, flipping midway.

5.   Divide stuffed salmon on plates and serve.

Enjoy the recipe!

The nutritional facts: calories 290, fat 15, fiber 3, carbs 12, protein 31

MUSTARD SALMON

Prep. time: 10 minutes

The cooking time: 10 minutes

The recipe servings: 1

Fixings:

1 major salmon filet, boneless

Salt and dark pepper to the taste 2 tablespoons mustard

1 tablespoon coconut oil

1   tablespoon maple separate

Guidelines:

1.   In a bowl, blend maple separate with mustard, whisk well, season salmon with salt and pepper and brush salmon with this blend.

2.   Spray some cooking splash over fish, place in the air fryer cooker and cook at 370 Deg. Fahrenheit for about 10 minutes, flipping midway.

3.   Serve with a delicious side plate of mixed greens.

Enjoy the recipe!

The nutritional facts: calories 300, fat 7, fiber 14, carbs 16, protein 20

SEASONED JAMAICAN SALMON

Prep. time: 10 minutes

The cooking time: 10 minutes

The recipe servings: 4

Fixings:

2 teaspoons sriracha sauce 4 teaspoons sugar

2   scallions, cleaved

Salt and dark pepper to the taste 2 teaspoons olive oil

3   teaspoons apple juice vinegar 3 teaspoons avocado oil

4 medium salmon fillets, boneless 4 cups child arugula

2 cups cabbage, destroyed

1   and ½ teaspoon Jamaican snap flavoring

¼ cup pepitas, toasted 2 cups radish, julienned

Guidelines:

1. In a bowl, blend sriracha with sugar, whisk and move 2 teaspoons to another bowl.

2. Combine 2 teaspoons sriracha blend in with the avocado oil, olive oil, vinegar, salt and pepper and whisk well.

3. Sprinkle twitch flavoring over salmon, rub with sriracha and sugar blend and season with salt and pepper.

4. Transfer to the air fryer cooker and cook at 360 Deg. Fahrenheit for about 10 minutes, flipping once.

5. In a bowl, blend radishes in with cabbage, arugula, salt, pepper, sriracha and vinegar blend and hurl well.

6. Divide salmon and radish blend on plates, sprinkle pepitas and scallions on top and serve.

Enjoy the recipe!

The nutritional facts: calories 290, fat 6, fiber 12, carbs 17, protein 10

SWORDFISH AND MANGO SALSA

Prep. time: 10 minutes

The cooking time: 6 minutes

The recipe servings: 2

Fixings:

2   medium swordfish steaks

Salt and dark pepper to the taste 2 teaspoons avocado oil

1 tablespoon cilantro, slashed 1 mango, cleaved

1 avocado, hollowed, stripped and slashed A spot of cumin

A spot of onion powder A touch of garlic powder

1 orange, stripped and cut

½ tablespoon balsamic vinegar

Guidelines:

1.   Season fish steaks with salt, pepper, garlic powder, onion powder and cumin and rub with half of the oil, place in the air fryer cooker and cook at 360 Deg. Fahrenheit for about 6 minutes, flipping midway.

2.   Meanwhile, in a bowl, blend avocado in with mango, cilantro, balsamic vinegar, salt, pepper and the remainder of the oil and mix well.

3.   Divide fish on plates, top with mango salsa and present with orange cuts as an afterthought.

Enjoy the recipe!

The nutritional facts: calories 200, fat 7, fiber 2, carbs 14, protein 14

SALMON AND ORANGE MARMALADE

Prep. time: 10 minutes

The cooking time: 15 minutes

The recipe servings: 4

Fixings:

1 pound wild salmon, skinless, boneless and cubed 2 lemons, cut

¼ cup balsamic vinegar

¼ cup squeezed orange

1/3 cup orange preserves

A spot of salt and dark pepper

Guidelines:

1.   Heat up a pot with the vinegar over medium heat, include preserves and squeezed orange, mix, bring to a stew, cook for 1 moment and take off heat.

2.   Thread salmon shapes and lemon cuts on sticks, season with salt and dark pepper, brush them with half of the orange preserves blend, mastermind in the air fryer cooker's crate and cook at 360 Deg. Fahrenheit for about 3 minutes on each side.

3.   Brush sticks with the remainder of the vinegar blend, separate among plates and serve immediately with a side serving of mixed greens.

Enjoy the recipe!

The nutritional facts: calories 240, fat 9, fiber 12, carbs 14, protein 10

STEW SALMON

Prep. time: 10 minutes

The cooking time: 15 minutes

The recipe servings: 12

Fixings:

1   and ¼ cups coconut, destroyed 1 pound salmon, cubed

1/3 cup flour

A touch of salt and dark pepper 1 egg

1   tablespoons olive oil

¼ cup water

4 red chilies, hacked 3 garlic cloves, minced

¼ cup balsamic vinegar

½ cup HONNEY

Guidelines:

1.   In a bowl, blend flour in with a touch of salt and mix.

2.   In another bowl, blend egg in with dark pepper and whisk.

3.   Put coconut in a third bowl.

4.   Dip salmon shapes in flour, egg and coconut, put them in the air fryer cooker's container, cook at 370 Deg. Fahrenheit for about 8 minutes, shaking midway and partition among plates.

5.   Heat up a skillet with the water over medium high heat, include chilies, cloves, vinegar and HONNEY, mix well overall, heat to the point of boiling, stew for several minutes, shower over salmon and serve.

Enjoy the recipe!

The nutritional facts: calories 220, fat 12, fiber 2, carbs 14, protein 13

SALMON AND LEMON RELISH

Prep. time: 10 minutes

The cooking time: 30 minutes

The recipe servings: 2

Fixings:

2 salmon fillets, boneless

Salt and dark pepper to the taste 1 tablespoon of olive oil

For the relish:

1 tablespoon lemon juice 1 shallot, hacked

1 Meyer lemon, cut in wedges and afterward cut 2 tablespoons parsley, hacked

¼ cup olive oil

Guidelines:

1.   Season the salmon recipes with little salt and pepper, then, rub with 1 tablespoon oil, place in the air fryer cooker's bin and cook at 320 Deg. Fahrenheit for about 20 minutes, flipping the fish midway.

2.   Meanwhile, in a bowl, blend shallot in with the lemon squeeze, a spot of salt and dark pepper, mix and leave aside for 10 minutes.

3.   In a different bowl, blend marinated shallot with lemon cuts, salt, pepper, parsley and ¼ cup oil and whisk well.

4.   Divide salmon on plates, top with lemon relish and serve.

Enjoy the recipe!

The nutritional facts: calories 200, fat 3, fiber 3, carbs 23, protein 19

SALMON AND AVOCADO SAUCE

Prep. time: 10 minutes

The cooking time: 10 minutes

The recipe servings: 4

Fixings:

1 avocado, hollowed, stripped and cleaved 4 salmon fillets, boneless

¼ cup cilantro, cleaved 1/3 cup coconut milk

1 tablespoon lime juice

1 tablespoon lime pizzazz, ground 1 teaspoon onion powder

1 teaspoon garlic powder

Salt and dark pepper to the taste

Guidelines:

1.   Season salmon fillets with salt, dark pepper and lime pizzazz, rub well, put in the air fryer cooker, cook at 350 Deg. Fahrenheit for about 9 minutes, flipping once and partition among plates.

2.   In your food processor, blend avocado in with cilantro, garlic powder, onion powder, lime juice, salt, pepper and coconut milk, mix well, sprinkle over salmon and serve immediately.

Enjoy the recipe!

The nutritional facts: calories 260, fat 7, fiber 20, carbs 28, protein 18

CRUSTED SALMON

Prep. time: 10 minutes

The cooking time: 10 minutes

The recipe servings: 4

Fixings:

•   1 cup pistachios, hacked 4 salmon fillets

¼ cup lemon juice

1   tablespoons HONNEY

1 teaspoon dill, hacked

Salt and dark pepper to the taste 1 tablespoon mustard

Guidelines:

1.   In a bowl, blend pistachios in with mustard, HONNEY, lemon juice, salt, dark pepper and dill, whisk and spread over salmon.

2.   Put in the air fryer cooker and cook at 350 Deg. Fahrenheit for about 10 minutes.

3.   Divide among plates and present with a side serving of mixed greens.

Enjoy the recipe!

The nutritional facts: calories 300, fat 17, fiber 12, carbs 20, protein 22

STUFFED CALAMARI

Prep. time: 10 minutes

The cooking time: 25 minutes

The recipe servings: 4

Fixings:

•   big calamari, limbs isolated and slashed and tubes held 2 tablespoons parsley, hacked

4   ounces kale, cleaved 2 garlic cloves, minced

1   red ringer pepper, slashed 1 tablespoon of olive oil

2   ounces canned tomato puree 1 yellow onion, cleaved

Salt and dark pepper to the taste

Guidelines:

1.   Heat up a container with the oil over medium heat, include onion and garlic, mix and cook for 2 minutes.

2.   Add ringer pepper, tomato puree, calamari arms, kale, salt and pepper, mix, cook for 10 minutes and take off heat. mix and cook for 3 minutes.

3.   Stuff calamari tubes with this blend, secure with toothpicks, put in the air fryer cooker and cook at 360 Deg. Fahrenheit for about 20 minutes.

4.   Divide calamari on plates, sprinkle parsley all finished and serve.

Enjoy the recipe!

The nutritional facts: calories 322, fat 10, fiber 14, carbs 14, protein 22

SALMON AND CHIVES VINAIGRETTE

Prep. time: 10 minutes

The cooking time: 12 minutes

The recipe servings: 4

Fixings:

2 tablespoons dill, hacked 4 salmon fillets, boneless

2 tablespoons chives, hacked 1/3 cup maple syrup

1 tablespoon of olive oil

3 tablespoons balsamic vinegar Salt and dark pepper to the taste

Guidelines:

1.   Season fish with salt and pepper, rub with the oil, place in the air fryer cooker and cook at 350 Deg. Fahrenheit for about 8 minutes, flipping once.

2.   Heat up a little pot with the vinegar over medium heat, include maple syrup, chives and dill, mix and cook for 3 minutes.

3.   Divide fish on plates and present with chives vinaigrette on top.

Enjoy the recipe!

The nutritional facts: calories 270, fat 3, fiber 13, carbs 25, protein 10

ROASTED COD AND PROSCIUTTO

Prep. time: 10 minutes

The cooking time: 10 minutes

The recipe servings: 4

Fixings:

1 tablespoon parsley, cleaved 4 medium cod fillets

¼ cup margarine, liquefied

1   garlic cloves, minced

2   tablespoons lemon juice

3   tablespoons prosciutto, slashed 1 teaspoon Dijon mustard

1   shallot, slashed

Salt and dark pepper to the taste

Guidelines:

1.   In a bowl, blend mustard in with spread, garlic, parsley, shallot, lemon juice, prosciutto, salt and pepper and whisk well.

2.   Season fish with salt and pepper, spread prosciutto blend all finished, put in the air fryer cooker and cook at 390 Deg. Fahrenheit for about 10 minutes.

3.   Divide among plates and serve.

Enjoy the recipe!

The nutritional facts: calories 200, fat 4, fiber 7, carbs 12, protein 6

HALIBUT AND SUN DRIED TOMATOES MIX

Prep. time: 10 minutes

The cooking time: 10 minutes

The recipe servings: 2

Fixings:

2   medium halibut fillets 2 garlic cloves, minced 2 teaspoons olive oil

Salt and dark pepper to the taste 6 sun dried tomatoes, slashed

2 little red onions, cut 1 fennel bulb, cut

9 dark olives, hollowed and cut 4 rosemary springs, slashed

½ teaspoon red pepper drops, squashed

Guidelines:

1.　　　Season fish with salt, pepper, rub with garlic and oil and put in a heat confirmation dish that accommodates the air fryer cooker.

2.　　　Add onion cuts, sun dried tomatoes, fennel, olives, rosemary and sprinkle pepper chips, move to the air fryer cooker and cook at 380 Deg. Fahrenheit for about 10 minutes.

3.　　　Divide fish and veggies on plates and serve.

Enjoy the recipe!

The nutritional facts: calories 300, fat 12, fiber 9, carbs 18, protein 30

DARK COD AND PLUM SAUCE

Prep. time: 10 minutes The cooking time: 15 minutes The recipe servings: 2

Fixings:

1 egg white

½ cup red quinoa, effectively cooked 2 teaspoons entire wheat flour

4 teaspoons lemon juice

½ teaspoon smoked paprika 1 teaspoon olive oil

2 medium dark cod fillets, skinless and boneless 1 red plum, hollowed and cleaved

2 teaspoons crude HONNEY

¼ teaspoon dark peppercorns, squashed 2 teaspoons parsley

¼ cup water

Guidelines:

1.	In a bowl, blend 1 teaspoon lemon juice with egg white, flour and ¼ teaspoon paprika and whisk well.

2.	Put quinoa in a bowl and blend it in with 1/3 of egg white blend.

3.	Put the fish into the bowl with the rest of the egg white blend and hurl to cover.

4.	Dip fish in quinoa blend, coat well and leave aside for 10 minutes.

5.	Heat up a skillet with 1 teaspoon oil over medium heat, include peppercorns, HONNEY and plum, mix, bring to a stew and cook for 1 moment.

6.	Add the remainder of the lemon squeeze, the remainder of the paprika and the water, mix well and stew for 5 minutes.

7.	Add parsley, mix, take sauce off heat and leave aside until further notice.

8.	Put fish in the air fryer cooker and cook at 380 Deg. Fahrenheit for about 10 minutes

9.	Arrange fish on plates, sprinkle plum sauce on top and serve.

Enjoy the recipe!

The nutritional facts: calories 324, fat 14, fiber 22, carbs 27, protein 22

FISH AND COUSCOUS

Prep. time: 10 minutes

The cooking time: 15 minutes

The recipe servings: 4

Fixings:

2 red onions, slashed Cooking splash

2 little fennel bulbs, cored and cut

¼ cup almonds, toasted and cut Salt and dark pepper to the taste 2 and ½ pounds ocean bass, gutted

5 teaspoons fennel seeds

¾ cup entire wheat couscous, cooked

Guidelines:

1. Season fish with salt and pepper, shower with cooking splash, place in the air fryer cooker and cook at 350 Deg. Fahrenheit for about 10 minutes.

2. Meanwhile, shower a dish with some cooking oil and heat it up over medium heat.

3. Add fennel seeds to this skillet, mix and toast them for 1 moment.

4. Add onion, salt, pepper, fennel bulbs, almonds and couscous, mix, cook for 2-3 minutes and partition among plates.

5. Add fish by couscous blend and serve immediately.

Enjoy the recipe!

The nutritional facts: calories 354, fat 7, fiber 10, carbs 20, protein 30

CHINESE COD

Prep. time: 10 minutes

The cooking time: 10 minutes

The recipe servings: 2

Fixings:

2 medium cod fillets, boneless 1 teaspoon peanuts, squashed

2 teaspoons garlic powder

1 tablespoon light soy sauce

½ teaspoon ginger, ground

Guidelines:

1.   Put fish fillets in a heat confirmation dish that accommodates the air fryer cooker, include garlic powder, soy sauce and ginger, hurl well, put in the air fryer cooker and cook at 350 Deg. Fahrenheit for about 10 minutes.

2.   Divide fish on plates, sprinkle peanuts on top and serve.

Enjoy the recipe!

The nutritional facts: calories 254, fat 10, fiber 11, carbs 14, protein 23

COD WITH PEARL ONIONS

Prep. time: 10 minutes

The cooking time: 15 minutes

The recipe servings: 4

Fixings:

14 ounces pearl onions 2 medium cod fillets

1 tablespoon parsley, dried 1 teaspoon thyme, dried Black pepper to the taste

8 ounces mushrooms, cut

Guidelines:

1.   Put fish in a heat verification dish that accommodates the air fryer cooker, include onions, parsley, mushrooms, thyme and dark pepper, hurl well, put in the air fryer cooker and cook at 350 degrees F and cook for 15 minutes.

2.   Divide everything on plates and serve.

Enjoy the recipe!

The nutritional facts: calories 270, fat 14, fiber 8, carbs 14, protein 22

HAWAIIAN SALMON

Prep. time: 10 minutes

The cooking time: 10 minutes

The recipe servings: 2

Fixings:

20 ounces canned pineapple pieces and squeeze

½ teaspoon ginger, ground 2 teaspoons garlic powder 1 teaspoon onion powder

1   tablespoon balsamic vinegar

2   medium salmon fillets, boneless Salt and dark pepper to the taste

Guidelines:

1.   Season salmon with garlic powder, onion powder, salt and dark pepper, rub well, move to a heat evidence dish that accommodates the air fryer cooker, include ginger and pineapple pieces and hurl them actually tenderly.

2.   Drizzle the vinegar all finished, put in the air fryer cooker and cook at 350 Deg. Fahrenheit for about 10 minutes.

3.   Divide everything on plates and serve..

Enjoy the recipe!

The nutritional facts: calories 200, fat 8, fiber 12, carbs 17, protein 20

SALMON AND AVOCADO SALAD

Prep. time: 10 minutes

The cooking time: 20 minutes

The recipe servings: 4

Fixings:

2 medium salmon fillets

¼ cup dissolved spread

4 ounces mushrooms, cut

Ocean salt and dark pepper to the taste 12 cherry tomatoes, split

2 tablespoons olive oil

8 ounces lettuce leaves, torn

1 avocado, hollowed, stripped and cubed 1 jalapeno pepper, hacked

5 cilantro springs, hacked

2 tablespoons white wine vinegar 1 ounce feta cheddar, disintegrated

Guidelines:

1.   Place salmon on a lined preparing sheet, brush with 2 tablespoons dissolved spread, season with salt and pepper, cook for 15 minutes over medium heat and afterward keep warm.

2.   Meanwhile, heat up a container with the remainder of the spread over medium heat, include mushrooms, mix and cook for a couple of moments.

3.   Put tomatoes in a bowl, include salt, pepper and 1 tablespoon of olive oil and hurl to cover.

4.   In a serving of mixed greens bowl, blend salmon in with mushrooms, lettuce, avocado, tomatoes, jalapeno and cilantro.

5.   Add the remainder of the oil, vinegar, salt and pepper, sprinkle cheddar on top and serve.

Enjoy the recipe!

The nutritional facts: calories 235, fat 6, fiber 8, carbs 19, protein 5

SALMON AND GREEK YOGURT SAUCE

Prep. time: 10 minutes The cooking time: 20 minutes The recipe servings: 2

Ingredients:

2 medium salmon fillets

1   tablespoon basil, cleaved 6 lemon cuts

Ocean salt and dark pepper to the taste 1 cup Greek yogurt

2   teaspoons curry powder A spot of cayenne pepper 1 garlic clove, minced

½ teaspoon cilantro, cleaved

½ teaspoon mint, cleaved

directions:

1. Place every salmon filet on a material paper piece, make 3 parts in each, and stuff them with basil.

2. Season the recipe with salt and pepper and top each filet with 3 lemon cuts, overlay material, seal edges, present in the oven at 400 degrees F, and heat for 20 minutes.

3. Meanwhile, in a bowl, blend yogurt in with cayenne pepper, salt to the taste, garlic, curry, mint, and cilantro and whisk well.

4. Transfer fish to plates, shower the yogurt sauce you've quite recently arranged on top, and serve immediately!

Enjoy the recipe!

The nutritional facts: calories 242, fat 1, fiber 2, carbs 3, protein 3

EXTRAORDINARY SALMON

Prep. time: 10 minutes The cooking time: 25 minutes The recipe servings: 4

Fixings:

1 pound medium beets, cut 6 tablespoons olive oil

1 and ½ pounds salmon fillets, skinless and boneless Salt and pepper to the taste

1 tablespoon chives, slashed 1 tablespoon parsley, cleaved

1 tablespoon crisp tarragon, slashed 3 tablespoon shallots, hacked

1 tablespoon ground lemon pizzazz

¼ cup lemon juice

4 cups blended infant greens

Guidelines:

1.   In a bowl, blend beets in with ½ tablespoon oil and hurl to cover.

2.   Season them with salt and pepper, orchestrate them on a heating sheet, present in the oven at 450 degrees F, and prepare for 20 minutes.

3.   Take beets out of the oven, including salmon top, brush it with the rest of the oil and season with salt and pepper.

4.   In a bowl, blend chives in with parsley and tarragon and sprinkle one tablespoon of this blend over salmon.

5.   Introduce in the oven again and prepare for 15 minutes.

6.   Meanwhile, in an overflow with shallots with lemon strip, salt, pepper, and lemon juice and the remainder of the herbs blend and mix tenderly.

7.	Combine 2 tablespoons of shallots dressing with blended greens and hurl delicately.

8.	Take salmon out of the oven, mastermind on plates, include beets and greens the side, sprinkle the remainder of the shallot dressing on top, and serve immediately.

Enjoy the recipe!

The nutritional facts: calories 312, fat 2, fiber 2, carbs 2, protein 4

SPANISH SALMON

Prep. time: 10 minutes The cooking time: 15 minutes The recipe servings: 6

Fixings:

2	cups bread garnishes

3	red onions, cut into medium wedges

¾ cup green olives pitted

3 red ringer peppers, cut into medium wedges

½ teaspoon smoked paprika

Salt and dark pepper to the taste 5 tablespoons olive oil

6 medium salmon fillets, skinless and boneless 2 tablespoons parsley, slashed

Guidelines:

1.   In a heat confirmation dish that accommodates the air fryer cooker, blend bread garnishes with onion wedges, chime pepper ones, olives, salt, pepper, paprika, and 3 tablespoons olive oil, hurl well, place in the air fryer cooker and cook at 356 Deg. Fahrenheit for about 7 minutes.

2.   Rub salmon with the remainder of the oil, include over veggies and cook at 360 Deg. Fahrenheit for about 8 minutes.

3.   Divide fish and veggie blend on plates sprinkle parsley all finished and serve.

Enjoy the recipe!

The nutritional facts: calories 321, fat 8, fiber 14, carbs 27, protein 22

MARINATED SALMON

Prep. time: 1 hour The cooking time: 20 minutes The recipe servings: 6

Fixings:

1 entire salmon

1 tablespoon dill, hacked

1 tablespoon tarragon, hacked 1 tablespoon garlic, minced Juice from 2 lemons

1 lemon, cut

A touch of salt and dark pepper

Guidelines:

1.   In a vast fish, blend fish in with salt, pepper, and lemon juice, hurl well and keep in the cooler for 60 minutes.

2.   Stuff salmon with garlic and lemon cuts, place in the air fryer cooker's crate, and cook at 320 Deg. Fahrenheit for about 25 minutes.

3.   Divide among plates and present with a delicious coleslaw as an afterthought. Enjoy the recipe!

The nutritional facts: calories 300, fat 8, fiber 9, carbs 19, protein 27

DELIGHTFUL RED SNAPPER

Prep. time: 30 minutes

The cooking time: 15 minutes

The recipe servings: 4

Fixings:

1 major red snapper, cleaned and scored Salt and dark pepper to the taste

3 garlic cloves, minced 1 jalapeno, cleaved

¼ pound okra, cleaved 1 tablespoon margarine

2 tablespoons olive oil

1   red chime pepper, cleaved 2 tablespoons white wine

2   tablespoons parsley, cleaved

Guidelines:

1.   In a bowl, blend jalapeno, wine with garlic, mix well and rub snapper with this blend.

2.   Season fish with salt and pepper and leave it aside for 30 minutes.

3.   Meanwhile, heat up a container with 1 tablespoon margarine over medium heat, include ringer pepper and okra, mix and cook for 5 minutes.

4.   Stuff red snapper's gut with this blend, likewise include parsley and rub with the olive oil.

5.   Place in the preheated air fryer and cook at 400 Deg. Fahrenheit for about 15 minutes, flipping the fish midway.

6.   Divide among plates and serve. Enjoy the recipe!

The nutritional facts: calories 261, fat 7, fiber 18, carbs 28, protein 18

SNAPPER FILLETS AND VEGGIES

Prep. time: 10 minutes

The cooking time: 14 minutes

The recipe servings: 2

Fixings:

2 red snapper fillets, boneless 1 tablespoon of olive oil

½ cup red chime pepper, cleaved

½ cup green chime pepper, cleaved

½ cup leeks, cleaved

Salt and dark pepper to the taste 1 teaspoon tarragon, dried

A sprinkle of white wine

Guidelines:

1.   In a heat verification dish that accommodates the air fryer cooker, blend fish fillets with salt, pepper, oil, green ringer pepper, red chime pepper, leeks, tarragon and wine, hurl well everything, present in preheated air fryer at 350 degrees F and cook for 14 minutes, flipping fish fillets midway.

2.   Divide fish and veggies on plates and serve warm. Enjoy the recipe!

The nutritional facts: calories 300, fat 12, fiber 8, carbs 29, protein 12

AIR FRIED BRANZINO

Prep. time: 10 minutes

The cooking time: 10 minutes

The recipe servings: 4

Fixings:

Pizzazz from 1 lemon, ground Zest from 1 orange, ground Juice from ½ lemon

Juice from ½ orange

Salt and dark pepper to the taste

4 medium branzino fillets, boneless

½ cup parsley, slashed 2 tablespoons olive oil

A spot of red pepper drops, squashed

Guidelines:

1.	In an enormous bowl, blend fish fillets with lemon get-up-and-go, orange pizzazz, lemon juice, squeezed orange, salt, pepper, oil and pepper chips, hurl truly well, move fillets to your preheated air fryer at 350 degrees F and prepare for 10 minutes, flipping fillets once.

2.	Divide fish on plates, sprinkle with parsley and serve immediately. Enjoy the recipe!

The nutritional facts: calories 261, fat 8, fiber 12, carbs 21, protein 12

LEMON SOLE AND SWISS CHARD

Prep. time: 10 minutes

The cooking time: 14 minutes

The recipe servings: 4

Fixings:

1 teaspoon lemon get-up-and-go, ground 4 white bread cuts, quartered

¼ cup pecans, hacked

¼ cup parmesan, ground 4 tablespoons olive oil 4 sole fillets, boneless

Salt and dark pepper to the taste 4 tablespoons spread

¼ cup lemon juice

3 tablespoons tricks

2 garlic cloves, minced

2 packs Swiss chard, cleaved

Guidelines:

1.   In your food processor, blend bread in with pecans, cheddar and lemon pizzazz and heartbeat well.

2.   Add portion of the olive oil, beat truly well again and leave aside for the present.

3.   Heat up a container with the margarine over medium heat, include lemon juice, salt, pepper and tricks, mix well, include fish and hurl it.

4.   Transfer fish to your preheated air fryer's bushel, top with bread blend you've made toward the start and cook at 350 Deg. Fahrenheit for about 14 minutes.

5.   Meanwhile, heat another skillet with the remainder of the oil, include garlic, Swiss chard, salt and pepper, mix tenderly, cook for 2 minutes and take off heat.

6.   Divide fish on plates and present with sautéed chard as an afterthought. Enjoy the recipe!

The nutritional facts: calories 321, fat 7, fiber 18, carbs 27, protein 12

SALMON AND BLACKBERRY GLAZE

Prep. time: 33 minutes

The cooking time: 10 minutes

The recipe servings: 4

Fixings:

1 cup water

1 inch ginger piece, ground Juice from ½ lemon

12 ounces blackberries 1 tablespoon of olive oil

¼ cup sugar

4 medium salmon fillets, skinless Salt and dark pepper to the taste

Guidelines:

1.   Heat up a pot with the water over medium high heat, include ginger, lemon squeeze and blackberries, mix, heat to the point of boiling, cook for 4-5 minutes, take off heat, strain into a bowl, come back to dish and join with sugar.

2.   Stir this blend, bring to a stew over medium low heat and cook for 20 minutes.

3.   Leave blackberry sauce to chill off, brush salmon with it, season with salt and pepper, shower olive oil all finished and rub fish well.

4.   Place fish in your preheated air fryer at 350 degrees F and cook for 10 minutes, flipping fish fillets once.

5.   Divide among plates, sprinkle a portion of the rest of the blackberry sauce all finished and serve.

Enjoy the recipe!

The nutritional facts: calories 312, fat 4, fiber 9, carbs 19, protein 14

ORIENTAL FISH

Prep. time: 10 minutes

The cooking time: 12 minutes

The recipe servings: 4

Fixings:

2 pounds red snapper fillets, boneless Salt and dark pepper to the taste

2   garlic cloves, minced 1 yellow onion, hacked

1 tablespoon tamarind glue

1   tablespoon oriental sesame oil 1 tablespoon ginger, ground

2   tablespoons water

½ teaspoon cumin, ground 1 tablespoon lemon juice

3   tablespoons mint, hacked

Guidelines:

1.   In your food processor, blend garlic in with onion, salt, pepper, tamarind glue, sesame oil, ginger, water and cumin, beat well and rub fish with this blend.

2.   Place fish in your preheated air fryer at 320 degrees F and cook for 12 minutes, flipping fish midway.

3.   Divide fish on plates, shower lemon squeeze all finished, sprinkle mint and serve immediately.

Enjoy the recipe!

The nutritional facts: calories 241, fat 8, fiber 16, carbs 17, protein 12

SCRUMPTIOUS FRENCH COD

Prep. time: 10 minutes

The cooking time: 22 minutes

The recipe servings: 4

Fixings:

2 tablespoons olive oil

1   yellow onion, cleaved

½ cup white wine

2   garlic cloves, minced

14 ounces canned tomatoes, stewed 3 tablespoons parsley, cleaved

2 pounds cod, boneless

Salt and dark pepper to the taste 2 tablespoons margarine

Guidelines:

1.   Heat up a container with the oil over medium heat, include garlic and onion, mix and cook for 5 minutes.

2.   Add wine, mix and cook for brief more.

3.   Add tomatoes, mix, heat to the point of boiling, cook for 2 minutes, include parsley, mix again and take off heat.

4.   Pour this blend into a heat verification dish that accommodates the air fryer cooker, include fish, seasoned with salt and pepper then cook in your fryer at 350 Deg. Fahrenheit for about 14 minutes.

5.   Divide fish and tomatoes blend on plates and serve. Enjoy the recipe!

The nutritional facts: calories 231, fat 8, fiber 12, carbs 26, protein 14

EXTRAORDINARY CATFISH FILLETS

Prep. time: 10 minutes

The cooking time: 10 minutes

The recipe servings: 4

Fixings:

2 catfish fillets

½ teaspoon garlic, minced 2 ounces margarine

4 ounces Worcestershire sauce

½ teaspoon yank flavoring 1 teaspoon mustard

1 tablespoon balsamic vinegar

¾ cup catsup

Salt and dark pepper to the taste 1 tablespoon parsley, slashed

Guidelines:

1.	Heat up a skillet with the spread over medium heat, include Worcestershire sauce, garlic, yank flavoring, mustard, catsup, vinegar, salt and pepper, mix well, take off heat and include fish fillets.

2.	Toss well, leave aside for 10 minutes, channel fillets, move them to your preheated air fryer's container at 350 degrees F and cook for 8 minutes, flipping fillets midway.

3.	Divide among plates, sprinkle parsley on top and serve immediately. Enjoy the recipe!

The nutritional facts: calories 351, fat 8, fiber 16, carbs 27, protein 17

COCONUT TILAPIA

Prep. time: 10 minutes

The cooking time: 10 minutes

The recipe servings: 4

Fixings:

4 medium tilapia fillets

Salt and dark pepper to the taste

½ cup coconut milk

1 teaspoon ginger, ground

½ cup cilantro, slashed 2 garlic cloves, hacked

½ teaspoon garam masala Cooking shower

½ jalapeno, slashed

Guidelines:

1.   In your food processor, blend coconut milk with salt, pepper, cilantro, ginger, garlic, jalapeno and garam masala and beat truly well.

2.   Spray fish with cooking shower, spread coconut blend all finished, rub well, move to the air fryer cooker's bin and cook at 400 Deg. Fahrenheit for about 10 minutes.

3.   Divide among plates and serve hot. Enjoy the recipe!

The nutritional facts: calories 200, fat 5, fiber 6, carbs 25, protein 26

TILAPIA AND CHIVES SAUCE

Prep. time: 10 minutes

The cooking time: 8 minutes

The recipe servings: 4

Fixings:

4 medium tilapia fillets Cooking shower

Salt and dark pepper to the taste 2 teaspoons HONNEY

¼ cup Greek yogurt Juice from 1 lemon

2 tablespoons chives, cleaved

Guidelines:

1.   Season fish with salt and pepper, shower with cooking splash, place in preheated air fryer 350 degrees F and cook for 8 minutes, flipping midway.

2.   Meanwhile, in a bowl, blend yogurt in with HONNEY, salt, pepper, chives and lemon squeeze and whisk truly well.

3.   Divide air fryer fish on plates, shower yogurt sauce all finished and serve immediately.

Enjoy the recipe!

The nutritional facts: calories 261, fat 8, fiber 18, carbs 24, protein 21

HONNEY SEA BASS

Prep. time: 10 minutes

The cooking time: 10 minutes

The recipe servings: 2

Fixings:

2 ocean bass fillets

Get-up-and-go from ½ orange, ground Juice from ½ orange

A touch of salt and dark pepper 2 tablespoons mustard

2 teaspoons HONNEY

2 tablespoons olive oil

½ pound canned lentils, depleted A little pack of dill, cleaved 2 ounces watercress

A little pack of parsley, cleaved

Guidelines:

1.   Season fish fillets with salt and pepper, include orange get-up-and-go and squeeze, rub with 1 tablespoon oil, with HONNEY and mustard, rub, move to the air fryer cooker and cook at 350 Deg. Fahrenheit for about 10 minutes, flipping midway.

2.   Meanwhile, put lentils in a little pot, warm it up over medium heat, include the remainder of the oil, watercress, dill and parsley, mix well and gap among plates.

3.   Add fish fillets and serve immediately. Enjoy the recipe!

The nutritional facts: calories 212, fat 8, fiber 12, carbs 9, protein 17

DELICIOUS POLLOCK

Prep. time: 10 minutes

The cooking time: 15 minutes

The recipe servings: 6

Fixings:

½ cup sharp cream

4 Pollock fillets, boneless

¼ cup parmesan, ground

2 tablespoons spread, softened

Salt and dark pepper to the taste Cooking splash

Guidelines:

1.   In a bowl, blend sharp cream in with margarine, parmesan, salt and pepper and whisk well.

2.   Spray fish with cooking splash and season with salt and pepper.

3.   Spread sharp cream blend on one side of every Pollock filet, orchestrate them in your preheated air fryer at 320 degrees F and cook them for 15 minutes.

4.   Divide Pollock fillets on plates and present with a delicious side serving of mixed greens. Enjoy the recipe!

The nutritional facts: calories 300, fat 13, fiber 3, carbs 14, protein 44

AIR FRYER POULTRY RECIPES

CREAMY COCONUT CHICKEN

Prep. time: 2 hours The cooking time: 25 minutes The recipe servings: 4

Fixings:

- 4   big chicken legs

- 5   teaspoons turmeric powder 2 tablespoons ginger, ground

- Salt and dark pepper to the taste 4 tablespoons coconut cream

Guidelines:

1.   In a bowl, blend cream in with turmeric, ginger, salt and pepper, whisk, include chicken pieces, hurl them well and leave aside for 2 hours.

2.   Transfer chicken to your preheated air fryer, cook at 370 Deg. Fahrenheit for about 25 minutes, partition among plates and present with a side serving of mixed greens.

Enjoy the recipe!

The nutritional facts: calories 300, fat 4, fiber 12, carbs 22, protein 20

CHINESE CHICKEN WINGS

Prep. time: 2 hours The cooking time: 15 minutes The recipe servings: 6

Fixings:

16 chicken wings

2 tablespoons HONNEY

2 tablespoons soy sauce

Salt and dark pepper to the taste

¼ teaspoon white pepper 3 tablespoons lime juice

Guidelines:

1.   In a bowl, blend HONNEY in with soy sauce, salt, highly contrasting pepper and lime juice, whisk well, include chicken pieces, hurl to cover and keep in the ice chest for 2 hours.

2.   Transfer chicken to the air fryer cooker, cook at 370 Deg. Fahrenheit for about 6 minutes on each side, increment heat to 400 degrees F and cook for 3 minutes more.

3.   Serve hot.

Enjoy the recipe!

The nutritional facts: calories 372, fat 9, fiber 10, carbs 37, protein 24

HERBED CHICKEN

Prep. time: 30 minutes

The cooking time: 40 minutes

The recipe servings: 4

Fixings:

1 entire chicken

Salt and dark pepper to the taste 1 teaspoon garlic powder

1 teaspoon onion powder

½ teaspoon thyme, dried

1   teaspoon rosemary, dried 1 tablespoon lemon juice

2   tablespoons olive oil

Guidelines:

1.   Seasoned the chicken with pepper and salt, then rub with thyme, rosemary, garlic powder and onion powder, rub with lemon juice and olive oil and leave aside for 30 minutes.

2. Put chicken in the air fryer cooker and cook at 360 Deg. Fahrenheit for about 20 minutes on each side.

3. Leave chicken aside to chill off, cut and serve.

Enjoy the recipe!

The nutritional facts: calories 390, fat 10, fiber 5, carbs 22, protein 20

CHICKEN PARMESAN

Prep. time: 10 minutes

The cooking time: 15 minutes

The recipe servings: 4

Fixings:

2 cups panko bread morsels

¼ cup parmesan, ground

½ teaspoon garlic powder 2 cups white flour

1 egg, whisked

1 and ½ pounds chicken cutlets, skinless and boneless Salt and dark pepper to the taste

1 cup mozzarella, ground 2 cups tomato sauce

3 tablespoons basil, slashed

Guidelines:

1.   In a bowl, blend panko with parmesan and garlic powder and mix.

2.   Put flour in a subsequent bowl and the egg in a third.

3.   Season chicken with salt and pepper, plunge in flour, at that point in egg blend and in panko.

4.   Put chicken pieces in the air fryer cooker and cook them at 360 Deg. Fahrenheit for about 3 minutes on each side.

5.   Transfer chicken to a preparing dish that accommodates the air fryer cooker, include tomato sauce and top with mozzarella, present in the air fryer cooker and cook at 375 Deg. Fahrenheit for about 7 minutes.

6.   Divide among plates, sprinkle basil on top and serve.

Enjoy the recipe!

The nutritional facts: calories 304, fat 12, fiber 11, carbs 22, protein 15

MEXICAN CHICKEN

Prep. time: 10 minutes

The cooking time: 20 minutes

The recipe servings: 4

Fixings:

16 ounces salsa verde 1 tablespoon of olive oil

Salt and dark pepper to the taste

1 pound chicken bosom, boneless and skinless 1 and ½ cup Monterey Jack cheddar, ground

¼ cup cilantro, hacked 1 teaspoon garlic powder

Guidelines:

1.   Pour salsa verde in a preparing dish that accommodates the air fryer cooker, season chicken with salt, pepper, garlic powder, brush with olive oil and spot it over your salsa verde.

2.   Introduce in the air fryer cooker and cook at 380 Deg. Fahrenheit for about 20 minutes.

3.   Sprinkle cheddar on top and cook for 2 minutes more.

4.   Divide among plates and serve hot.

Enjoy the recipe!

The nutritional facts: calories 340, fat 18, fiber 14, carbs 32, protein 18

CREAMY CHICKEN, RICE AND PEAS

Prep. time: 10 minutes

The cooking time: 30 minutes

The recipe servings: 4

Fixings:

1 pound chicken bosoms, skinless, boneless and cut into quarters 1 cup white rice, effectively cooked

Salt and dark pepper to the taste 1 tablespoon of olive oil

3 garlic cloves, minced 1 yellow onion, cleaved

½ cup white wine

¼ cup substantial cream 1 cup chicken stock

¼ cup parsley, cleaved 2 cups peas, solidified

1 and ½ cups parmesan, ground

Guidelines:

1.   Season chicken bosoms with salt and pepper, sprinkle half of the oil over them, rub well, put in the air fryer cooker's bushel and cook them at 360 Deg. Fahrenheit for about 6 minutes.

2.   Heat up a container with the remainder of the oil over medium high heat, include garlic, onion, wine, stock, salt, pepper and overwhelming cream, mix, bring to a stew and cook for 9 minutes.

3.   Transfer chicken bosoms to a heat confirmation dish that accommodates the air fryer cooker, include peas, rice and cream blend over them, hurl, sprinkle parmesan and parsley all finished, place in the air fryer cooker and cook at 420 Deg. Fahrenheit for about 10 minutes.

4.   Divide among plates and serve hot.

Enjoy the recipe!

The nutritional facts: calories 313, fat 12, fiber 14, carbs 27, protein 44

ITALIAN CHICKEN

Prep. time: 10 minutes

The cooking time: 16 minutes

The recipe servings: 4

Fixings:

5 chicken thighs

1 tablespoon thyme, hacked

½ cup overwhelming cream

¾ cup chicken stock

1   teaspoon red pepper chips, squashed

¼ cup parmesan, ground

½ cup sun dried tomatoes

2   tablespoons basil, hacked Salt and dark pepper to the taste

Guidelines:

1.   Season the chicken with pepper and then salt, rub with half of the oil, place in your preheated air fryer at 350 degrees F and cook for 4 minutes.

2.   Meanwhile, heat up a container with the remainder of the oil over medium high heat, include thyme garlic, pepper drops, sun dried tomatoes, substantial cream, stock, parmesan, salt and pepper, mix, bring to a stew, take off heat and move to a dish that accommodates the air fryer cooker.

3.   Add chicken thighs on top, present in the air fryer cooker and cook at 320 Deg. Fahrenheit for about 12 minutes.

4.   Divide among plates and present with basil sprinkled on top.

Enjoy the recipe!

The nutritional facts: calories 272, fat 9, fiber 12, carbs 37, protein 23

HONNEY DUCK BREASTS

Prep. time: 10 minutes

The cooking time: 22 minutes

The recipe servings: 4

Fixings:

1 smoked duck bosom, divided 1 teaspoon HONNEY

1   teaspoon tomato glue 1 tablespoon mustard

½ teaspoon apple vinegar

Guidelines:

1.   In a bowl, blend HONNEY in with tomato glue, mustard and vinegar, whisk well, include duck bosom pieces, hurl to cover well, move to the air fryer cooker and cook at 370 Deg. Fahrenheit for about 15 minutes.

2.   Take duck bosom out of the fryer, add to HONNEY blend, hurl once more, come back to air fryer and cook at 370 Deg. Fahrenheit for about 6 minutes more.

3.   Divide among plates and present with a side serving of mixed greens.

Enjoy the recipe!

The nutritional facts: calories 274, fat 11, fiber 13, carbs 22, protein 13

CHINESE DUCK LEGS

Arrangement time:10 minutes

The cooking time: 36 minutes

The recipe servings: 2

2duck legs

2 dried chilies, hacked 1 tablespoon of olive oil

2 star anise

1 pack spring onions, slashed 4 ginger cuts

1 tablespoon shellfish sauce 1 tablespoon soy sauce

1 teaspoon sesame oil 14 ounces water

1 tablespoon rice wine

Guidelines:

1.   Heat up a dish with the oil over medium high heat, include bean stew, star anise, sesame oil, rice wine, ginger, clam sauce, soy sauce and water, mix and cook for 6 minutes.

2.   Add spring onions and duck legs, hurl to cover, move to a dish that accommodates the air fryer cooker, put in the air fryer cooker and cook at 370 Deg. Fahrenheit for about 30 minutes.

3.   Divide among plates and serve.

Enjoy the recipe!

The nutritional facts: calories 300, fat 12, fiber 12, carbs 26, protein 18

CHINESE STUFFED CHICKEN

Prep. time: 10 minutes

The cooking time: 35 minutes

The recipe servings: 8

Fixings:

1 entire chicken

10 wolfberries

2 red chilies, hacked 4 ginger cuts

1 cubed yam

1 teaspoon of soy sauce

Add Salt and the grinded white pepper to the taste

3 teaspoons sesame oil

Guidelines:

1.   Season the chicken with salt, pepper, rub with soy sauce and sesame oil and stuff with wolfberries, yam 3D squares, chilies and ginger.

2.   Place in the air fryer cooker, cook at 400 Deg. Fahrenheit for about 20 minutes and afterward at 360 Deg. Fahrenheit for about 15 minutes.

3.   Carve chicken, separate among plates and serve.

Enjoy the recipe!

The nutritional facts: calories 320, fat 12, fiber 17, carbs 22, protein 12

SIMPLE CHICKEN THIGHS AND BABY POTATOES

Prep. time: 10 minutes

The cooking time: 30 minutes

The recipe servings: 4

Fixings:

2 tablespoons olive oil

1   pound child potatoes, divided 2 teaspoons oregano, dried

2   teaspoons rosemary, dried

½ teaspoon sweet paprika

Salt and dark pepper to the taste 2 garlic cloves, minced

1   red onion, hacked

2   teaspoons thyme, hacked

Guidelines:

1.   In a bowl, blend chicken thighs in with potatoes, salt, pepper, thyme, paprika, onion, rosemary, garlic, oregano and oil.

2.   Toss to cover, spread everything in a heat verification dish that accommodates the air fryer cooker and cook at 400 Deg. Fahrenheit for about 30 minutes, shaking midway.

3.   Divide among plates and serve.

Enjoy the recipe!

The nutritional facts: calories 364, fat 14, fiber 13, carbs 21, protein 34

CHICKEN AND CAPERS

Prep. time: 10 minutes

The cooking time: 20 minutes

The recipe servings: 2

Fixings:

3 tablespoons tricks

3   garlic cloves, minced

3   tablespoons spread, softened

Salt and dark pepper to the taste

½ cup chicken stock 1 lemon, cut

4   green onions, hacked

Guidelines:

1.   Brush chicken with spread, sprinkle salt and pepper to the taste, place them in a heating dish that accommodates the air fryer cooker.

2.   Also include tricks, garlic, chicken stock and lemon cuts, hurl to cover, present in the air fryer cooker and cook at 370 Deg. Fahrenheit for about 20 minutes, shaking midway.

3.   Sprinkle green onions, separate among plates and serve.

Enjoy the recipe!

The nutritional facts: calories 200, fat 9, fiber 10, carbs 17, protein 7

CHICKEN AND CREAMY MUSHROOMS

Prep. time: 10 minutes

The cooking time: 30 minutes

The recipe servings: 8

Fixings:

Salt and dark pepper to the taste

8 ounces cremini mushrooms, split 3 garlic cloves, minced

3 tablespoons spread, softened 1 cup chicken stock

¼ cup overwhelming cream

½ teaspoon basil, dried

½ teaspoon thyme, dried

½ teaspoon oregano, dried 1 tablespoon mustard

¼ cup parmesan, ground

Guidelines:

1.   Rub chicken pieces with 2 tablespoons spread, season with salt and pepper, put in the air fryer cooker's container, cook at 370 Deg. Fahrenheit for about 5 minutes and leave aside in a bowl for the time being.

2.   Meanwhile, heat up a container with the remainder of the margarine over medium high heat, include mushrooms and garlic, mix and cook for 5 minutes.

3.   Add salt, pepper, stock, oregano, thyme and basil, mix well and move to a heat verification dish that accommodates the air fryer cooker.

4.   Add chicken, hurl everything, put in the air fryer cooker and cook at 370 Deg. Fahrenheit for about 20 minutes.

5.   Add mustard, parmesan and substantial cream, hurl everything once more, cook for 5 minutes more, partition among plates and serve.

Enjoy the recipe!

The nutritional facts: calories 340, fat 10, fiber 13, carbs 22, protein 12

DODGE AND PLUM SAUCE

Prep. time: 10 minutes The cooking time: 32 minutes The recipe servings: 2

Fixings:

2 duck bosoms

1 tablespoon margarine, liquefied 1 star anise

1 tablespoon of olive oil 1 shallot, slashed

9 ounces red plumps, stoned, cut into little wedges 2 tablespoons sugar

2 tablespoons red wine 1 cup hamburger stock

Guidelines:

1.   Heat up the skillet together with the olive oil over medium heat, include shallot, mix and cook for 5 minutes,

2.   Add sugar and plums, mix and cook until sugar breaks down.

3.   Add stock and wine, mix, cook for 15 minutes, take off heat and save warm for the time being.

4.	Score duck bosoms, season with salt and pepper, rub with softened margarine, move to a heat evidence dish that accommodates the air fryer cooker, include star anise and plum sauce, present in the air fryer cooker and cook at 360 Deg. Fahrenheit for about 12 minutes.

5.	Divide everything on plates and serve.

Enjoy the recipe!

The nutritional facts: calories 400, fat 25, fiber 12, carbs 29, protein 44

AIR FRIED JAPANESE DUCK BREASTS

Prep. time: 10 minutes

The cooking time: 20 minutes

The recipe servings: 6

Fixings:

6 duck bosoms, boneless 4 tablespoons soy sauce

1 and ½ teaspoon five zest powder 2 tablespoons HONNEY

Salt and dark pepper to the taste 20 ounces chicken stock

4 ginger cuts

4 tablespoons of hoisin sauce & 1 teaspoon of sesame oil

Guidelines:

1.   In a bowl, blend five zest powder with soy sauce, salt, pepper and HONNEY, whisk, include duck bosoms, hurl to cover and leave aside for the time being.

2.   Heat up a container with the stock over medium high heat, hoisin sauce, ginger and sesame oil, mix well, cook for 2-3 minutes more, take off heat and leave aside.

3.   Put duck bosoms in the air fryer cooker and cook them at 400 Deg. Fahrenheit for about 15 minutes.

4.   Divide among plates, sprinkle hoisin and ginger sauce all over them and serve.

Enjoy the recipe!

The nutritional facts: calories 336, fat 12, fiber 1, carbs 25, protein 33

SIMPLE DUCK BREASTS

Prep. time: 10 minutes

The cooking time: 40 minutes

The recipe servings: 6

Fixings:

6 duck bosoms, divided

Salt and dark pepper to the taste 3 tablespoons flour

6 tablespoons margarine, liquefied 2 cups chicken stock

½ cup white wine

¼ cup parsley, slashed

2 cups mushrooms, slashed

Guidelines:

1.   Season duck bosoms with salt and pepper, place them in a bowl, include softened margarine, hurl and move to another bowl.

2.   Combine softened margarine with flour, wine, salt, pepper and chicken stock and mix well.

3.   Arrange duck bosoms in a heating dish that accommodates the air fryer cooker, pour the sauce over them, include parsley and mushrooms, present in the air fryer cooker and cook at 350 Deg. Fahrenheit for about 40 minutes.

4.   Divide among plates and serve.

Enjoy the recipe!

The nutritional facts: calories 320, fat 28, fiber 12, carbs 12, protein 42

DUCK BREASTS WITH ENDIVES

Prep. time: 10 minutes

The cooking time: 25 minutes

The recipe servings: 4

Fixings:

2 duck bosoms

Salt and dark pepper to the taste 1 tablespoon sugar

1   tablespoon of olive oil 6 endives, julienned

2   tablespoons cranberries 8 ounces white wine

1 tablespoons garlic, minced 2 tablespoons substantial cream

Guidelines:

1.   Score duck bosoms and season them with salt and pepper, put in preheated air fryer and cook at 350 deg. F for about 20 minutes, flipping them midway.

2.   Meanwhile, heat up a dish with the oil over medium heat, include sugar and endives, mix and cook for 2 minutes.

3.   Add salt, pepper, wine, garlic, cream and cranberries, mix and cook for 3 minutes.

4. Divide duck bosoms on plates, shower the endives sauce all finished and serve.

Enjoy the recipe!

The nutritional facts: calories 400, fat 12, fiber 32, carbs 29, protein 28

CHICKEN BREASTS AND TOMATOES SAUCE

Prep. time: 10 minutes

The cooking time: 20 minutes

The recipe servings: 4

Fixings:

1 red onion, slashed

4 chicken bosoms, skinless and boneless

¼ cup balsamic vinegar

14 ounces canned tomatoes, slashed Salt and dark pepper to the taste

¼ cup parmesan, ground

¼ teaspoon garlic powder Cooking shower

Guidelines:

1.   Spray a heating dish that accommodates the air fryer cooker with cooking oil, include chicken, season with salt, pepper, balsamic vinegar, garlic powder, tomatoes and cheddar, hurl, present in the air fryer cooker and cook at 400 Deg. Fahrenheit for about 20 minutes.

2.   Divide among plates and serve hot.

Enjoy the recipe!

The nutritional facts: calories 250, fat 12, fiber 12, carbs 19, protein 28

CHICKEN AND ASPARAGUS

Prep. time: 10 minutes

The cooking time: 20 minutes

The recipe servings: 4

Fixings:

8 chicken wings, divided 8 asparagus lances

Salt and dark pepper to the taste 1 tablespoon rosemary, slashed 1 teaspoon cumin, ground

Guidelines:

1.	Pat dry chicken wings, season with salt, pepper, cumin and rosemary, put them in the air fryer cooker's container and cook at 360 Deg. Fahrenheit for about 20 minutes.

2.	Meanwhile, heat up a skillet over medium heat, include asparagus, add water to cover, steam for a couple of moments, move to a bowl loaded up with ice water, deplete and organize on plates.

3.	Add chicken wings as an afterthought and serve.

Enjoy the recipe!

The nutritional facts: calories 270, fat 8, fiber 12, carbs 24, protein 22

CHICKEN THIGHS AND APPLE MIX

Prep. time: 12 hours The cooking time: 30 minutes The recipe servings: 4

Fixings:

8 chicken thighs, bone in and skin on Salt and dark pepper to the taste

1 tablespoon apple juice vinegar 3 tablespoons onion, slashed

1 tablespoon ginger, ground

½ teaspoon thyme, dried

3 apples, cored and cut into quarters

¾ cup squeezed apple

½ cup maple syrup

Guidelines:

1.   In a bowl, blend chicken in with salt, pepper, vinegar, onion, ginger, thyme, squeezed apple and maple syrup, hurl well, spread and keep in the refrigerator for 12 hours.

2.   Transfer this entire blend to a heating dish that accommodates the air fryer cooker, include apple pieces, place in the air fryer cooker and cook at 350 Deg. Fahrenheit for about 30 minutes.

3.   Divide among plates and serve warm.

Enjoy the recipe!

The nutritional facts: calories 314, fat 8, fiber 11, carbs 34, protein 22

CHICKEN AND PARSLEY SAUCE

Prep. time: 10 minutes

The cooking time: 25 minutes

The recipe servings: 6

Fixings:

1 cup parsley, slashed

1 teaspoon oregano, dried

½ cup olive oil

¼ cup red wine 4 garlic cloves A spot of salt

A sprinkle of maple syrup 12 chicken thighs

Guidelines:

1.   In your food processor, blend parsley in with oregano, garlic, salt, oil, wine and maple syrup and heartbeat truly well.

2.   In a bowl, blend chicken in with parsley sauce, hurl well and keep in the ice chest for 30 minutes.

3.   Drain chicken, move to the air fryer cooker's crate and cook at 380 Deg. Fahrenheit for about 25 minutes, flipping chicken once.

4.   Divide chicken on plates, shower parsley sauce all finished and serve.

Enjoy the recipe!

The nutritional facts: calories 354, fat 10, fiber 12, carbs 22, protein 17

CHICKEN AND LENTILS CASSEROLE

Prep. time: 10 minutes

The cooking time: 60 minutes

The recipe servings: 8

Fixings:

1   and ½ cups green lentils 3 cups chicken stock

2   pound chicken bosoms, skinless, boneless and hacked Salt and cayenne pepper to the taste

3   teaspoons cumin, ground Cooking splash

5 garlic cloves, minced 1 yellow onion, hacked

2 red chime peppers, slashed

14 ounces canned tomatoes, hacked 2 cups corn

2 cups cheddar, destroyed

2 tablespoons jalapeno pepper, hacked 1 tablespoon garlic powder

1 cup cilantro, hacked

Guidelines:

1.   Put the stock in a pot, include some salt, include lentils, mix, heat to the point of boiling over medium heat, spread and stew for 35 minutes.

2.   Meanwhile, shower chicken pieces with some cooking splash, season with salt, cayenne pepper and 1 teaspoon cumin, put them in the air fryer cooker's container and cook them at 370 degrees for 6 minutes, flipping midway.

3.   Transfer chicken to a heat verification dish that accommodates the air fryer cooker, include ringer peppers, garlic, tomatoes, onion, salt, cayenne and 1 teaspoon cumin.

4.   Drain lentils and add them to the chicken blend too.

5.   Add jalapeno pepper, garlic powder, the remainder of the cumin, corn, half of the cheddar and half of the cilantro, present in the air fryer cooker and cook at 320 Deg. Fahrenheit for about 25 minutes.

Enjoy the recipe!

6.   Sprinkle the remainder of the cheddar and the rest of the cilantro, isolate chicken meal on plates and serve.

The nutritional facts: calories 344, fat 11, fiber 12, carbs 22, protein 33

FALL AIR FRIED CHICKEN MIX

Prep. time: 10 minutes

The cooking time: 20 minutes

The recipe servings: 8

Fixings:

3 pounds chicken bosoms, skinless and boneless 1 yellow onion, hacked

1 garlic clove, minced

Salt and dark pepper to the taste 10 white mushrooms, split

1 tablespoon of olive oil

1   red chime pepper, cleaved 1 green ringer pepper

2   tablespoons mozzarella cheddar, destroyed Cooking splash

Guidelines:

1.   Seasoned the chicken with pepper and salt, rub with garlic, splash with cooking shower, place in your preheated air fryer and cook at 390 Deg. Fahrenheit for about 12 minutes.

2.   Meanwhile, heat up a container with the oil over medium heat, include onion, mix and sauté for 2 minutes.

3.   Add mushrooms, garlic and chime peppers, mix and cook for 8 minutes.

4.   Divide chicken on plates, include mushroom blend the side, sprinkle cheddar while chicken is as yet hot and serve immediately.

Enjoy the recipe!

The nutritional facts: calories 305, fat 12, fiber 11, carbs 26, protein 32

CHICKEN SALAD

Prep. time: 10 minutes

The cooking time: 10 minutes

The recipe servings: 4

Fixings:

1 pound chicken bosom, boneless, skinless and split Cooking shower

Salt and dark pepper to the taste

½ cup feta cheddar, cubed 2 tablespoons lemon juice

1 and ½ teaspoons mustard 1 tablespoon of olive oil

1 and ½ teaspoons red wine vinegar

½ teaspoon anchovies, minced

¾ teaspoon garlic, minced 1 tablespoon water

8 cups lettuce leaves, cut into strips 4 tablespoons parmesan, ground

Guidelines:

1.   Spray chicken bosoms with cooking oil, season with salt and pepper, present in the air fryer cooker's crate and cook at 370 Deg. Fahrenheit for about 10 minutes, flipping midway.

2.   Transfer chicken brutes to a cutting load up, shred utilizing 2 forks, put in a serving of mixed greens bowl and blend in with lettuce leaves.

3.   In your blender, blend feta cheddar with lemon juice, olive oil, mustard, vinegar, garlic, anchovies, water and half of the parmesan and mix quite well.

4.   Add this over chicken blend, hurl, sprinkle the remainder of the parmesan and serve.

Enjoy the recipe!

The nutritional facts: calories 312, fat 6, fiber 16, carbs 22, protein 26

CHICKEN AND GREEN ONIONS SAUCE

Prep. time: 10 minutes

The cooking time: 16 minutes

The recipe servings: 4

Fixings:

10 green onions, generally hacked 1 inch piece ginger root, cleaved 4 garlic cloves, minced

1 teaspoon Chinese five flavor 10 chicken drumsticks

1 cup coconut milk

Salt and dark pepper to the taste 1 teaspoon spread, dissolved

¼ cup cilantro, hacked 1 tablespoon lime juice

Guidelines:

1.   In your food processor, blend green onions in with ginger, garlic, soy sauce, fish sauce, five zest, salt, pepper, margarine and coconut milk and heartbeat well.

2.   In a bowl, blend chicken in with green onions blend, hurl well, move everything to a skillet that accommodates the air fryer cooker and cook at 370 Deg. Fahrenheit for about 16 minutes, shaking the fryer once.

3.   Divide among plates, sprinkle cilantro on top, shower lime squeeze and present with a side serving of mixed greens.

Enjoy the recipe!

The nutritional facts: calories 321, fat 12, fiber 12, carbs 22, protein 20

CHICKEN CACCIATORE

Prep. time: 10 minutes

The cooking time: 20 minutes

The recipe servings: 4

Fixings:

Salt and dark pepper to the taste 8 chicken drumsticks, bone-in

1 narrows leaf

1 teaspoon garlic powder 1 yellow onion, cleaved

28 ounces canned tomatoes and juice, squashed 1 teaspoon oregano, dried

½ cup dark olives, hollowed and cut

Guidelines:

1.   In a heat verification dish that accommodates the air fryer cooker, blend chicken in with salt, pepper, garlic powder, narrows leaf, onion, tomatoes and juice, oregano and olives, hurl, present in your preheated air fryer and cook at 365 Deg. Fahrenheit for about 20 minutes.

2.   Divide among plates and serve. Enjoy the recipe!

The nutritional facts: calories 300, fat 12, fiber 8, carbs 20, protein 24

CHICKEN WINGS AND MINT SAUCE

Prep. time: 10 minutes

The cooking time: 16 minutes

The recipe servings: 4

Fixings:

18 chicken wings, divided

1 tablespoon turmeric powder 1 tablespoon cumin, ground

1 tablespoon ginger, ground

1 tablespoon coriander, ground 1 tablespoon sweet paprika

Salt and dark pepper to the taste 2 tablespoons olive oil

For the mint sauce:

Juice from ½ lime 1 cup mint leaves

1 little ginger piece, cleaved

¾ cup cilantro

1 tablespoon of olive oil 1 tablespoon water

Salt and dark pepper to the taste 1 Serrano pepper, cleaved

Guidelines:

1.   In a bowl, blend 1 tablespoon ginger with cumin, coriander, paprika, turmeric, salt, pepper, cayenne and 2 tablespoons oil and mix well.

2.   Add chicken wings pieces to this blend, hurl to cover well and keep in the refrigerator for 10 minutes.

3.   Transfer chicken to the air fryer cooker's bin and cook at 370 Deg. Fahrenheit for about 16 minutes, flipping them midway.

4.   In your blender, blend mint in with cilantro, 1 little ginger pieces, juice from ½ lime, 1 tablespoon of olive oil, salt, pepper, water and Serrano pepper and mix quite well.

5.   Divide chicken wings on plates, sprinkle mint sauce all finished and serve.

Enjoy the recipe!

The nutritional facts: calories 300, fat 15, fiber 11, carbs 27, protein 16

LEMON CHICKEN

Prep. time: 10 minutes

The cooking time: 30 minutes

The recipe servings: 6

Fixings:

1 entire chicken, cut into medium pieces 1 tablespoon of olive oil

Salt and dark pepper to the taste Juice from 2 lemons

Pizzazz from 2 lemons, ground

Guidelines:

1.   Season chicken with salt, pepper, rub with oil and lemon get-up-and-go, shower lemon juice, put in the air fryer cooker and cook at 350 Deg. Fahrenheit for about 30 minutes, flipping chicken pieces midway.

2.   Divide among plates and present with a side serving of mixed greens.

Enjoy the recipe!

The nutritional facts: calories 334, fat 24, fiber 12, carbs 26, protein 20

CHICKEN AND SIMPLE COCONUT SAUCE

Prep. time: 10 minutes

The cooking time: 12 minutes

The recipe servings: 6

Fixings:

1 tablespoon of olive oil

3 and ½ pounds chicken bosoms 1 cup chicken stock

1   and ¼ cups yellow onion, cleaved 1 tablespoon lime juice

¼ cup coconut milk

2   teaspoons sweet paprika

1   teaspoon red pepper pieces

2   tablespoons green onions, cleaved Salt and dark pepper to the taste

Guidelines:

1.   Heat up a container that accommodates the air fryer cooker with the oil over medium high heat, include onions, mix and cook for 4 minutes.

2.   Add stock, coconut milk, pepper chips, paprika, lime squeeze, salt and pepper and mix well.

3.   Add chicken to the dish, include increasingly salt and pepper, hurl, present in the air fryer cooker and cook at 360 Deg. Fahrenheit for about 12 minutes.

4.   Divide chicken and sauce on plates and serve.

Enjoy the recipe!

The nutritional facts: calories 320, fat 13, fiber 13, carbs 32, protein 23

CHICKEN AND BLACK OLIVES SAUCE

Prep. time: 10 minutes

The cooking time: 8 minutes

The recipe servings: 2

Fixings:

1 chicken bosom cut into 4 pieces 2 tablespoons olive oil

3 garlic cloves, minced

For the sauce:

1 cup dark olives, pitted

Salt and dark pepper to the taste 2 tablespoons olive oil

¼ cup parsley, cleaved

1 tablespoons lemon juice

Guidelines:

1.	In your food processor, blend olives in with salt, pepper, 2 tablespoons olive oil, lemon juice and parsley, mix well overall and move to a bowl.

2.	Season the chicken sauce1with salt and pepper, rub with the oil and garlic, place in your preheated air fryer and cook at 370 deg. F for about 8 minutes.

3.	Divide chicken on plates, top with olives sauce and serve.

Enjoy the recipe!

The nutritional facts: calories 270, fat 12, fiber 12, carbs 23, protein 22

CHEDDAR CRUSTED CHICKEN

Prep. time: 10 minutes

The cooking time: 15 minutes

The recipe servings: 4

Fixings:

4 bacon cuts, cooked and disintegrated

4 chicken bosoms, skinless and boneless 1 tablespoon water

½ cup avocado oil 1 egg, whisked

Salt and dark pepper to the taste 1 cup asiago cheddar, destroyed

¼ teaspoon garlic powder

1 cup parmesan cheddar, ground

Guidelines:

1.   In a bowl, blend parmesan in with garlic, salt and pepper and mix.

2.   In another bowl, blend egg in with water and whisk well.

3.   Season chicken with salt and pepper and dunk every piece into egg and afterward into cheddar blend.

4.   Add chicken to the air fryer cooker and cook at 320 Deg. Fahrenheit for about 15 minutes.

5.   Divide chicken on plates, sprinkle bacon and asiago cheddar on top and serve.

Enjoy the recipe!

The nutritional facts: calories 400, fat 22, fiber 12, carbs 32, protein 47

PEPPERONI CHICKEN

Prep. time: 10 minutes

The cooking time: 22 minutes

The recipe servings: 6

Fixings:

14 ounces tomato glue 1 tablespoon of olive oil

4 medium chicken bosoms, skinless and boneless Salt and dark pepper to the taste

1   teaspoon oregano, dried 6 ounces mozzarella, cut 1 teaspoon garlic powder

2   ounces pepperoni, cut

Guidelines:

1.   In a bowl, blend chicken in with salt, pepper, garlic powder and oregano and hurl.

2.   Put chicken in the air fryer cooker, cook at 350 Deg. Fahrenheit for about 6 minutes and move to a skillet that accommodates the air fryer cooker.

3.   Add mozzarella cuts on top, spread tomato glue, top with pepperoni cuts, present in the air fryer cooker and cook at 350 Deg. Fahrenheit for about 15 minutes more.

4.   Divide among plates and serve.

Enjoy the recipe!

The nutritional facts: calories 320, fat 10, fiber 16, carbs 23, protein 27

CHICKEN AND CREAMY VEGGIE MIX

Prep. time: 10 minutes

The cooking time: 30 minutes

The recipe servings: 6

Fixings:

2 cups whipping cream

40 ounces chicken pieces, boneless and skinless 3 tablespoons margarine, dissolved

½ cup yellow onion, slashed

¾ cup red peppers, slashed 29 ounces chicken stock

Salt and dark pepper to the taste 1 cove leaf

8 ounces mushrooms, slashed 17 ounces asparagus, cut 3 teaspoons thyme, hacked

Guidelines:

1.   Heat up a skillet with the spread over medium heat, include onion and peppers, mix and cook for 3 minutes.

2.		Add stock, cove leaf, salt and pepper, heat to the point of boiling and stew for 10 minutes.

3.		Add asparagus, mushrooms, chicken, cream, thyme, salt and pepper to the taste, mix, present in the air fryer cooker and cook at 360 Deg. Fahrenheit for about 15 minutes.

4.		Divide chicken and veggie blend on plates and serve.

Enjoy the recipe!

The nutritional facts: calories 360, fat 27, fiber 13, carbs 24, protein 47

TURKEY QUARTERS AND VEGGIES

Prep. time: 10 minutes

The cooking time: 34 minutes

The recipe servings: 4

Fixings:

1 yellow onion, hacked 1 carrot, slashed

3 garlic cloves, minced 2 pounds turkey quarters 1 celery stalk, hacked 1 cup chicken stock

2 tablespoons olive oil 2 sound leaves

½ teaspoon rosemary, dried

½ teaspoon wise, dried

½ teaspoon thyme, dried

Salt and dark pepper to the taste

Guidelines:

1.   Rub turkey quarters with salt, pepper, half of the oil, thyme, sage, rosemary and thyme, put in the air fryer cooker and cook at 360 Deg. Fahrenheit for about 20 minutes.

2.   In a dish that accommodates the air fryer cooker, blend onion in with carrot, garlic, celery, the remainder of the oil, stock, cove leaves, salt and pepper and hurl.

3.   Add turkey, present everything in the air fryer cooker and cook at 360 Deg. Fahrenheit for about 14 minutes more.

4.   Divide everything on plates and serve.

Enjoy the recipe!

The nutritional facts: calories 362, fat 12, fiber 16, carbs 22, protein 17

CHICKEN AND GARLIC SAUCE

Prep. time: 10 minutes

The cooking time: 34 minutes

The recipe servings: 4

Fixings:

1 tablespoon margarine, dissolved

4 chicken bosoms, skin on and bone-in 1 tablespoon of olive oil

Salt and dark pepper to the taste

40 garlic cloves, stripped and slashed 2 thyme springs

¼ cup chicken stock

2 tablespoons parsley, slashed

¼ cup dry white wine

Guidelines:

1.   Season chicken bosoms with salt and pepper, rub with the oil, place in the air fryer cooker, cook at 360 Deg. Fahrenheit for about 4 minutes on each side and move to a heat confirmation dish that accommodates the air fryer cooker.

2.   Add softened spread, garlic, thyme, stock, wine and parsley, hurl, present in the air fryer cooker and cook at 350 Deg. Fahrenheit for about 15 minutes more.

3.   Divide everything on plates and serve. Enjoy the recipe!

The nutritional facts: calories 227, fat 9, fiber 13, carbs 22, protein 12

TURKEY, PEAS, AND MUSHROOMS CASSEROLE

Prep. time: 10 minutes

The cooking time: 20 minutes

The recipe servings: 4

Fixings:

2 pounds turkey bosoms, skinless, boneless Salt and dark pepper to the taste

1 yellow onion, slashed 1 celery stalk, hacked

½ cup peas

1 cup chicken stock

1   cup cream of mushrooms soup 1 cup bread blocks

Guidelines:

1.   In a skillet that accommodates the air fryer cooker, blend turkey in with salt, pepper, onion, celery, peas and stock, present in the air fryer cooker and cook at 360 Deg. Fahrenheit for about 15 minutes.

2.   Add bread blocks and cream of mushroom soup, mix hurl and cook at 360 Deg. Fahrenheit for about 5 minutes more.

3.   Divide among plates and serve hot. Enjoy the recipe!

The nutritional facts: calories 271, fat 9, fiber 9, carbs 16, protein 7

SCRUMPTIOUS CHICKEN THIGHS

Prep. time: 10 minutes

The cooking time: 20 minutes

The recipe servings: 6

Fixings:

2 ½ pounds chicken thighs Salt and dark pepper to the taste 5 green onions, slashed

2 tablespoons sesame oil 1 tablespoon sherry wine

½ teaspoon white vinegar 1 tablespoon soy sauce

¼ teaspoon sugar

Guidelines:

1.   Season chicken with salt and pepper, rub with half of the sesame oil, add to the air fryer cooker and cook at 360 Deg. Fahrenheit for about 20 minutes.

2.   Meanwhile, heat up a skillet with the remainder of the oil over medium high heat, include green onions, sherry wine, vinegar, soy sauce and sugar, hurl, spread and cook for 10 minutes

3.   Shred chicken utilizing 2 forks isolate among plates, shower sauce all finished and serve.

Enjoy the recipe!

The nutritional facts: calories 321, fat 8, fiber 12, carbs 36, protein 24

CHICKEN FINGERS AND THE FLAVORED SAUCE

Prep. time: 10 minutes

The cooking time: 10 minutes

The recipe servings: 6

Fixings:

1teaspoon bean stew powder 2 teaspoon garlic powder 1 teaspoon onion powder 1 teaspoon sweet paprika

Salt and dark pepper to the taste 2 tablespoons margarine

1   tablespoons olive oil

2 pounds chicken fingers 2 tablespoons cornstarch

½ cup chicken stock 2 cups substantial cream 2 tablespoons water

2 tablespoons parsley, cleaved

Guidelines:

1.   In a bowl, blend garlic powder with onion powder, bean stew, salt, pepper and paprika, mix, include chicken and hurl.

2.   Rub chicken fingers with oil, place in the air fryer cooker and cook at 360 Deg. Fahrenheit for about 10 minutes.

3.   Meanwhile, heat up a skillet with the margarine over medium high heat, include cornstarch, stock, cream, water and parsley, mix, spread and cook for 10 minutes.

4.   Divide chicken on plates, sprinkle sauce all finished and serve. Enjoy the recipe!

The nutritional facts: calories 351, fat 12, fiber 9, carbs 20, protein 17

DUCK AND VEGGIES

Prep. time: 10 minutes

The cooking time: 20 minutes

The recipe servings: 8

Fixings:

1 duck, cleaved in medium pieces 3 cucumbers, hacked

3 tablespoon white wine 2 carrots, cleaved

1 cup chicken stock

1 little ginger piece, ground

Salt and dark pepper to the taste

Guidelines:

1.   In a container that accommodates the air fryer cooker, blend duck pieces with cucumbers, wine, carrots, ginger, stock, salt and pepper, hurl, present in the air fryer cooker and cook at 370 Deg. Fahrenheit for about 20 minutes.

2.   Divide everything on plates and serve.

Enjoy the recipe!

The nutritional facts: calories 200, fat 10, fiber 8, carbs 20, protein 22

CHICKEN AND APRICOT SAUCE

Prep. time: 10 minutes

The cooking time: 20 minutes

The recipe servings: 4

Fixings:

1 entire chicken, cut into medium pieces Salt and dark pepper to the taste

1   tablespoon of olive oil

½ teaspoon smoked paprika

¼ cup white wine

½ teaspoon marjoram, dried

¼ cup chicken stock

2   tablespoons white vinegar

¼ cup apricot jam

1 and ½ teaspoon ginger, ground 2 tablespoons HONNEY

Guidelines:

1.   Season chicken with salt, pepper, marjoram and paprika, hurl to cover, include oil, rub well, place in the air fryer cooker and cook at 360 Deg. Fahrenheit for about 10 minutes.

2.   Transfer chicken to a skillet that accommodates the air fryer cooker, include stock, wine, vinegar, ginger, apricot jelly and HONNEY, hurl, put in the air fryer cooker and cook at 360 Deg. Fahrenheit for about 10 minutes more.

3.   Divide chicken and apricot sauce on plates and serve.

Enjoy the recipe!

The nutritional facts: calories 200, fat 7, fiber 19, carbs 20, protein 14

CHICKEN AND CAULIFLOWER RICE MIX

Prep. time: 10 minutes

The cooking time: 20 minutes

The recipe servings: 6

Fixings:

3 bacon cuts, slashed 3 carrots, hacked

3 pounds chicken thighs, boneless and skinless 2 cove leaves

¼ cup red wine vinegar 4 garlic cloves, minced

Salt and dark pepper to the taste 4 tablespoons olive oil

1 tablespoon garlic powder

1 tablespoon Italian flavoring 24 ounces cauliflower rice

1   teaspoon turmeric powder 1 cup hamburger stock

Guidelines:

1.   Heat up a skillet that accommodates the air fryer cooker over medium high heat, include bacon, carrots, onion and garlic, mix and cook for 8 minutes.

2.   Add chicken, oil, vinegar, turmeric, garlic powder, Italian flavoring and cove leaves, mix, present in the air fryer cooker and cook at 360 Deg. Fahrenheit for about 12 minutes.

3.   Add cauliflower rice and stock, mix, cook for 6 minutes more, isolate among plates and serve.

Enjoy the recipe!

The nutritional facts: calories 340, fat 12, fiber 12, carbs 16, protein 8

CHICKEN AND SPINACH SALAD

Prep. time: 10 minutes

The cooking time: 12 minutes

The recipe servings: 2

Fixings:

2 teaspoons parsley, dried

2 chicken bosoms, skinless and boneless

½ teaspoon onion powder 2 teaspoons sweet paprika

½ cup lemon juice

Salt and dark pepper to the taste 5 cups child spinach

8 strawberries, cut

1   small red onion, cut

2   tablespoons balsamic vinegar

1 avocado, hollowed, stripped and hacked

¼ cup olive oil

1 tablespoon tarragon, hacked

Guidelines:

1.   Put chicken in a bowl, include lemon juice, parsley, onion powder and paprika and hurl.

2.   Transfer chicken to the air fryer cooker and cook at 360 Deg. Fahrenheit for about 12 minutes.

3.   In a bowl, blend spinach, onion, strawberries and avocado and hurl.

4.   In another bowl, blend oil in with vinegar, salt, pepper and tarragon, whisk well, add to the plate of mixed greens and hurl.

5.   Divide chicken on plates, include spinach serving of mixed greens the side and serve. Enjoy the recipe!

The nutritional facts: calories 240, fat 5, fiber 13, carbs 25, protein 22

CHICKE N AND CHESTNUTS MIX

Prep. time: 10 minutes The cooking time: 12 minutes The recipe servings: 2

Fixings:

½ pound chicken pieces

1 little yellow onion, slashed 2 teaspoons garlic, minced

A spot of ginger, ground A touch of allspice, ground

4 tablespoons water chestnuts 2 tablespoons soy sauce

2 tablespoons chicken stock

2 tablespoons balsamic vinegar 2 tortillas for serving

Guidelines:

1.   In a skillet that accommodates the air fryer cooker, blend chicken meat in with onion, garlic, ginger, allspice, chestnuts, soy sauce, stock and vinegar, mix, move to the air fryer cooker and cook at 360 deg. F for about 12 minutes.

2.   Divide everything on plates and serve.

The nutritional facts: calories 301, fat 12, fiber 7, carbs 24, protein 12

JUICE GLAZED CHICKEN

Prep. time: 10 minutes

The cooking time: 14 minutes

The recipe servings: 4

Fixings:

1 sweet potato, cubed

1   apples, cored and cut 1 tablespoon of olive oil

1 tablespoon rosemary, cleaved Salt and dark pepper to the taste

6 chicken thighs, bone inside of it and skin on 2/3 cup apple juice

1   tablespoon mustard

2   tablespoons HONNEY

1 tablespoon margarine

Guidelines:

1.   Heat up a container that accommodates the air fryer cooker with half of the oil over medium high heat, include juice, HONNEY, spread and mustard, whisk well, bring to a stew, take off heat, include chicken and hurl truly well.

2.   In a bowl, blend potato blocks with rosemary, apples, salt, pepper and the remainder of the oil, hurl well and add to chicken blend.

3.   Place dish in the air fryer cooker and cook at 390 Deg. Fahrenheit for about 14 minutes.

4.   Divide everything on plates and serve.

Enjoy the recipe!

The nutritional facts: calories 241, fat 7, fiber 12, carbs 28, protein 22

VEGGIE STUFFED CHICKEN BREASTS

Prep. time: 10 minutes

The cooking time: 15 minutes

The recipe servings: 4

Fixings:

4 chicken bosoms, skinless and boneless 2 tablespoons olive oil

Salt and dark pepper to the taste 1 zucchini, cleaved

1   teaspoon Italian flavoring

2   yellow ringer peppers, slashed 3 tomatoes, cleaved

1 red onion, cleaved

1   cup mozzarella, destroyed

Guidelines:

1.   Mix a cut on every chicken bosom making a pocket, season with salt and pepper and rub them with olive oil.

2.   In a bowl, blend zucchini in with Italian flavoring, ringer peppers, tomatoes and onion and mix.

3.   Stuff chicken bosoms with this blend, sprinkle mozzarella over them, place them in the air fryer cooker's crate and cook at 350 Deg. Fahrenheit for about 15 minutes.

4.   Divide among plates and serve.

Enjoy the recipe!

The nutritional facts: calories 300, fat 12, fiber 7, carbs 22, protein 18

GREEK CHICKEN

Prep. time: 10 minutes

The cooking time: 15 minutes

The recipe servings: 4

Fixings:

2tablespoons olive oil Juice from 1 lemon

1 teaspoon of oregano, dried 3 garlic cloves, minced

1   pound chicken thighs

Salt and dark pepper to the taste

½ pound asparagus, cut 1 zucchini, generally cleaved 1 lemon cut

Guidelines:

1.   In a heat verification dish that accommodates the air fryer cooker, blend chicken pieces in with oil, lemon juice, the oregano, the garlic, salt, pepper, asparagus, zucchini and lemon cuts, hurl, present in preheated air fryer and cook at 380 deg. F for about 15 minutes.

2.	Divide everything on plates and serve. Enjoy the recipe!

The nutritional facts: calories 300, fat 8, fiber 12, carbs 20, protein 18

THE DUCK BREASTS AND RED WINE AND ORANGE SAUCE

Prep. time: 10 minutes

The cooking time: 35 minutes

The recipe servings: 4

Fixings:

½ cup HONNEY

2	cups squeezed orange 4 cups red wine

2 tablespoons sherry vinegar 2 cups chicken stock

2 teaspoons pumpkin pie zest 2 tablespoons margarine

2 duck bosoms, skin on and divided 2 tablespoons olive oil

Salt and dark pepper to the taste

Guidelines:

1.	Heat up a container with the squeezed orange over medium heat, include HONNEY, mix well and cook for 10 minutes.

2.	Add wine, vinegar, stock, pie zest and margarine, mix well, cook for 10 minutes more and take off heat.

3.	Season duck bosoms with salt and pepper, rub with olive oil, place in preheated air fryer at 370 degrees F and cook for 7 minutes on each side.

4.	Divide duck bosoms on plates, sprinkle wine and squeezed orange all finished and serve immediately.

Enjoy the recipe!

The nutritional facts: calories 300, fat 8, fiber 12, carbs 24, protein 11

DUCK BREAST WITH FIG SAUCE

Prep. time: 10 minutes

The cooking time: 20 minutes

The recipe servings: 4

Fixings:

2duck bosoms, skin on, split 1 tablespoon of olive oil

½ teaspoon thyme, hacked

½ teaspoon garlic powder

¼ teaspoon sweet paprika

Salt and dark pepper to the taste 1 cup meat stock

2   tablespoons spread, softened 1 shallot, slashed

½ cup port wine

3   tablespoons fig jelly 1 tablespoon white flour

Guidelines:

1.   Season duck bosoms with salt and pepper, sprinkle half of the dissolved spread, rub well, put in the air fryer cooker's crate and cook at 350 Deg. Fahrenheit for about 5 minutes on each side.

2.   Meanwhile, heat up a skillet with the olive oil and the remainder of the spread over medium high heat, include shallot, mix and cook for 2 minutes.

3.   Add thyme, garlic powder, paprika, stock, salt, pepper, wine and figs, mix and cook for 7-8 minutes.

4.   Add flour, mix well, cook until sauce thickens a piece and take off heat.

5.   Divide duck bosoms on plates, sprinkle figs sauce all finished and serve. Enjoy the recipe!

The nutritional facts: calories 246, fat 12, fiber 4, carbs 22, protein 3

DUCK BREASTS AND RASPBERRY SAUCE

Prep. time: 10 minutes

The cooking time: 15 minutes

The recipe servings: 4

Fixings:

2 duck bosoms, skin on and scored Salt and dark pepper to the taste Cooking splash

½ teaspoon cinnamon powder

½ cup raspberries 1 tablespoon sugar

1 teaspoon red wine vinegar

½ cup water

Guidelines:

1.   Season duck bosoms with salt and pepper, splash them with cooking shower, put in preheated air fryer skin side down and cook at 350 Deg. Fahrenheit for about 10 minutes.

2.   Heat up a dish with the water over medium heat, include raspberries, cinnamon, sugar and wine, mix, bring to a stew, move to your blender, puree and come back to skillet.

3.   Add air fryer duck bosoms to container also, hurl to cover, isolate among plates and serve immediately.

Enjoy the recipe!

The nutritional facts: calories 456, fat 22, fiber 4, carbs 14, protein 45

DUCK AND CHERRIES

Prep. time: 10 minutes The cooking time: 20 minutes The recipe servings: 4

Fixings:

½ cup sugar

¼ cup HONNEY

1/3 cup balsamic vinegar 1 teaspoon garlic, minced

1 tablespoon ginger, ground 1 teaspoon cumin, ground

½ teaspoon clove, ground

½ teaspoon cinnamon powder 4 sage leaves, cleaved

1   jalapeno, cleaved

2   cups rhubarb, cut

½ cup yellow onion, cleaved 2 cups fruits, pitted

4 duck bosoms, boneless, skin on and scored Salt and dark pepper to the taste

Guidelines:

1.   Season duck bosom with salt and pepper, put in the air fryer cooker and cook at 350 Deg. Fahrenheit for about 5 minutes on each side.

2.   Meanwhile, heat up a container over medium heat, include sugar, HONNEY, vinegar, garlic, ginger, cumin, clove, cinnamon, sage, jalapeno, rhubarb, onion and fruits, mix, bring to a stew and cook for 10 minutes.

3.   Add duck bosoms, hurl well, partition everything on plates and serve. Enjoy the recipe!

The nutritional facts: calories 456, fat 13, fiber 4, carbs 64, protein 31

SIMPLE DUCK BREAST

Prep. time: 10 minutes

The cooking time: 15 minutes

The recipe servings: 4

Fixings:

4 duck bosoms, skinless and boneless

4 garlic heads, stripped, finishes cut off and quartered 2 tablespoons lemon juice

Salt and dark pepper to the taste

½ teaspoon lemon pepper

1   and ½ tablespoon of olive oil

Guidelines:

1.   In a bowl, blend duck bosoms with garlic, lemon juice, salt, pepper, lemon pepper and olive oil and hurl everything.

2.   Transfer duck and garlic to the air fryer cooker and cook at 350 Deg. Fahrenheit for about 15 minutes.

3.   Divide duck bosoms and garlic on plates and serve. Enjoy the recipe!

The nutritional facts: calories 200, fat 7, fiber 1, carbs 11, protein 17

DUCK AND TEA SAUCE

Prep. time: 10 minutes

The cooking time: 20 minutes

The recipe servings: 4

Fixings:

2 duck bosom parts, boneless 2 and ¼ cup chicken stock

¾ cup shallot, cleaved

1 and ½ cup squeezed orange

Salt and dark pepper to the taste 3 teaspoons duke dim tea leaves 3 tablespoons spread, softened

1   tablespoon HONNEY

Guidelines:

1.   Season duck bosom parts with salt and pepper, put in preheated air fryer and cook at 360 Deg. Fahrenheit for about 10 minutes.

2.   Meanwhile, heat up a container with the spread over medium heat, include shallot, mix and cook for 2-3 minutes.

3.   Add stock, mix and cook for one more moment.

4.   Add squeezed orange, tea leaves and HONNEY, mix, cook for 2-3 minutes more and strain into a bowl.

5.   Divide duck on plates, shower tea sauce all finished and serve. Enjoy the recipe!

The nutritional facts: calories 228, fat 11, fiber 2, carbs 20, protein 12

MARINATED DUCK BREASTS

Prep. time: 1 day The cooking time: 15 minutes The recipe servings: 2

Fixings:

2   duck bosoms

1   cup white wine

¼ cup soy sauce

2   garlic cloves, minced 6 tarragon springs

Salt and dark pepper to the taste 1 tablespoon margarine

¼ cup sherry wine

Guidelines:

1.   In a bowl, blend duck bosoms with white wine, soy sauce, garlic, tarragon, salt and pepper, hurl well and keep in the ice chest for 1 day.

2.   Transfer duck bosoms to your preheated air fryer at 350 degrees F and cook for 10 minutes, flipping midway.

3.   Meanwhile, pour the marinade in a dish, heat up over medium heat, include margarine and sherry, mix, bring to a stew, cook for 5 minutes and take off heat.

4.   Divide duck bosoms on plates, shower sauce all finished and serve. Enjoy the recipe!

The nutritional facts: calories 475, fat 12, fiber 3, carbs 10, protein 48

CHIKEN BREASTS WITH PASSION FRUIT SAUCE

Prep. time: 10 minutes

The cooking time: 10 minutes

The recipe servings: 4

Fixings:

4 chicken bosoms

Salt and dark pepper to the taste

4 enthusiasm natural products, split, deseeded and mash saved 1 tablespoon bourbon

2 star anise

2 ounces maple syrup

1   bunch chives, slashed

Guidelines:

1.   Heat up a skillet with the energy natural product mash over medium heat, include bourbon, star anise, maple syrup and chives, mix well, stew for 5-6 minutes and take off heat.

2.   Season the chicken, put in preheated air fryer and cook at 360 Deg. Fahrenheit for about 10 minutes, flipping midway.

3.   Divide chicken on plates, heat up the sauce a piece, sprinkle it over chicken and serve.

Enjoy the recipe!

The nutritional facts: calories 374, fat 8, fiber 22, carbs 34, protein 37

CHICKEN BREASTS AND BBQ CHILI SAUCE

Prep. time: 10 minutes

The cooking time: 20 minutes

The recipe servings: 6

2cups bean stew sauce 2 cups ketchup

1 cup pear jam

¼ cup HONNEY

½ teaspoon fluid smoke 1 teaspoon bean stew powder

1 teaspoonful of mustard powder & 1 teaspoonful of sweet paprika

Salt and dark pepper to the taste 1 teaspoon garlic powder

6 chicken bosoms, skinless and boneless

Guidelines:

1.	Season chicken bosoms with salt and pepper, put in preheated air fryer and cook at 350 Deg. Fahrenheit for about 10 minutes.

2.	Meanwhile, heat up a skillet with the stew sauce over medium heat, include ketchup, pear jam, HONNEY, fluid smoke, bean stew powder, mustard powder, sweet paprika, salt, pepper and the garlic powder, mix, bring to a stew and cook for 10 minutes.

3.	Add air fried chicken bosoms, hurl well, separate among plates and serve. Enjoy the recipe!

The nutritional facts: calories 473, fat 13, fiber 7, carbs 39, protein 33

DUCK BREASTS AND MANGO MIX

Prep. time: 1 hour The cooking time: 10 minutes The recipe servings: 4

Fixings:

4 duck bosoms

1   and ½ tablespoons lemongrass, hacked 3 tablespoons lemon juice

2   tablespoons olive oil

Salt and dark pepper to the taste 3 garlic cloves, minced

For the mango blend:

1 mango, stripped and cleaved

1 tablespoon coriander, cleaved 1 red onion, slashed

1 tablespoon sweet bean stew sauce 1 and ½ tablespoon lemon juice 1 teaspoon ginger, ground

¾ teaspoon sugar

Guidelines:

1.   In a bowl, blend duck bosoms with salt, pepper, lemongrass, 3 tablespoons lemon juice, olive oil and garlic, hurl well, keep in the refrigerator for 60 minutes, move to the air fryer cooker and cook at 360 Deg. Fahrenheit for about 10 minutes, flipping once.

2.   Meanwhile, in a bowl, blend mango in with coriander, onion, bean stew sauce, lemon squeeze, ginger and sugar and hurl well.

3.   Divide duck on plates, include mango blend the side and serve. Enjoy the recipe!

The nutritional facts: calories 465, fat 11, fiber 4, carbs 29, protein 38

BRISK CREAMY CHICKEN CASSEROLE

Prep. time: 10 minutes

The cooking time: 12 minutes

The recipe servings: 4

10 ounces spinach, cleaved 4 tablespoons margarine

3 tablespoons flour 1 and ½ cups milk

½ cup parmesan, ground

½ cup substantial cream

Salt and dark pepper to the taste

2 cup chicken bosoms, skinless, boneless and cubed 1 cup bread scraps

Guidelines:

1.   Heat up a container with the margarine over medium heat, include flour and mix well.

2.   Add milk, substantial cream and parmesan, mix well, cook for 1-2 minutes more and take off heat.

3.   In a container that accommodates the air fryer cooker, spread chicken and spinach.

4.   Add salt and pepper and hurl.

5.   Add cream blend and spread, sprinkle bread scraps on top, present in the air fryer cooker and cook at 350 for 12 minutes.

6.   Divide chicken and spinach blend on plates and serve. Enjoy the recipe!

The nutritional facts: calories 321, fat 9, fiber 12, carbs 22, protein 17

CHICKEN AND PEACHES

Prep. time: 10 minutes

The cooking time: 30 minutes

The recipe servings: 6

1 entire chicken, cut into medium pieces

¾ cup water 1/3 cup HONNEY

Salt and dark pepper to the taste

¼ cup olive oil

4 peaches, split

Guidelines:

1.   Put the water in a pot, bring to a stew over medium heat, include HONNEY, whisk truly well and leave aside.

2.   Rub chicken pieces with the oil, season with salt and pepper, place in the air fryer cooker's crate and cook at 350 Deg. Fahrenheit for about 10 minutes.

3.   Brush chicken with a portion of the HONNEY blend, cook for 6 minutes progressively, flip once more, brush once again with the HONNEY blend and cook for 7 minutes more.

4.   Divide chicken pieces on plates and keep warm.

5.   Brush peaches with what's left of the HONNEY marinade, place them in the air fryer cooker and cook them for 3 minutes.

6.   Divide among plates beside chicken pieces and serve.

Enjoy the recipe!

The nutritional facts: calories 430, fat 14, fiber 3, carbs 15, protein 20

TEA GLAZED CHICKEN

Prep. time: 10 minutes

The cooking time: 30 minutes

The recipe servings: 6

½ cup apricot jelly

½ cup pineapple jelly 6 chicken legs

1 cup hot water 6 dark tea packs

1 tablespoon soy sauce 1 onion, slashed

¼ teaspoon red pepper drops 1 tablespoon of olive oil

Salt and dark pepper to the taste 6 chicken legs

Guidelines:

1.   Put the hot water in a bowl, include tea packs, leave aside secured for 10 minutes, dispose of sacks toward the end and move tea to another bowl.

2.   Add soy sauce, pepper drops, apricot and pineapple jam, whisk truly well and take off heat.

3.   Season the chicken, rub with oil, put in the air fryer cooker and cook at 350 Deg. Fahrenheit for about 5 minutes.

4.   Spread onion on the base of a heating dish that accommodates the air fryer cooker, include chicken pieces, shower the tea coat on top, present in the air fryer cooker and cook at 320 Deg. Fahrenheit for about 25 minutes.

5.   Divide everything on plates and serve.

Enjoy the recipe!

The nutritional facts: calories 298, fat 14, fiber 1, carbs 14, protein 30

CHICKEN AND RADDISH MIX

Prep. time: 10 minutes

The cooking time: 30 minutes

The recipe servings: 4

4 chicken things, bone-in

Salt and dark pepper to the taste 1 tablespoon of olive oil

1 cup chicken stock 6 radishes, divided

1 teaspoon sugar

3 carrots, cut into flimsy sticks 2 tablespoon chives, slashed

Guidelines:

1.   Heat up a skillet that accommodates the air fryer cooker over medium heat, include stock, carrots, sugar and radishes, mix delicately, decrease heat to medium, spread pot somewhat and stew for 20 minutes.

2.   Season the recipe, put in the air fryer cooker and cook at 350 Deg. Fahrenheit for about 4 minutes.

3.   Add chicken to radish blend, hurl, present everything in the air fryer cooker, cook for 4 minutes more, separate among plates and serve.

Enjoy the recipe!

The nutritional facts: calories 237, fat 10, fiber 4, carbs 19, protein 29

AIR FRYER MEAT RECIPES

ENRICHED RIB EYE STEAK

Prep. time: 10 minutes The cooking time: 20 minutes The recipe servings: 4

Fixings:

2   pounds rib eye steak

Salt and dark pepper to the taste 1 tablespoons olive oil

For the rub:

3   tablespoons sweet paprika 2 tablespoons onion powder 2 tablespoons garlic powder 1 tablespoon dark colored sugar

2 tablespoons oregano, dried 1 tablespoon cumin, ground 1 tablespoon rosemary, dried

Guidelines:

1.   In a bowl, blend paprika in with onion and garlic powder, sugar, oregano, rosemary, salt, pepper and cumin, mix and rub steak with this blend.

2.   Season steak with salt and pepper, rub again with the oil, put in the air fryer cooker and cook at 400 Deg. Fahrenheit for about 20 minutes, flipping them midway.

3.   Transfer steak to a cutting board, cut and present with a side plate of mixed greens.

Enjoy the recipe!

The nutritional facts: calories 320, fat 8, fiber 7, carbs 22, protein 21

CHINESE STEAK AND BROCCOLI

Prep. time: 10 minutes

The cooking time: 12 minutes

The recipe servings: 4

¾ pound round steak, cut into strips 1 pound broccoli florets

1/3 cup shellfish sauce

2 teaspoons sesame oil 1 teaspoon soy sauce 1 teaspoon sugar

1/3 cup sherry

1 tablespoonful of olive oil, and 1 garlic clove, minced

Guidelines:

1.   In a bowl, blend sesame oil with shellfish sauce, soy sauce, sherry and sugar, mix well, include hamburger, hurl and leave aside for 30 minutes.

2.   Transfer hamburger to a container that accommodates the air fryer cooker, likewise include broccoli, garlic and oil, hurl everything and cook at 380 Deg. Fahrenheit for about 12 minutes.

3.   Divide among plates and serve.

Enjoy the recipe!

The nutritional facts: calories 330, fat 12, fiber 7, carbs 23, protein 23

PROVENCAL PORK

Prep. time: 10 minutes

The cooking time: 15 minutes

The recipe servings: 2

1 red onion, cut

1   yellow chime pepper, cut into strips 1 green ringer pepper, cut into strips Salt and dark pepper to the taste

2   teaspoons Provencal herbs

½ tablespoon mustard 1 tablespoon of olive oil

7 ounces pork tenderloin

Guidelines:

1.   In a preparing dish that accommodates the air fryer cooker, blend yellow chime pepper with green ringer pepper, onion, salt, pepper, Provencal herbs and half of the oil and hurl well.

2.   Season pork with salt, pepper, mustard and the remainder of the oil, hurl well and add to veggies.

3.   Introduce everything in the air fryer cooker, cook at 370 Deg. Fahrenheit for about 15 minutes, separate among plates and serve.

Enjoy the recipe!

The nutritional facts: calories 300, fat 8, fiber 7, carbs 21, protein 23

MEAT STRIPS WITH SNOW PEAS AND MUSHROOMS

Prep. time: 10 minutes

The cooking time: 22 minutes

The recipe servings: 2

2 meat steaks, cut into strips

Salt and dark pepper to the taste 7 ounces snow peas

8 ounces white mushrooms, split 1 yellow onion, cut into rings

2   tablespoons soy sauce 1 teaspoon olive oil

Guidelines:

1.   In a bowl, blend olive oil in with soy sauce, whisk, include meat strips and hurl.

2.   In another bowl, blend snow peas, onion and mushrooms with salt, pepper and the oil, hurl well, put in a container that accommodates the air fryer cooker and cook at 350 Deg. Fahrenheit for about 16 minutes.

3.   Add hamburger strips to the skillet also and cook at 400 Deg. Fahrenheit for about 6 minutes more.

4.   Divide everything on plates and serve.

Enjoy the recipe!

The nutritional facts: calories 235, fat 8, fiber 2, carbs 22, protein 24

GARLIC LAMB CHOPS

Prep. time: 10 minutes

The cooking time: 10 minutes

The recipe servings: 4

3 tablespoons olive oil 8 lamb cleaves

Salt and dark pepper to the taste 4 garlic cloves, minced

1 tablespoon oregano, cleaved 1 tablespoon coriander, slashed

Guidelines:

1.   In a bowl, blend oregano in with salt, pepper, oil, garlic and lamb cleaves and hurl to cover.

2.   Transfer lamb hacks to the air fryer cooker and cook at 400 Deg. Fahrenheit for about 10 minutes.

3.   Divide lamb hacks on plates and present with a side serving of mixed greens.

Enjoy the recipe!

The nutritional facts: calories 231, fat 7, fiber 5, carbs 14, protein 23

FIRM LAMB

Prep. time: 10 minutes

The cooking time: 30 minutes

The recipe servings: 4

1tablespoon bread pieces

1   tablespoons macadamia nuts, toasted and squashed 1 tablespoon of olive oil

1 garlic clove, minced 28 ounces rack of lamb

Salt and dark pepper to the taste 1 egg,

1 tablespoon rosemary, hacked

Guidelines:

1.   In a bowl, blend oil in with garlic and mix well.

2.   Season lamb with salt, pepper and brush with the oil.

3.   In another bowl, blend nuts in with breadcrumbs and rosemary.

4.   Put the egg in a different bowl and whisk well.

5.   Dip lamb in egg, at that point in macadamia blend, place them in the air fryer cooker's bushel, cook at 360 degrees F and cook for 25 minutes, increment heat to 400 degrees F and cook for 5 minutes more.

6.   Divide among plates and serve immediately.

Enjoy the recipe!

The nutritional facts: calories 230, fat 2, fiber 2, carbs 10, protein 12

INDIAN PORK

Prep. time: 35 minutes

The cooking time: 10 minutes

The recipe servings: 4

1teaspoon ginger powder 2 teaspoons stew glue

1   garlic cloves, minced

14 ounces pork hacks, cubed 1 shallot, cleaved

1   teaspoon coriander, ground 7 ounces coconut milk

2   tablespoons olive oil

3   ounces peanuts, ground 3 tablespoons soy sauce

Salt and dark pepper to the taste

Guidelines:

1.   In a bowl, blend ginger in with 1 teaspoon bean stew glue, half of the garlic, whisk, include meat, hurl and leave aside for 10 minutes.

2.   Transfer meat to the air fryer cooker's bushel and cook at 400 Deg. Fahrenheit for about 12 minutes, turning midway.

3.   Meanwhile, heat up a dish with the remainder of the oil over medium high heat, include shallot, the remainder of the garlic, coriander, coconut milk, the remainder of the peanuts, the remainder of the bean stew glue and the remainder of the soy sauce, mix and cook for 5 minutes.

4.   Divide pork on plates, spread coconut blend on top and serve.

Enjoy the recipe!

The nutritional facts: calories 423, fat 11, fiber 4, carbs 42, protein 18

LAMB AND CREAMY BRUSSELS SPROUTS

Prep. time: 10 minutes

The cooking time: 1 hour and 10 minutes

The recipe servings: 4

Fixings:

2 pounds leg of lamb, scored 2 tablespoons olive oil

1 tablespoon rosemary, cleaved

1 tablespoon lemon thyme, cleaved 1 garlic clove, minced

1 and ½ pounds Brussels grows, cut 1 tablespoon margarine, liquefied

½ cup acrid cream

Salt and dark pepper to the taste

Guidelines:

1.   Season leg of lamb with salt, pepper, thyme and rosemary, brush with oil, place in the air fryer cooker's bin, cook at 300 Deg. Fahrenheit for about 60 minutes, move to a plate and keep warm.

2.   In a container that accommodates the air fryer cooker, blend Brussels grows with salt, pepper, garlic, spread and harsh cream, hurl, put in the air fryer cooker and cook at 400 Deg. Fahrenheit for about 10 minutes.

3.   Divide lamb on plates, include Brussels grows the side and serve.

Enjoy the recipe!

The nutritional facts: calories 440, fat 23, fiber 0, carbs 2, protein 49

MEAT FILLETS WITH GARLIC MAYO

Prep. time: 10 minutes

The cooking time: 40 minutes

The recipe servings: 8

1cup mayonnaise 1/3 cup sharp cream

1   garlic cloves, minced 3 pounds meat filet

2 tablespoons chives, cleaved 2 tablespoons mustard

2 tablespoons mustard

¼ cup tarragon, slashed

Salt and dark pepper to the taste

Guidelines:

1.   Season hamburger with salt and pepper to the taste, place in the air fryer cooker, cook at 370 Deg. Fahrenheit for about 20 minutes, move to a plate and leave aside for a couple of moments.

2.   In a bowl, blend garlic in with acrid cream, chives, mayo, some salt and pepper, whisk and leave aside.

3.   In another bowl, blend mustard in with Dijon mustard and tarragon, whisk, include meat, hurl, come back to the air fryer cooker and cook at 350 Deg. Fahrenheit for about 20 minutes more.

4.   Divide meat on plates, spread garlic mayo on top and serve.

Enjoy the recipe!

The nutritional facts: calories 400, fat 12, fiber 2, carbs 27, protein 19

MUSTARD MARINA TED BEEF

Prep. time: 10 minutes

The cooking time: 45 minutes

The recipe servings: 6

6 bacon strips

2   tablespoons spread

3   garlic cloves, minced

Salt and dark pepper to the taste 1 tablespoon horseradish

1 tablespoon mustard 3 pounds meat broil

1   and ¾ cup meat stock

¾ cup red wine

Guidelines:

1.   In a bowl, blend spread in with mustard, garlic, salt, pepper and horseradish, whisk and rub meat with this blend.

2.   Arrange bacon strips on a cutting board, place meat on top, crease bacon around hamburger, move to the air fryer cooker's crate, cook at 400 Deg. Fahrenheit for about 15 minutes and move to a container that accommodates your fryer.

3.   Add stock and wine to hamburger, present dish in the air fryer cooker and cook at 360 Deg. Fahrenheit for about 30 minutes more.

4.   Carve hamburger, separate among plates and present with a side serving of mixed greens.

Enjoy the recipe!

The nutritional facts: calories 500, fat 9, fiber 4, carbs 29, protein 36

CREAMY PORK

Prep. time: 10 minutes

The cooking time: 22 minutes

The recipe servings: 6

2pounds pork meat, boneless and cubed 2 yellow onions, cleaved

3 cups chicken stock

2   tablespoons sweet paprika

Salt and dark pepper to the taste 2 tablespoons white flour

1   and ½ cups acrid cream

2   tablespoons dill, cleaved

Guidelines:

1.   In a container that accommodates the air fryer cooker, blend pork in with salt, pepper and oil, hurl, present in the air fryer cooker and cook at 360 Deg. Fahrenheit for about 7 minutes.

2.   Add onion, garlic, stock, paprika, flour, harsh cream and dill, hurl and cook at 370 Deg. Fahrenheit for about 15 minutes more.

3.   Divide everything on plates and serve immediately.

Enjoy the recipe!

The nutritional facts: calories 300, fat 4, fiber 10, carbs 26, protein 34

MARINATED PORK CHOPS AND ONIONS

Prep. time: 24 hours The cooking time: 25 minutes The recipe servings: 6

Fixings:

2 pork hacks

¼ cup olive oil

2 yellow onions, cut 2 garlic cloves, minced 2 teaspoons mustard

1   teaspoon sweet paprika

Salt and dark pepper to the taste

½ teaspoon oregano, dried

½ teaspoon thyme, dried A touch of cayenne pepper

Guidelines:

1.   In a bowl, blend oil in with garlic, mustard, paprika, dark pepper, oregano, thyme and cayenne and whisk well.

2.   Combine onions with meat and mustard blend, hurl to cover, spread and keep in the ice chest for 1 day.

3.   Transfer meat and onions blend to a dish that accommodates the air fryer cooker and cook at 360 Deg. Fahrenheit for about 25 minutes.

4.   Divide everything on plates and serve.

Enjoy the recipe!

The nutritional facts: calories 384, fat 4, fiber 4, carbs 17, protein 25

STRAIGHTFORWARD BRAISED PORK

Prep. time: 40 minutes

The cooking time: 40 minutes

The recipe servings: 4

2pounds pork midsection broil, boneless and cubed 4 tablespoons margarine, liquefied

Salt and dark pepper to the taste 2 cups chicken stock

½ cup of the dry white wine 2 garlic cloves, minced

1 teaspoon thyme, hacked 1 thyme spring

1   bay leaf

½ yellow onion, hacked 2 tablespoons white flour

½ pound red grapes

Guidelines:

1.   Season pork 3D squares with salt and pepper, rub with 2 tablespoons liquefied margarine, put in the air fryer cooker and cook at 370 Deg. Fahrenheit for about 8 minutes.

2.   Meanwhile, heat up a dish that accommodates the air fryer cooker with 2 tablespoons spread over medium high heat, include garlic and onion, mix and cook for 2 minutes.

3.	Add wine, stock, salt, pepper, thyme, flour and inlet leaf, mix well, bring to a stew and take off heat.

4.	Add pork 3D shapes and grapes, hurl, present in the air fryer cooker and cook at 360 Deg. Fahrenheit for about 30 minutes more.

5.	Divide everything on plates and serve. Enjoy the recipe!

The nutritional facts: calories 320, fat 4, fiber 5, carbs 29, protein 38

PORK WITH COUSCOUS

Prep. time: 10 minutes

The cooking time: 35 minutes

The recipe servings: 6

2½ pounds pork midsection, boneless and cut

¾ cup chicken stock

2 tablespoons olive oil

½ tablespoon sweet paprika 2 and ¼ teaspoon wise, dried

½ tablespoon garlic powder

¼ teaspoon rosemary, dried

¼ teaspoon marjoram, dried 1 teaspoon basil, dried

1 teaspoon oregano, dried

Salt and dark pepper to the taste 2 cups couscous, cooked

Guidelines:

1.   In a bowl, blend oil in with stock, paprika, garlic powder, sage, rosemary, thyme, marjoram, oregano, salt and pepper to the taste, whisk well, include pork midsection, hurl well and leave aside for 60 minutes.

2.   Transfer everything to a container that accommodates the air fryer cooker and cook at 370 Deg. Fahrenheit for about 35 minutes.

3.   Divide among plates and present with couscous as an afterthought. Enjoy the recipe!

The nutritional facts: calories 310, fat 4, fiber 6, carbs 37, protein 34

STRAIGHTFORWARD AIR FRIED PORK SHOULDER

Prep. time: 30 minutes The cooking time: 1 hour and 20 minutes The recipe servings: 6

Fixings:

3   tablespoons garlic, minced 3 tablespoons olive oil

4   pounds pork shoulder

Salt and dark pepper to the taste

Guidelines:

1.   In a bowl, blend olive oil in with salt, pepper and oil, whisk well and brush pork shoulder with this blend.

2.   Place in preheated air fryer and cook at 390 Deg. Fahrenheit for about 10 minutes.

3.   Reduce heat to 300 degrees F and meal pork for 1 hour and 10 minutes.

4.   Slice pork shoulder, partition among plates and present with a side serving of mixed greens. Enjoy the recipe!

The nutritional facts: calories 221, fat 4, fiber 4, carbs 7, protein 10

FENNEL FLAVORED PORK ROAST

Prep. time: 10 minutes

The cooking time: 60 minutes

The recipe servings: 10

Fixings:

5   and ½ pounds pork midsection broil, cut Salt and dark pepper to the taste

3 garlic cloves, minced

2 tablespoons rosemary, cleaved 1 teaspoon fennel, ground

1   tablespoon fennel seeds

2   teaspoons red pepper, squashed

¼ cup olive oil

Guidelines:

1.   In your food processor blend garlic in with fennel seeds, fennel, rosemary, red pepper, some dark pepper and the olive oil and mix until you get a glue.

2.   Spread 2 tablespoons garlic glue on pork midsection, rub well, season with salt and pepper, present in your preheated air fryer and cook at 350 Deg. Fahrenheit for about 30 minutes.

3.   Reduce the intensity of the heat to 300 deg. F and cook for 15 minutes more.

4.   Slice pork, separate among plates and serve. Enjoy the recipe!

The nutritional facts: calories 300, fat 14, fiber 9, carbs 26, protein 22

MEAT BRISKET AND ONION SAUCE

Prep. time:10 minnutes

The cooking time: 2 hours

The recipe servings: 6

Fixings:

1 pound yellow onion, slashed 4 pounds meat brisket

1 pound carrot, slashed 8 duke dim tea packs

½ pound celery, slashed

Salt and dark pepper to the taste 4 cups water

For the sauce:

16 ounces canned tomatoes, slashed

½ pound celery, slashed 1 ounce garlic, minced

4 ounces vegetable oil

1 pound sweet onion, slashed 1 cup dark colored sugar

8 lord dim tea sacks 1 cup white vinegar

Guidelines:

1.	Put the water in a heat confirmation dish that accommodates the air fryer cooker, include 1 pound onion, 1 pound carrot, ½ pound celery, salt and pepper, mix and bring to a stew over medium high heat.

2.	Add hamburger brisket and 8 tea packs, mix, move to the air fryer cooker and cook at 300 Deg. Fahrenheit for about 1 hour and 30 minutes.

3.	Meanwhile, heat up a skillet with the vegetable oil over medium high heat, include 1 pound onion, mix and sauté for 10 minutes.

4.	Add garlic, ½ pound celery, tomatoes, sugar, vinegar, salt, pepper and 8 tea packs, mix, bring to a stew, cook for 10 minutes and dispose of tea sacks.

5.	Transfer hamburger brisket to a cutting board, cut, isolate among plates, sprinkle onion sauce all finished and serve.

Enjoy the recipe!

The nutritional facts: calories 400, fat 12, fiber 4, carbs 38, protein 34

HAMBURGER AND GREEN ONIONS MARINADE

Prep. time: 10 minutes

The cooking time: 20 minutes

The recipe servings: 4

1 cup green onion, cleaved 1 cup soy sauce

½ cup water

¼ cup dark colored sugar

¼ cup sesame seeds

5 garlic cloves, minced 1 teaspoon dark pepper 1 pound lean hamburger

Guidelines:

1.   In a bowl, blend onion in with soy sauce, water, sugar, garlic, sesame seeds and pepper, whisk, include meat, hurl and leave aside for 10 minutes.

2.   Drain hamburger, move to your preheated air fryer and cook at 390 Deg. Fahrenheit for about 20 minutes.

3.   Slice, isolate among plates and present with a side serving of mixed greens. Enjoy the recipe!

The nutritional facts: calories 329, fat 8, fiber 12, carbs 26, protein 22

GARLIC AND BELL PEPPER BEEF

Prep. time: 10 minutes

The cooking time: 30 minutes

The recipe servings: 4

11 ounces steak fillets, cut 4 garlic cloves, minced

2 tablespoons olive oil

1 red ringer pepper, slice into strips Black pepper to the taste

1   tablespoon sugar

2   tablespoons fish sauce 2 teaspoons corn flour

½ cup hamburger stock

4 green onions, cut

Guidelines:

1.   In a skillet that accommodates the air fryer cooker blend meat in with oil, garlic, dark pepper and ringer pepper, mix, spread and keep in the refrigerator for 30 minutes.

2.   Put the container in your preheated air fryer and cook at 360 Deg. Fahrenheit for about 14 minutes.

3.   In a bowl, blend sugar in with fish sauce, mix well, pour over meat and cook at 360 Deg. Fahrenheit for about 7 minutes more.

4.   Add stock blended in with corn flour and green onions, hurl and cook at 370 Deg. Fahrenheit for about 7 minutes more.

5.   Divide everything on plates and serve. Enjoy the recipe!

The nutritional facts: calories 343, fat 3, fiber 12, carbs 26, protein 38

MARINATED LAMB AND VEGGIES

Prep. time: 10 minutes

The cooking time: 30 minutes

The recipe servings: 4

1 carrot, hacked

1 onion, cut

½ tablespoon of olive oil 3 ounces bean grows

8 ounces lamb midsection, cut

For the marinade:

1 garlic clove, minced

½ apple, ground

Salt and dark pepper to the taste 1 little yellow onion, ground

1 tablespoon ginger, ground 5 tablespoons soy sauce

1   tablespoons sugar

2   tablespoons squeezed orange

Guidelines:

1.   In a bowl, blend 1 ground onion with the apple, garlic, 1 tablespoon ginger, soy sauce, squeezed orange, sugar and dark pepper, whisk well, include lamb and leave aside for 10 minutes.

2.   Heat up a dish that accommodates the air fryer cooker with the olive oil over medium high heat, include 1 cut onion, carrot and bean sprouts, mix and cook for 3 minutes.

3.   Add lamb and the marinade, move dish to your preheated air fryer and cook at 360 Deg. Fahrenheit for about 25 minutes.

4.   Divide everything into bowls and serve. Enjoy the recipe!

The nutritional facts: calories 265, fat 3, fiber 7, carbs 18, protein 22

CREAMY LAMB

Prep. time: 1 day The cooking time: 1 hour The recipe servings: 8

Fixings:

5 pounds leg of lamb

2 cups low fat buttermilk 2 tablespoons mustard

½ cup spread

2 tablespoons basil, hacked 2 tablespoons tomato glue 2 garlic cloves, minced

Salt and dark pepper to the taste 1 cup white wine

1 tablespoon cornstarch blended in with 1 tablespoon water

½ cup sharp cream

Guidelines:

1.   Put lamb broil in a major dish, include buttermilk, hurl to cover, spread and keep in the cooler for 24 hours.

2.   Pat dry lamb and put in a dish that accommodates the air fryer cooker.

3.   In a bowl, blend margarine in with tomato glue, mustard, basil, rosemary, salt, pepper and garlic, whisk well, spread over lamb, present everything in the air fryer cooker and cook at 300 Deg. Fahrenheit for about 60 minutes.

4.   Slice lamb, isolate among plates, leave aside for the time being and heat up cooking juices from the dish on your stove.

5.   Add wine, cornstarch blend, salt, pepper and harsh cream, mix, take off heat, sprinkle this sauce over lamb and serve.

Enjoy the recipe!

The nutritional facts: calories 287, fat 4, fiber 7, carbs 19, protein 25

AIR FRYER LAMB SHANKS

Prep. time: 10 minutes The cooking time: 45 minutes The recipe servings: 4

Fixings:

4 lamb shanks

1 yellow onion, slashed 1 tablespoon of olive oil

4 teaspoons coriander seeds, squashed 2 tablespoons white flour

4 cove leaves

2 teaspoons HONNEY 5 ounces dry sherry

2 and ½ cups chicken stock Salt and pepper to the taste

Guidelines:

1.   Season lamb shanks with salt and pepper, rub with half of the oil, put in the air fryer cooker and cook at 360 Deg. Fahrenheit for about 10 minutes.

2.   Heat up a skillet that accommodates the air fryer cooker with the remainder of the oil over medium high heat, include onion and coriander, mix and cook for 5 minutes.

3.   Add flour, sherry, stock, HONNEY and cove leaves, salt and pepper, mix, bring to a stew, include lamb, present everything in the air fryer cooker and cook at 360 Deg. Fahrenheit for about 30 minutes.

4.   Divide everything on plates and serve. Enjoy the recipe!

The nutritional facts: calories 283, fat 4, fiber 2, carbs 17, protein 26

LAMB ROAST AND POTATOES

Prep. time: 10 minutes The cooking time: 45 minutes The recipe servings: 6

Fixings:

4 pounds lamb broil 1 spring rosemary

3   garlic cloves, minced 6 potatoes, split

½ cup lamb stock 4 sound leaves

Salt and dark pepper to the taste

Guidelines:

1.   Put potatoes in a dish that accommodates the air fryer cooker, include lamb, garlic, rosemary spring, salt, pepper, sound leaves and stock, hurl, present in the air fryer cooker and cook at 360 Deg. Fahrenheit for about 45 minutes.

2.   Slice lamb, separate among plates and present with potatoes and cooking juices.

Enjoy the recipe!

The nutritional facts: calories 273, fat 4, fiber 12, carbs 25, protein 29

Lemony Lamb Leg

Prep. time: 10 minutes The cooking time: 1 hour The recipe servings: 6

Fixings:

4   pounds lamb leg

2 tablespoons olive oil

2 springs rosemary, hacked

2 tablespoons parsley, hacked 2 tablespoons oregano, cleaved Salt and dark pepper to the taste 1 tablespoon lemon skin, ground 3 garlic cloves, minced

2 tablespoons lemon juice 2 pounds child potatoes

1   cup meat stock

Guidelines:

1.   Make little cuts all over lamb, embed rosemary springs and season with salt and pepper.

2.   In a bowl, blend 1 tablespoon oil with oregano, parsley, garlic, lemon juice and skin, mix and rub lamb with this blend.

3.   Heat up a skillet that accommodates the air fryer cooker with the remainder of the oil over medium high heat, include potatoes, mix and cook for 3 minutes.

4.   Add lamb and stock, mix, present in the air fryer cooker and cook at 360 Deg. Fahrenheit for about 60 minutes.

5.   Divide everything on plates and serve. Enjoy the recipe!

The nutritional facts: calories 264, fat 4, fiber 12, carbs 27, protein 32

HAMBURGER CURRY

Prep. time: 10 minutes

The cooking time: 45 minutes

The recipe servings: 4

2pounds hamburger steak, cubed 2 tablespoons olive oil

2   potatoes, cubed

1   tablespoon wine mustard

2   and ½ tablespoons curry powder 2 yellow onions, slashed

2 garlic cloves, minced

10 ounces canned coconut milk 2 tablespoons tomato sauce

Salt and dark pepper to the taste

Guidelines:

1.   Heat up a skillet that accommodates the air fryer cooker with the oil over medium high heat, include onions and garlic, mix and cook for 4 minutes.

2.   Add potatoes and mustard, mix and cook for 1 moment.

3.   Add hamburger, curry powder, salt, pepper, coconut milk and tomato sauce, mix, move to the air fryer cooker and cook at 360 Deg. Fahrenheit for about 40 minutes.

4.   Divide into bowls and serve.

Enjoy the recipe!

The nutritional facts: calories 432, fat 16, fiber 4, carbs 20, protein 27

HAMBURGER ROAST AND WINE SAUCE

Prep. time: 10 minutes

The cooking time: 45 minutes

The recipe servings: 6

3 pounds hamburger broil

Salt and dark pepper to the taste 17 ounces hamburger stock

3   ounces red wine

½ teaspoon chicken salt

½ teaspoon smoked paprika 1 yellow onion, slashed

4   garlic cloves, minced 3 carrots, slashed

5   potatoes, slashed

Guidelines:

1.   In a bowl, blend salt, pepper, chicken salt and paprika, mix, rub hamburger with this blend and put it in a major skillet that accommodates the air fryer cooker.

2.   Add onion, garlic, stock, wine, potatoes and carrots, present in the air fryer cooker and cook at 360 Deg. Fahrenheit for about 45 minutes.

3.   Divide everything on plates and serve.

Enjoy the recipe!

The nutritional facts: calories 304, fat 20, fiber 7, carbs 20, protein 32

MEAT AND CABBAGE MIX

Prep. time: 10 minutes

The cooking time: 40 minutes

The recipe servings: 6

2 and ½ pounds meat brisket 1 cup hamburger stock

2   bay leaves

3   garlic cloves, cleaved 4 carrots, hacked

1 cabbage head, cut into medium wedges Salt and dark pepper to the taste

3   turnips, cut into quarters

Guidelines:

1.   Put meat brisket and stock in a huge skillet that accommodates the air fryer cooker, season hamburger with salt and pepper, include garlic and inlet leaves, carrots, cabbage, potatoes and turnips, hurl, present in the air fryer cooker and cook at 360 degrees F and cook for 40 minutes.

2.   Divide among plates and serve.

Enjoy the recipe!

The nutritional facts: calories 353, fat 16, fiber 7, carbs 20, protein 24

LAMB SHANKS AND CARROTS

Prep. time: 10 minutes The cooking time: 45 minutes The recipe servings: 4

Fixings:

4   lamb shanks

2 tablespoons olive oil

1   yellow onion, finely cleaved 6 carrots, generally hacked

2   garlic cloves, minced

2 tablespoons tomato glue 1 teaspoon oregano, dried 1 tomato, generally cleaved 2 tablespoons water

4 ounces red wine

Salt and dark pepper to the taste

Guidelines:

1.   Season lamb with salt and pepper, rub with oil, put in the air fryer cooker and cook at 360 Deg. Fahrenheit for about 10 minutes.

2.   In a container that accommodates the air fryer cooker, blend onion in with carrots, garlic, tomato glue, tomato, oregano, wine and water and hurl.

3.   Add lamb, hurl, present in the air fryer cooker and cook at 370 Deg. Fahrenheit for about 35 minutes.

4.   Divide everything on plates and serve.

Enjoy the recipe!

The nutritional facts: calories 432, fat 17, fiber 8, carbs 17, protein 43

SCRUMPTIOUS LAMB RIBS

Prep. time: 15 minutes

The cooking time: 40 minutes

The recipe servings: 8

8 lamb ribs

4 garlic cloves, minced 2 carrots, slashed

2 cups veggie stock

1   tablespoon rosemary, slashed

2   tablespoons additional virgin olive oil Salt and dark pepper to the taste 3 tablespoons white flour

Guidelines:

1.   Season lamb ribs with salt and pepper, rub with oil and garlic, put in preheated air fryer and cook at 360 Deg. Fahrenheit for about 10 minutes.

2.   In a heat confirmation dish that accommodates your fryer, blend stock in with flour and whisk well.

3.   Add rosemary, carrots and lamb ribs, place in the air fryer cooker and cook at 350 Deg. Fahrenheit for about 30 minutes.

4.   Divide lamb blend on plates and serve hot.

Enjoy the recipe!

The nutritional facts: calories 302, fat 7, fiber 2, carbs 22, protein 27

ORIENTAL AIR FRIED LAMB

Prep. time: 10 minutes

The cooking time: 42 minutes

The recipe servings: 8

2and ½ pounds lamb shoulder, slashed 3 tablespoons HONNEY

2   ounces almonds, stripped and slashed 9 ounces plumps, pitted

8 ounces veggie stock

2 yellow onions, slashed 2 garlic cloves, minced

Salt and dark pepper to the preferences 1 teaspoon cumin powder

1 teaspoonful of the turmeric powder, and 1 teaspoonful of ginger powder

1   teaspoon cinnamon powder 3 tablespoons olive oil

Guidelines:

1.   In a bowl, blend cinnamon powder with ginger, cumin, turmeric, garlic, olive oil and lamb, hurl to cover, place in your preheated air fryer and cook at 350 Deg. Fahrenheit for about 8 minutes.

2.   Transfer meat to a dish that accommodates the air fryer cooker, include onions, stock, HONNEY and plums, mix, present in the air fryer cooker and cook at 350 Deg. Fahrenheit for about 35 minutes.

3.   Divide everything on plates and present with almond sprinkled on top.

Enjoy the recipe!

The nutritional facts: calories 432, fat 23, fiber 6, carbs 30, protein 20

SHORT RIBS AND SPECIAL SAUCE

Prep. time: 10 minutes

The cooking time: 36 minutes

The recipe servings: 4

2green onions, slashed 1 teaspoon vegetable oil 3 garlic cloves, minced 3 ginger cuts

4 pounds short ribs

½ cup water

½ cup soy sauce

¼ cup rice wine

¼ cup pear juice

2 teaspoons sesame oil

Guidelines:

1.   Heat up a skillet that accommodates the air fryer cooker with the oil over medium heat, include green onions, ginger and garlic, mix and cook for 1 moment.

2.   Add ribs, water, wine, soy sauce, sesame oil and pear juice, mix, present in the air fryer cooker and cook at 350 Deg. Fahrenheit for about 35 minutes.

3.   Divide ribs and sauce on plates and serve.

Enjoy the recipe!

The nutritional facts: calories 321, fat 12, fiber 4, carbs 20, protein 14

SHORT RIBS AND BEER SAUCE

Prep. time: 10 minutes

The cooking time: 45 minutes

The recipe servings: 6

4 pounds short ribs, cut into little pieces 1 yellow onion, cleaved

Salt and dark pepper to the taste

¼ cup tomato glue 1 cup dull lager

1 cup chicken stock 1 inlet leaf

6 thyme springs, hacked

1   Portobello mushroom, dried

Guidelines:

1.   Heat up a dish that accommodates the air fryer cooker over medium heat, include tomato glue, onion, stock, lager, mushroom, narrows leaves and thyme and bring to a stew.

2.   Add ribs, present in the air fryer cooker and cook at 350 Deg. Fahrenheit for about 40 minutes.

3.   Divide everything on plates and serve.

Enjoy the recipe!

The nutritional facts: calories 300, fat 7, fiber 8, carbs 18, protein 23

ROASTED PORK BELLY AND APPLE SAUCE

Prep. time: 10 minutes

The cooking time:40 minutes

The recipe servings: 6

2tablespoons sugar

1 tablespoon lemon juice 1 quart water

17 ounces apples, cored and cut into wedges 2 pounds pork gut, scored

Salt and dark pepper to the taste A sprinkle of olive oil

Guidelines:

1.   In your blender, blend water in with apples, lemon squeeze and sugar, beat well, move to a bowl, include meat, hurl well, channel, put in the air fryer cooker and cook at 400 Deg. Fahrenheit for about 40 minutes.

2.   Pour the sauce in a pot, heat up over medium heat and stew for 15 minutes.

3.   Slice pork stomach, partition among plates, sprinkle the sauce all finished and serve.

Enjoy the recipe!

The nutritional facts: calories 456, fat 34, fiber 4, carbs 10, protein 25

STUFFED PORK STEAKS

Prep. time: 10 minutes

The cooking time: 20 minutes

The recipe servings: 4

Get-up-and-go from 2 limes, ground Zest from 1 orange, ground Juice from 1 orange

Juice from 2 limes

4 teaspoons garlic, minced

¾ cup olive oil

1 cup cilantro, cleaved 1 cup mint, hacked

1 teaspoon oregano, dried

Salt and dark pepper to the taste 2 teaspoons cumin, ground

4 pork midsection steaks 2 pickles, hacked

4 ham cuts

6 Swiss cheddar cuts 2 tablespoons mustard

Guidelines:

1.   In your food processor, blend lime get-up-and-go and squeeze with orange get-up-and-go and squeeze, garlic, oil, cilantro, mint, oregano, cumin, salt and pepper and mix well.

2.   Season the steaks with salt & pepper, place them into a bowl, add marinade and hurl to cover.

3.   Place steaks on a working surface, separate pickles, cheddar, mustard and ham on them, roll and secure with toothpicks.

4.   Put stuffed pork steaks in the air fryer cooker and cook at 340 Deg. Fahrenheit for about 20 minutes.

5.   Divide among plates and present with a side serving of mixed greens.

Enjoy the recipe!

The nutritional facts: calories 270, fat 7, fiber 2, carbs 13, protein 20

PORK CHOPS AND MUSHROOMS MIX

Prep. time: 10 minutes

The cooking time: 40 minutes

The recipe servings: 3

- 8 ounces mushrooms, cut 1 teaspoon garlic powder

- 1 yellow onion, hacked 1 cup mayonnaise

  - pork hacks, boneless 1 teaspoon nutmeg

- 1 tablespoon balsamic vinegar

- ½ cup olive oil

Guidelines:

1.   Heat up a dish that accommodates the air fryer cooker with the oil over medium heat, include mushrooms and onions, mix and cook for 4 minutes.

2.   Add pork hacks, nutmeg and garlic powder and dark colored on the two sides.

3.   Introduce dish the air fryer cooker at 330 degrees F and cook for 30 minutes.

4.   Add vinegar and mayo, mix, separate everything on plates and serve.

Enjoy the recipe!

The nutritional facts: calories 600, fat 10, fiber 1, carbs 8, protein 30

MEAT STUFFED SQUASH

Prep. time: 10 minutes

The cooking time: 40 minutes

The recipe servings: 2

1 spaghetti squash, pricked 1 pound meat, ground

Salt and dark pepper to the taste 3 garlic cloves, minced

1 yellow onion, hacked

1 Portobello mushroom, cut

28 ounces canned tomatoes, hacked 1 teaspoon oregano, dried

¼ teaspoon cayenne pepper

½ teaspoon thyme, dried

1 green chime pepper, hacked

Guidelines:

1.   Put spaghetti squash in the air fryer cooker, cook at 350 Deg. Fahrenheit for about 20 minutes, move to a cutting board, and cut into equal parts and dispose of seeds.

2.   Heat up a dish over medium high heat, include meat, garlic, onion and mushroom, mix and cook until meat tans.

3.   Add salt, pepper, thyme, oregano, cayenne, tomatoes and green pepper, mix and cook for 10 minutes.

4.   Stuff squash with this meat blend, present in the fryer and cook at 360 Deg. Fahrenheit for about 10 minutes.

5.   Divide among plates and serve.

Enjoy the recipe!

The nutritional facts: calories 260, fat 7, fiber 2, carbs 14, protein 10

GREEK BEEF MEATBALLS SALAD

Prep. time: 10 minutes

The cooking time: 10 minutes

The recipe servings: 6

¼ cup milk

17 ounces meat, ground 1 yellow onion, ground 5 bread cuts, cubed

1   egg, whisked

¼ cup parsley, cleaved

Salt and dark pepper to the taste 2 garlic cloves, minced

¼ cup mint, cleaved

2   and ½ teaspoons oregano, dried 1 tablespoon of olive oil

Cooking splash

7 ounces cherry tomatoes, split 1 cup infant spinach

1   and ½ tablespoons lemon juice 7 ounces Greek yogurt

Guidelines:

1.   Put torn bread in a bowl, include milk, drench for a couple of moments, crush and move to another bowl.

2.	Add hamburger, egg, salt, pepper, oregano, mint, parsley, garlic and onion, mix and shape medium meatballs out of this blend.

3.	Spray them with cooking splash, place them in the air fryer cooker and cook at 370 Deg. Fahrenheit for about 10 minutes.

Enjoy the recipe!

4.	In a plate of mixed greens bowl, blend spinach in with cucumber and tomato.

5.	Add meatballs, the oil, some salt, pepper, lemon juice and yogurt, hurl and serve.

The nutritional facts: calories 200, fat 4, fiber 8, carbs 13, protein 27

HAMBURGER PATTIES AND MUSHROOM SAUCE

Prep. time: 10 minutes The cooking time: 25 minutes The recipe servings: 6;

Fixings:

2	pounds hamburger, ground

Salt and dark pepper to the taste

½ teaspoon garlic powder 1 tablespoon soy sauce

¼ cup hamburger stock

¾ cup flour

1 tablespoon parsley, cleaved 1 tablespoon onion drops

For the sauce:

1   cup yellow onion, cleaved 2 cups mushrooms, cut

2   tablespoons bacon fat 2 tablespoons margarine

½ teaspoon soy sauce

¼ cup acrid cream

½ cup hamburger stock

Salt and dark pepper to the taste

Guidelines:

1.   In a bowl, blend hamburger in with salt, pepper, garlic powder, 1 tablespoon soy sauce, ¼ cup meat stock, flour, parsley and onion pieces, mix well, shape 6 patties, place them in the air fryer cooker and cook at 350 Deg. Fahrenheit for about 14 minutes.

2.   Meanwhile, heat up a container with the margarine and the bacon fat over medium heat, include mushrooms, mix and cook for 4 minutes.

3.   Add onions, mix and cook for 4 minutes more.

4.   Add ½ teaspoon soy sauce, acrid cream and ½ cup stock, mix well, bring to a stew and take off heat.

5.   Divide hamburger patties on plates and present with mushroom sauce on top.

Enjoy the recipe!

The nutritional facts: calories 435, fat 23, fiber 4, carbs 6, protein 32

HAMBURGER CASSEROLE

Prep. time: 30 minutes The cooking time: 35 minutes The recipe servings: 12

Fixings:

1   tablespoon of olive oil 2 pounds hamburger, ground

2   cups eggplant, cleaved

Salt and dark pepper to the taste 2 teaspoons mustard

2 teaspoons gluten free Worcestershire sauce 28 ounces canned tomatoes, cleaved

2 cups mozzarella, ground 16 ounces tomato sauce

2 tablespoons parsley, cleaved 1 teaspoon oregano, dried

Guidelines:

1.   In a bowl, blend eggplant in with salt, pepper and oil and hurl to cover.

2.   In another bowl, blend meat in with salt, pepper, mustard and Worcestershire sauce, mix well and spread on the base of a skillet that accommodates the air fryer cooker.

3.   Add eggplant blend, tomatoes, tomato sauce, parsley, oregano and sprinkle mozzarella toward the end.

4.   Introduce in the air fryer cooker and cook at 360 Deg. Fahrenheit for about 35 minutes

5.   Divide among plates and serve hot.

Enjoy the recipe!

The nutritional facts: calories 200, fat 12, fiber 2, carbs 16, protein 15

LAMB AND SPINACH MIX

Prep. time: 10 minutes

The cooking time: 35 minutes

The recipe servings: 6

2 tablespoons ginger, ground 2 garlic cloves, minced

2 teaspoons cardamom, ground 1 red onion, hacked

1   pound lamb meat, cubed 2 teaspoons cumin powder 1 teaspoon garam masala

½ teaspoon stew powder 1 teaspoon turmeric

2   teaspoons coriander, ground 1 pound spinach

14 ounces canned tomatoes, hacked

Guidelines:

1.   In a heat evidence dish that accommodates the air fryer cooker, blend lamb in with spinach, tomatoes, ginger, garlic, onion, cardamom, cloves, cumin, garam masala, stew, turmeric and coriander, mix, present in preheated air fryer and cook at 360 Deg. Fahrenheit for about 35 minutes

2.   Divide into bowls and serve.

Enjoy the recipe!

The nutritional facts: calories 160, fat 6, fiber 3, carbs 17, protein 20

LAMB AND LEMON SAUCE

Prep. time: 10 minutes

The cooking time: 30 minutes

The recipe servings: 4

2 lamb shanks

Salt and dark pepper to the taste 2 garlic cloves, minced

4 tablespoons olive oil Juice from ½ lemon Zest from ½ lemon

½ teaspoon oregano, dried

Guidelines:

1.   Season lamb with salt, pepper, rub with garlic, put in the air fryer cooker and cook at 350 Deg. Fahrenheit for about 30 minutes.

2.   Meanwhile, in a bowl, blend lemon squeeze in with lemon get-up-and-go, some salt and pepper, the olive oil and oregano and whisk well overall.

3.   Shred lamb, dispose of bone, partition among plates, shower the lemon dressing all finished and serve.

Enjoy the recipe!

The nutritional facts: calories 260, fat 7, fiber 3, carbs 15, protein 12

LAMB AND GREEN PESTO

Prep. time: 1 hour The cooking time: 45 minutes The recipe servings: 4

Fixings:

1 cup parsley

1 cup mint

1 little yellow onion, generally slashed 1/3 cup pistachios, hacked

1 teaspoon lemon pizzazz, ground 5 tablespoons olive oil

Salt and dark pepper to the taste 2 pounds lamb riblets

½ onion, slashed

5 garlic cloves, minced Juice from 1 orange

Guidelines:

1.   In your food processor, blend parsley in with mint, onion, pistachios, lemon pizzazz, salt, pepper and oil and mix quite well.

2.   Rub lamb with this blend, place in a bowl, spread and leave in the refrigerator for 60 minutes.

3.   Transfer lamb to a preparing dish that accommodates the air fryer cooker, likewise include garlic, sprinkle squeezed orange and cook in the air fryer cooker at 300 Deg. Fahrenheit for about 45 minutes.

4.   Divide lamb on plates and serve.

Enjoy the recipe!

The nutritional facts: calories 200, fat 4, fiber 6, carbs 15, protein 7

LAMB RACK S AND FENNEL MIX

Prep. time: 10 minutes The cooking time: 16 minutes The recipe servings: 4

Fixings:

12 ounces lamb racks 2 fennel bulbs, cut

Salt and dark pepper to the taste 2 tablespoons olive oil

4 figs, cut into equal parts

1/8 cup apple juice vinegar 1 tablespoon dark colored sugar

Guidelines:

1.   In a bowl, blend fennel in with figs, vinegar, sugar and oil, hurl to cover well, move to a preparing dish that accommodates the air fryer cooker, present in the air fryer cooker and cook at 350 Deg. Fahrenheit for about 6 minutes.

2.   Season lamb with salt and pepper, add to the preparing dish with the fennel blend and air fry for 10 minutes more.

3.   Divide everything on plates and serve.

Enjoy the recipe!

The nutritional facts: calories 240, fat 9, fiber 3, carbs 15, protein 12

BURGUNDY BEEF MIX

Prep. time: 10 minutes The cooking time: 1 hour The recipe servings: 7

Fixings:

2 pounds meat toss broil, cubed

15 ounces canned tomatoes, hacked 4 carrots, slashed

Salt and dark pepper to the taste

½ pounds mushrooms, cut 2 celery ribs, hacked

2 yellow onions, hacked 1 cup hamburger stock

1   tablespoon thyme, hacked

½ teaspoonful of the mustard powder, & 3 tablespoons almond flour 1 cup water

Guidelines:

1.   Heat up a heat evidence pot that accommodates the air fryer cooker over medium high heat, include hamburger, mix and dark colored them for two or three minutes.

2.   Add the tomatoes, the mushrooms, the onions, the carrots, the celery, salt, the pepper mustard, stock and thyme and mix.

3.   In a bowl blend water in with flour, mix well, add this to the pot, hurl, present in the air fryer cooker and cook at 300 Deg. Fahrenheit for about 60 minutes.

4.   Divide into bowls and serve.

Enjoy the recipe!

The nutritional facts: calories 275, fat 13, fiber 4, carbs 17, protein 28

MEXICAN BEEF MIX

Prep. time:10 minutes

The cooking time: 1 hour and 10 minutes

The recipe servings: 8

Fixings:

2   yellow onions, cleaved 2 tablespoons olive oil

2 pounds hamburger broil, cubed

2 green ringer peppers, hacked 1 habanero pepper, cleaved 4 jalapenos, slashed

14 ounces canned tomatoes, cleaved 2 tablespoons cilantro, hacked

6 garlic cloves, minced

½ cup water

Salt and dark pepper to the taste 1 and ½ teaspoons cumin, ground

½ cup dark olives, hollowed and cleaved 1 teaspoon oregano, dried

Guidelines:

1.	In a container that accommodates the air fryer cooker, consolidate meat with oil, green ringer peppers, onions, jalapenos, habanero pepper, tomatoes, garlic, water, cilantro, oregano, cumin, salt and pepper, mix, put in the air fryer cooker and cook at 300 Deg. Fahrenheit for about 1 hour and 10 minutes.

2.	Add olives, mix, partition into bowls and serve.

Enjoy the recipe!

The nutritional facts: calories 305, fat 14, fiber 4, carbs 18, protein 25

CREAMY HAM AND CAULIFLOWER MIX

Prep. time: 10 minutes

The cooking time: 4 hours

The recipe servings: 6

Fixings:

8 ounces cheddar, ground 4 cups ham, cubed

14 ounces chicken stock

½ teaspoon garlic powder

½ teaspoon onion powder

Salt and dark pepper to the taste 4 garlic cloves, minced

¼ cup substantial cream

16 ounces cauliflower florets

Guidelines:

1.   In a pot that accommodates the air fryer cooker, blend ham in with stock, cheddar, cauliflower, garlic powder, onion powder, salt, pepper, garlic and substantial cream, mix, put in the air fryer cooker and cook at 300 Deg. Fahrenheit for about 60 minutes.

2.   Divide into bowls and serve.

Enjoy the recipe!

The nutritional facts: calories 320, fat 20, fiber 3, carbs 16, protein 23

AIR FRIED SAUSAGE AND MUSHROOMS

Prep. time: 10 minutes

The cooking time: 40 minutes

The recipe servings: 6

3 red chime peppers, hacked

2 pounds pork hotdog, cut Salt and dark pepper to the taste

2 pounds Portobello mushrooms, cut 2 sweet onions, hacked

1 tablespoon darker sugar 1 teaspoon olive oil

Guidelines:

1.   In a heating dish that accommodates the air fryer cooker, blend frankfurter cuts with oil, salt, pepper, ringer pepper, mushrooms, onion and sugar, hurl, present in the air fryer cooker and cook at 300 Deg. Fahrenheit for about 40 minutes.

2.   Divide among plates and serve immediately.

Enjoy the recipe!

The nutritional facts: calories 130, fat 12, fiber 1, carbs 13, protein 18

HOTDOG AND KALE

Prep. time: 10 minutes

The cooking time: 20 minutes

The recipe servings: 4

1 cup yellow onion, hacked

1 and ½ pound Italian pork hotdog, cut

½ cup red chime pepper, slashed Salt and dark pepper to the taste 5 pounds kale, hacked

1   teaspoon garlic, minced

¼ cup scorching bean stew pepper, hacked 1 cup water

Guidelines:

1.   In a dish that accommodates the air fryer cooker, blend frankfurter in with onion, chime pepper, salt, pepper, kale, garlic, water and stew pepper, hurl, present in preheated air fryer and cook at 300 Deg. Fahrenheit for about 20 minutes.

2.   Divide everything on plates and serve.

Enjoy the recipe!

The nutritional facts: calories 150, fat 4, fiber 1, carbs 12, protein 14

SIRLON STEAKS AND PICO GALLO

Prep. time: 10 minutes

The cooking time: 10 minutes

The recipe servings: 4

2tablespoons bean stew powder 4 medium sirloin steaks

1 teaspoon cumin, ground

½ tablespoon sweet paprika 1 teaspoon onion powder

1 teaspoon garlic powder

Salt and dark pepper to the taste

For the Pico de gallo:

1   small red onion, slashed 2 tomatoes, hacked

1 little green chime pepper, slashed 1 jalapeno, hacked

¼ cup cilantro, hacked

¼ teaspoon cumin, ground

Guidelines:

1.   In a bowl, blend bean stew powder with a touch of salt, dark pepper, onion powder, garlic powder, paprika and 1 teaspoon cumin, mix well, season steaks with this blend, put them in the air fryer cooker and cook at 360 Deg. Fahrenheit for about 10 minutes.

2.   In a bowl, blend red onion in with tomatoes, garlic, lime juice, chime pepper, jalapeno, cilantro, dark pepper to the taste and ¼ teaspoon cumin and hurl.

3.   Top steaks with this blend and serve immediately

Enjoy the recipe!

The nutritional facts: calories 200, fat 12, fiber 4, carbs 15, protein 18

ESPRESSO FLAVORED STEAKS

Prep. time: 10 minutes

The cooking time: 15 minutes

The recipe servings: 4

1 and ½ tablespoons espresso, ground 4 rib eye steaks

½ tablespoon sweet paprika 2 tablespoons bean stew powder 2 teaspoons garlic powder 2 teaspoons onion powder

¼ teaspoon ginger, ground

¼ teaspoon, coriander, ground A touch of cayenne pepper Black pepper to the taste

Guidelines:

1.   In a bowl, blend espresso in with paprika, stew powder, garlic powder, onion powder, ginger, coriander, cayenne and dark pepper, mix, rub steaks with this blend, put in preheated air fryer and cook at 360 Deg. Fahrenheit for about 15 minutes.

2.   Divide steaks on plates and present with a side serving of mixed greens.

Enjoy the recipe!

The nutritional facts: calories 160, fat 10, fiber 8, carbs 14, protein 12

FILET MIGNON AND MUSHROOMS SAUCE

Prep. time: 10 minutes

The cooking time: 25 minutes

The recipe servings: 4

12 mushrooms, cut

1 shallot, cleaved

4 filet mignons

2 tablespoons of olive-oil

¼ cup Dijon mustard

¼ cup wine

1   and ¼ cup coconut cream

2   tablespoons parsley, slashed Salt and dark pepper to the taste

Guidelines:

1.   Heat up a skillet with the oil over medium high heat, include garlic and shallots, mix and cook for 3 minutes.

2.   Add mushrooms, mix and cook for 4 minutes more.

3.   Add wine, mix and cook until it vanishes.

4.   Add coconut cream, mustard, parsley, a spot of salt and dark pepper to the taste, mix, cook for 6 minutes more and take off heat.

5.   Season fillets with salt and pepper, put them in the air fryer cooker and cook at 360 Deg. Fahrenheit for about 10 minutes.

6.   Divide fillets on plates and present with the mushroom sauce on top.

Enjoy the recipe!

The nutritional facts: calories 340, fat 12, fiber 1, carbs 14, protein 23

HAMBURGER KABOBS

Prep. time: 10 minutes The cooking time: 10 minutes The recipe servings: 4

Fixings:

2 red ringer peppers, hacked

2 pounds sirloin steak, cut into medium pieces 1 red onion, slashed

1   zucchini, cut Juice structure 1 lime

2   tablespoons bean stew powder 2 tablespoon hot sauce

½ tablespoons cumin, ground

¼ cup olive oil

¼ cup salsa

Salt and dark pepper to the taste

Guidelines:

1.	In a bowl, blend salsa in with lime juice, oil, hot sauce, stew powder, cumin, salt and dark pepper and whisk well.

2.	Divide meat ringer peppers, zucchini and onion on sticks, brush kabobs with the salsa blend you made before, put them in your preheated air fryer and cook them for 10 minutes at 370 degrees F flipping kabobs midway.

3.	Divide among plates and present with a side serving of mixed greens.

Enjoy the recipe!

The nutritional facts: calories 170, fat 5, fiber 2, carbs 13, protein 16

MEDITERRANEAN STEAKS AND SCALLOPS

Prep. time: 10 minutes The cooking time: 14 minutes The recipe servings: 2

Fixings:

10 ocean scallops

2 meat steaks

4 garlic cloves, minced 1 shallot, hacked

2 tablespoons lemon juice

2 tablespoons parsley, hacked 2 tablespoons basil, slashed

1   teaspoon lemon get-up-and-go

¼ cup spread

¼ cup veggie stock

Salt and dark pepper to the taste

Guidelines:

1.   Season steaks with salt and pepper, put them in the air fryer cooker, cook at 360 Deg. Fahrenheit for about 10 minutes and move to a dish that fits the fryer.

2.   Add shallot, garlic, spread, stock, basil, lemon juice, parsley, lemon pizzazz and scallops, hurl everything delicately and cook at 360 Deg. Fahrenheit for about 4 minutes more.

3.   Divide steaks and scallops on plates and serve.

Enjoy the recipe!

The nutritional facts: calories 150, fat 2, fiber 2, carbs 14, protein 17

MEAT MEDALLIONS MIX

Prep. time: 2 hours The cooking time: 10 minutes The recipe servings: 4

Fixings:

2   teaspoons bean stew powder 1 cup tomatoes, squashed 4 hamburger emblems

2 teaspoons onion powder 2 tablespoons soy sauce

Salt and dark pepper to the taste 1 tablespoons hot pepper

2 tablespoons lime juice

Guidelines:

1.   In a bowl, blend tomatoes in with hot pepper, soy sauce, bean stew powder, onion powder, a spot of salt, dark pepper and lime squeeze and whisk well.

2.   Arrange hamburger emblems in a dish, pour sauce over them, hurl and leave them aside for 2 hours.

3.   Discard tomato marinade, put hamburger in your preheated air fryer and cook at 360 Deg. Fahrenheit for about 10 minutes.

4.   Divide steaks on plates and present with a side serving of mixed greens.

Enjoy the recipe!

The nutritional facts: calories 230, fat 4, fiber 1, carbs 13, protein 14

BALSAMIC BEEF

Prep. time: 10 minutes

The cooking time: 60 minutes

The recipe servings: 6

Fixings:

1 medium hamburger cook

1 tablespoon Worcestershire sauce

½ cup balsamic vinegar 1 cup hamburger stock

1 tablespoons HONNEY

Guidelines:

1.   In a heat verification dish that accommodates the air fryer cooker, blend broil in with cook with Worcestershire sauce, vinegar, stock, HONNEY, soy sauce and garlic, hurl well, present in the air fryer cooker and cook at 370 Deg. Fahrenheit for about 60 minutes.

2.   Slice dish, separate among plates, shower the sauce all finished and serve. Enjoy the recipe!

The nutritional facts: calories 311, fat 7, fiber 12, carbs 20, protein 16

PORK CHOPS AND ROASTED PEPPERS

Prep. time: 10 minutes

The cooking time: 16 minutes

The recipe servings: 4

3 tablespoons olive oil

3 tablespoons lemon juice

1 tablespoon smoked paprika 2 tablespoons thyme, cleaved 3 garlic cloves, minced

4 pork cleaves, bone in

Salta and dark pepper to the taste 2 cooked ringer peppers, cleaved

Guidelines:

1.   In a container that accommodates the air fryer cooker, blend pork slashes with oil, lemon juice, smoked paprika, thyme, garlic, ringer peppers, salt and pepper, hurl well, present in the air fryer cooker and cook at 400 Deg. Fahrenheit for about 16 minutes.

2.   Divide pork slashes and peppers blend on plates and serve immediately. Enjoy the recipe!

The nutritional facts: calories 321, fat 6, fiber 8, carbs 14, protein 17

PORK CHOPS AND GREEN BEANS

Prep. time: 10 minutes

The cooking time: 15 minutes

The recipe servings: 4

4 pork slashes, bone in 2 tablespoons olive oil

1 tablespoon savvy, hacked

Salt and dark pepper to the taste 16 ounces green beans

3 garlic cloves, minced

2 tablespoons parsley, slashed

Guidelines:

1.   In a skillet that accommodates the air fryer cooker, blend pork hacks with olive oil, savvy, salt, pepper, green beans, garlic and parsley, hurl, present in the air fryer cooker and cook at 360 Deg. Fahrenheit for about 15 minutes.

2.   Divide everything on plates and serve. Enjoy the recipe!

The nutritional facts: calories 261, fat 7, fiber 9, carbs 14, protein 20

PORK CHOPS AND SAGE SAUCE

Prep. time: 10 minutes

The cooking time: 15 minutes

The recipe servings: 4

2 pork slashes

Salt and dark pepper to the taste 1 tablespoon of olive oil

2 tablespoons margarine

1 shallot, cut

1   handful savvy, cleaved 1 teaspoon lemon juice

Guidelines:

1.   Season pork slashes with salt and pepper, rub with the oil, put in the air fryer cooker and cook at 370 Deg. Fahrenheit for about 10 minutes, flipping them midway.

2.   Meanwhile, heat up a skillet with the spread over medium heat, include shallot, mix and cook for 2 minutes.

3.   Add sage and lemon juice, mix well, cook for a couple of more minutes and take off heat.

4.   Divide pork slashes on plates, sprinkle sage sauce all finished and serve. Enjoy the recipe!

The nutritional facts: calories 265, fat 6, fiber 8, carbs 19, protein 12

DELICIOUS HAM AND GREENS

Prep. time: 10 minutes

The cooking time: 16 minutes

The recipe servings: 8

2tablespoons olive oil 4 cups ham, hacked 2 tablespoons flour

2   cups chicken stock

5 ounces onion, hacked

16 ounces collard greens, hacked

14 ounces canned dark looked at peas, depleted

½ teaspoon red pepper, squashed

Guidelines:

1.   Drizzle the oil in a dish that accommodates the air fryer cooker, include ham, stock and flour and whisk.

2.   Also include onion, dark looked at peas, red pepper and collard greens, present in the air fryer cooker and cook at 390 Deg. Fahrenheit for about 16 minutes.

3.   Divide everything on plates and serve. Enjoy the recipe!

The nutritional facts: calories 322, fat 6, fiber 8, carbs 12, protein 5

HAM AND VEGGIE AIR FRIED MIX

Prep. time: 10 minutes

The cooking time: 20 minutes

The recipe servings: 6

¼ cup spread

¼ cup flour 3 cups milk

½ teaspoon thyme, dried 2 cups ham, hacked

6 ounces sweet peas

4 ounces mushrooms, split 1 cup child carrots

Guidelines:

1.   Heat up a huge dish that accommodates the air fryer cooker with the margarine over medium heat, dissolve it, include flour and whisk well.

2.   Add milk and, well again and take off heat.

3.   Add thyme, ham, peas, mushrooms and child carrots, hurl, put in the air fryer cooker and cook at 360 Deg. Fahrenheit for about 20 minutes.

4.   Divide everything on plates and serve. Enjoy the recipe!

The nutritional facts: calories 311, fat 6, fiber 8, carbs 12, protein 7

AIR FRYER VEGETABLE RECIPES

SPINACH PIE

Prep. time: 10 minutes The cooking time: 15 minutes The recipe servings: 4

Fixings:

7 ounces flour

2 tablespoons spread 7ounces spinach

1   tablespoon of olive oil 2 eggs

2   tablespoons milk

3   ounces curds

Salt and dark pepper to the taste 1 yellow onion, hacked

Guidelines:

1.   In your food processor, blend flour in with spread, 1 egg, milk, salt and pepper, mix well, move to a bowl, massage, spread and leave for 10 minutes.

2.   Heat up a container with the oil over medium high heat, include onion and spinach, mix and cook for 2 minutes.

3.   Add salt, pepper, the rest of the egg and curds, mix well and take off heat.

4.   Divide mixture in 4 pieces, roll each piece, place on the base of a ramekin, include spinach filling over batter, place ramekins in the air fryer cooker's container and cook at 360 Deg. Fahrenheit for about 15 minutes.

5.   Serve warm,

Enjoy the recipe!

The nutritional facts: calories 250, fat 12, fiber 2, carbs 23, protein 12

BALSAMIC ARTICHOKES

Prep. time: 10 minutes The cooking time: 7 minutes The recipe servings: 4

Fixings:

4   big artichokes, cut

Salt and dark pepper to the taste 2 tablespoons lemon juice

¼ cup additional virgin olive oil

2 teaspoons of the balsamic vinegar

1 teaspoon of oregano, dried

2 garlic cloves, minced

Guidelines:

1.   Season the artichokes with pepper, then rub them with half of the oil and half of the lemon juice, put them in the air fryer cooker and cook at 360 Deg. Fahrenheit for about 7 minutes.

2.   Meanwhile, in a bowl, blend the remainder of the lemon juice with vinegar, the rest of the oil, salt, pepper, garlic and oregano and mix quite well.

3.   Arrange artichokes on a platter, shower the balsamic vinaigrette over them and serve.

Enjoy the recipe!

The nutritional facts: calories 200, fat 3, fiber 6, carbs 12, protein 4

CHEESY ARTICHOKES

Prep. time: 10 minutes The cooking time: 6 minutes The recipe servings: 6

Fixings:

14 ounces canned artichoke hearts 8 ounces cream cheddar

16 ounces parmesan cheddar, ground 10 ounces spinach

½ cup chicken stock

8 ounces mozzarella, destroyed

½ cup acrid cream

3 garlic cloves, minced

½ cup mayonnaise

1   teaspoon onion powder

Guidelines:

1.   In a container that accommodates the air fryer cooker, blend artichokes in with stock, garlic, spinach, cream cheddar, sharp cream, onion powder and mayo, hurl, present in the air fryer cooker and cook at 350 Deg. Fahrenheit for about 6 minutes.

2.   Add mozzarella and parmesan, mix well and serve.

Enjoy the recipe!

The nutritional facts: calories 261, fat 12, fiber 2, carbs 12, protein 15

ARTICHOKES AND SPECIAL SAUCE

Prep. time: 10 minutes The cooking time: 6 minutes The recipe servings: 2

Fixings:

2   artichokes, cut A sprinkle of olive oil

2 garlic cloves, minced

1 tablespoon lemon juice

For the sauce:

¼ cup coconut oil

¼ cup additional virgin olive oil 3 anchovy fillets

3   garlic cloves

Guidelines:

1.   In a bowl, blend artichokes in with oil, 2 garlic cloves and lemon juice, hurl well, move to the air fryer cooker, cook at 350 Deg. Fahrenheit for about 6 minutes and separation among plates.

2.   In your food processor, blend coconut oil with anchovy, 3 garlic cloves and olive oil, mix quite well, shower over artichokes and serve.

Enjoy the recipe!

The nutritional facts: calories 261, fat 4, fiber 7, carbs 20, protein 12

BEET SALAD AND PARSLEY DRESSING

Prep. time: 10 minutes

The cooking time: 14 minutes

The recipe servings: 4

4beets

2 tablespoons balsamic vinegar A lot of parsley, hacked Salt and dark pepper to the taste

1   tablespoon additional virgin olive oil 1 garlic clove, hacked

2   tablespoons tricks

Guidelines:

1.   Put beets in the air fryer cooker and cook them at 360 Deg. Fahrenheit for about 14 minutes.

2.   Meanwhile, in a bowl, blend parsley in with garlic, salt, pepper, olive oil and tricks and mix quite well.

3.   Transfer beets to a cutting load up, leave them to chill off, strip them, cut put them in a serving of mixed greens bowl.

4.   Add vinegar, sprinkle the parsley dressing all finished and serve.

Enjoy the recipe!

The nutritional facts: calories 70, fat 2, fiber 1, carbs 6, protein 4

BEETS AND BLUE CHEESE SALAD

Prep. time: 10 minutes

The cooking time: 14 minutes

The recipe servings: 6

6beets, stripped and quartered Salt and dark pepper to the taste

¼ cup blue cheddar, disintegrated 1 tablespoon of olive oil

Guidelines:

1.   Put beets in the air fryer cooker, cook them at 350 Deg. Fahrenheit for about 14 minutes and move them to a bowl.

2.   Add blue cheddar, salt, pepper and oil, hurl and serve.

Enjoy the recipe!

The nutritional facts: calories 100, fat 4, fiber 4, carbs 10, protein 5

BEETS AND ARGULA SALAD

Prep. time: 10 minutes

The cooking time: 10 minutes

The recipe servings: 4

1and ½ pounds beets, stripped and quartered A sprinkle of olive oil

1   teaspoons orange pizzazz, ground 2 tablespoons juice vinegar

½ cup squeezed orange

2 tablespoons dark colored sugar 2 scallions, hacked

2 teaspoons mustard

2 cups arugula

Guidelines:

1.   Rub beets with the oil and squeezed orange, place them in the air fryer cooker and cook at 350 Deg. Fahrenheit for about 10 minutes.

2.   Transfer beet quarters to a bowl, include scallions, arugula and orange pizzazz and hurl.

3.   In a different bowl, blend sugar in with mustard and vinegar, whisk well, add to plate of mixed greens, hurl and serve.

Enjoy the recipe!

The nutritional facts: calories 121, fat 2, fiber 3, carbs 11, protein 4

BEET, TOMATO AND GOAT CHEESE MIX

Prep. time: 30 minutes

The cooking time: 14 minutes

The recipe servings: 8

8 little beets, cut, stripped and divided 1 red onion, cut

4 ounces goat cheddar, disintegrated 1 tablespoon balsamic vinegar Salt and dark pepper to the taste 2 tablespoons sugar

1   pint blended cherry tomatoes, divided 2 ounces walnuts

2   tablespoons olive oil

Guidelines:

1.   Put beets in the air fryer cooker, season them with salt and pepper, cook at 350 Deg. Fahrenheit for about 14 minutes and move to a serving of mixed greens bowl.

2.   Add onion, cherry tomatoes and walnuts and hurl.

3.   In another bowl, blend vinegar in with sugar and oil, whisk well until sugar breaks up and add to serving of mixed greens.

4.   Also include goat cheddar, hurl and serve.

Enjoy the recipe!

The nutritional facts: calories 124, fat 7, fiber 5, carbs 12, protein 6

BROCCOLI SALAD

Prep. time: 10 minutes

The cooking time: 8 minutes

The recipe servings: 4

Fixings:

1 broccoli head, florets isolated 1 tablespoon nut oil

6 garlic cloves, minced

1 tablespoon of the chinese rice wine vinegar Salt and dark pepper to the taste

Guidelines:

1.   In a bowl, blend broccoli in with salt, pepper and half of the oil, hurl, move to the air fryer cooker and cook at 350 Deg. Fahrenheit for about 8 minutes, shaking the fryer midway.

2.   Transfer broccoli to a plate of mixed greens bowl, include the remainder of the nut oil, garlic and rice vinegar, hurl truly well and serve.

Enjoy the recipe!

The nutritional facts: calories 121, fat 3, fiber 4, carbs 4, protein 4

BRUSSELS SPROUTS AND TOMATOES MIX

Prep. time: 5 minutes

The cooking time: 10 minutes

The recipe servings: 4

Salt and dark pepper to the taste 6 cherry tomatoes, split

¼ cup green onions, cleaved 1 tablespoon of olive oil

Guidelines:

1.   Season Brussels grows with salt and pepper, put them in the air fryer cooker and cook at 350 Deg. Fahrenheit for about 10 minutes.

2.   Transfer them to a bowl, include salt, pepper, cherry tomatoes, green onions and olive oil, hurl well and serve.

Enjoy the recipe!

The nutritional facts: calories 121, fat 4, fiber 4, carbs 11, protein 4

BRUSSELS SPROUTS AND BUTTER SAUCE

Prep. time: 4 minutes

The cooking time: 10 minutes

The recipe servings: 4

Salt and dark pepper to the taste

½ cup bacon, cooked and hacked 1 tablespoon mustard

1   tablespoon spread

2   tablespoons dill, finely hacked

Guidelines:

1.   Put Brussels grows in the air fryer cooker and cook them at 350 Deg. Fahrenheit for about 10 minutes.

2.   Heat up a dish with the spread over medium high heat, include bacon, mustard and dill and whisk well.

3.   Divide Brussels grows on plates, shower spread sauce all finished and serve.

Enjoy the recipe!

The nutritional facts: calories 162, fat 8, fiber 8, carbs 14, protein 5

MUSHY BRUSSELS SPROUTS

Prep. time: 10 minutes The cooking time: 8 minutes The recipe servings: 4

Fixings:

1 pound Brussels grows, washed Juice of 1 lemon

Salt and dark pepper to the taste 2 tablespoons margarine

3 tablespoons parmesan, ground

Guidelines:

1.   Put Brussels grows in the air fryer cooker, cook them at 350 Deg. Fahrenheit for about 8 minutes and move them to a bowl.

2.   Heat up a container with the margarine over medium heat, include lemon squeeze, salt and pepper, whisk well and add to Brussels grows.

3.   Add parmesan, hurl until parmesan melts and serve.

Enjoy the recipe!

The nutritional facts: calories 152, fat 6, fiber 6, carbs 8, protein 12

FIERY CABBAGE

Prep. time: 10 minutes

The cooking time: 8 minutes

The recipe servings: 4

Fixings:

1 cabbage, cut into 8 wedges 1 tablespoon sesame seed oil 1 carrots, ground

¼ cup apple juice vinegar

¼ cups squeezed apple

½ teaspoon cayenne pepper

1   teaspoon red pepper drops, squashed

Guidelines:

1.   In a skillet that accommodates the air fryer cooker, join cabbage with oil, carrot, vinegar, squeezed apple, cayenne and pepper chips, hurl, present in preheated air fryer and cook at 350 Deg. Fahrenheit for about 8 minutes.

2.   Divide cabbage blend on plates and serve.

Enjoy the recipe!

The nutritional facts: calories 100, fat 4, fiber 2, carbs 11, protein 7

SWEET BABY CARROTS DISH

Prep. time: 10 minutes

The cooking time: 10 minutes

The recipe servings: 4

2cups infant carrots

A spot of salt and dark pepper 1 tablespoon darker sugar

½ tablespoon margarine, softened

Guidelines:

3.   In a dish that accommodates the air fryer cooker, blend infant carrots with margarine, salt, pepper and sugar, hurl, present in the air fryer cooker and cook at 350 Deg. Fahrenheit for about 10 minutes.

4.   Divide among plates and serve.

Enjoy the recipe!

The nutritional facts: calories 100, fat 2, fiber 3, carbs 7, protein 4

COLLARD GREENS MIX

Prep. time: 10 minutes

The cooking time: 10 minutes

The recipe servings: 4

1   1bunch collard greens, cut 2 tablespoons olive oil

2   tablespoons tomato puree 1 yellow onion, hacked

3   garlic cloves, minced

Salt and dark pepper to the taste 1 tablespoon balsamic vinegar

1 teaspoon sugar

Guidelines:

1.   In a dish that accommodates the air fryer cooker, blend oil, garlic, vinegar, onion and tomato puree and whisk.

2.   Add collard greens, salt, pepper and sugar, hurl, present in the air fryer cooker and cook at 320 Deg. Fahrenheit for about 10 minutes.

3.   Divide collard greens blend on plates and serve.

Enjoy the recipe!

The nutritional facts: calories 121, fat 3, fiber 3, carbs 7, protein 3

COLLARD GREENS AND TURKEY WINGS

Prep. time: 10 minutes

The cooking time: 20 minutes

The recipe servings: 6

Fixings:

1   sweet onion, hacked 2 smoked turkey wings 2 tablespoons olive oil 3 garlic cloves, minced

2   and ½ pounds collard greens, hacked Salt and dark pepper to the taste

2 tablespoons apple juice vinegar 1 tablespoon dark colored sugar

½ teaspoon squashed red pepper

Guidelines:

1.   Heat up a dish that accommodates the air fryer cooker with the oil over medium high heat, include onions, mix and cook for 2 minutes.

2.   Add garlic, greens, vinegar, salt, pepper, squashed red pepper, sugar and smoked turkey, present in preheated air fryer and cook at 350 Deg. Fahrenheit for about 15 minutes.

3.   Divide greens and turkey on plates and serve.

Enjoy the recipe!

The nutritional facts: calories 262, fat 4, fiber 8, carbs 12, protein 4

HERBED EGGPLANT AND ZUCCHINI MIX

Prep. time: 10 minutes

The cooking time: 8 minutes

The recipe servings: 4

Fixings:

1 eggplant, generally cubed 3 zucchinis, generally cubed 2 tablespoons lemon juice

Salt and dark pepper to the taste 1 teaspoon thyme, dried

1   teaspoon oregano, dried 3 tablespoons olive oil

Guidelines:

1.   Put eggplant in a dish that accommodates the air fryer cooker, include zucchinis, lemon juice, salt, pepper, thyme, oregano and olive oil, hurl, present in the air fryer cooker and cook at 360 Deg. Fahrenheit for about 8 minutes.

2.   Divide among plates and serve immediately.

Enjoy the recipe!

The nutritional facts: calories 152, fat 5, fiber 7, carbs 19, protein 5

SEASONED FENNEL

Prep. time: 10 minutes

The cooking time: 8 minutes

The recipe servings: 4

Fixings:

2   fennel bulbs, cut into quarters 3 tablespoons olive oil

Salt and dark pepper to the taste 1 garlic clove, minced

1 red bean stew pepper, hacked

¾ cup veggie stock Juice from ½ lemon

¼ cup white wine

¼ cup parmesan, ground

Guidelines:

1.   Heat up a container that accommodates the air fryer cooker with the oil over medium high heat, include garlic and stew pepper, mix and cook for 2 minutes.

2.   Add fennel, salt, pepper, stock, wine, lemon juice, and parmesan, hurl to cover, present in the air fryer cooker and cook at 350 Deg. Fahrenheit for about 6 minutes.

3.   Divide among plates and serve immediately.

Enjoy the recipe!

The nutritional facts: calories 100, fat 4, fiber 8, carbs 4, protein 4

OKRA AND CORN SALAD

Prep. time: 10 minutes

The cooking time: 12 minutes

The recipe servings: 6

Fixings:

1 pound okra, cut 6 scallions, slashed

3 green ringer peppers, slashed Salt and dark pepper to the taste 2 tablespoons olive oil

1 teaspoon sugar

28 ounces canned tomatoes, slashed 1 cup con

Guidelines:

1.   Heat up a skillet that accommodates the air fryer cooker with the oil over medium high heat, include scallions and ringer peppers, mix and cook for 5 minutes.

2.   Add okra, salt, pepper, sugar, tomatoes and corn, mix, present in the air fryer cooker and cook at 360 Deg. Fahrenheit for about 7 minutes.

3.   Divide okra blend on plates and serve warm.

Enjoy the recipe!

The nutritional facts: calories 152, fat 4, fiber 3, carbs 18, protein 4

AIR FRIED LEEKS

Prep. time: 10 minutes

The cooking time: 7 minutes

The recipe servings: 4

Fixings:

4 leeks, washed, closes cut off and divided Salt and dark pepper to the taste

1 tablespoon margarine, softened 1 tablespoon lemon juice

Guidelines:

1.   Rub leeks with dissolved spread, season with salt and pepper, put in the air fryer cooker and cook at 350 Deg. Fahrenheit for about 7 minutes.

2.   Arrange on a platter, shower lemon squeeze all finished and serve.

Enjoy the recipe!

The nutritional facts: calories 100, fat 4, fiber 2, carbs 6, protein 2

FIRM POTATOES AND PARSLEY

Prep. time: 10 minutes

The cooking time: 10 minutes

The recipe servings: 4

Fixings:

1   pound gold potatoes, cut into wedges Salt and dark pepper to the taste

2   tablespoons olive Juice from ½ lemon

¼ cup parsley leaves, hacked

Guidelines:

1.   Rub potatoes with salt, pepper, lemon juice and olive oil, put them in the air fryer cooker and cook at 350 Deg. Fahrenheit for about 10 minutes.

2.   Divide among plates, sprinkle parsley on top and serve.

Enjoy the recipe!

The nutritional facts: calories 152, fat 3, fiber 7, carbs 17, protein 4

INDIAN TURNIPS SALAD

Prep. time: 10 minutes

The cooking time: 12 minutes

The recipe servings: 4

20 ounces turnips, stripped and slashed 1 teaspoon garlic, minced

1 teaspoon ginger, ground 2 yellow onions, slashed 2 tomatoes, cleaved

1 teaspoon cumin, ground

1 teaspoon coriander, ground 2 green chilies, slashed

½ teaspoon turmeric powder 2 tablespoons margarine

Salt and dark pepper to the taste

A bunch coriander leaves, slashed

Guidelines:

1.   Heat up a skillet that accommodates the air fryer cooker with the margarine, liquefy it, include green chilies, garlic and ginger, mix and cook for 1 moment.

2.   Add onions, salt, pepper, tomatoes, turmeric, cumin, ground coriander and turnips, mix, present in the air fryer cooker and cook at 350 Deg. Fahrenheit for about 10 minutes.

3.   Divide among plates, sprinkle new coriander on top and serve.

Enjoy the recipe!

The nutritional facts: calories 100, fat 3, fiber 6, carbs 12, protein 4

STRAIGHTFORWARD STUFFED TOMATOES

Prep. time: 10 minutes

The cooking time: 15 minutes

The recipe servings: 4

4 tomatoes, finishes cut off and mash scooped and hacked Salt and dark pepper to the taste

1   yellow onion, cleaved 1 tablespoon spread

2   tablespoons celery, cleaved

½ cup mushrooms, cleaved 1 tablespoon bread pieces 1 cup curds

¼ teaspoon caraway seeds

1 tablespoon parsley, cleaved

Guidelines:

1.   Heat up a container with the spread over medium heat, liquefy it, include onion and celery, mix and cook for 3 minutes.

2.   Add tomato mash and mushrooms, mix and cook for brief more.

3.   Add salt, pepper, disintegrated bread, cheddar, caraway seeds and parsley, mix, cook for 4 minutes more and take off heat.

4.   Stuff tomatoes with this blend, place them in the air fryer cooker and cook at 350 Deg. Fahrenheit for about 8 minutes.

5.   Divide stuffed tomatoes on plates and serve.

Enjoy the recipe!

The nutritional facts: calories 143, fat 4, fiber 6, carbs 4, protein 4

INDIAN POTATOES

Prep. time: 10 minutes

The cooking time: 12 minutes

The recipe servings: 4

1 tablespoon of the coriander seeds

1 tablespoon of the cumin seeds

Salt and dark pepper to the taste

½ teaspoon turmeric powder

½ teaspoon red bean stew powder

1 teaspoon pomegranate powder

1 tablespoon cured mango, hacked 2 teaspoons fenugreek, dried

5 potatoes, bubbled, stripped and cubed 2 tablespoons olive oil

Guidelines:

1.	Heat up a container that accommodates the air fryer cooker with the oil over medium heat, include coriander and cumin seeds, mix and cook for 2 minutes.

2.	Add salt, pepper, turmeric, bean stew powder, pomegranate powder, mango, fenugreek and potatoes, hurl, present in the air fryer cooker and cook at 360 Deg. Fahrenheit for about 10 minutes.

3.	Divide among plates and serve hot. Enjoy the recipe!

The nutritional facts: calories 251, fat 7, fiber 4, carbs 12, protein 7

BROCCOLI AND TOMATOES AIR FRIED STEW

Prep. time: 10 minutes

The cooking time: 20 minutes

The recipe servings: 4

1 broccoli head, florets isolated 2 teaspoons coriander seeds

1 tablespoon of olive oil

1 yellow onion, hacked

Salt and dark pepper to the taste A touch of red pepper, squashed

1 little ginger piece, hacked 1 garlic clove, minced

28 ounces canned tomatoes, pureed

Guidelines:

1.   Heat up a dish that accommodates the air fryer cooker with the oil over medium heat, include onions, salt, pepper and red pepper, mix and cook for 7 minutes.

2.   Add ginger, garlic, coriander seeds, tomatoes and broccoli, mix, present in the air fryer cooker and cook at 360 Deg. Fahrenheit for about 12 minutes.

3.   Divide into bowls and serve.

Enjoy the recipe!

The nutritional facts: calories 150, fat 4, fiber 2, carbs 7, protein 12

COLLARD GREENS AND BACON

Prep. time: 10 minutes

The cooking time: 12 minutes

The recipe servings: 4

1pound collard greens 3 bacon strips, hacked

¼ cup cherry tomatoes, split 1 tablespoon apple juice vinegar 2 tablespoons chicken stock

Salt and dark pepper to the taste

Guidelines:

1.   Heat up a dish that accommodates the air fryer cooker over medium heat, include bacon, mix and cook 1-2 minutes

2.   Add tomatoes, collard greens, vinegar, stock, salt and pepper, mix, present in the air fryer cooker and cook at 320 Deg. Fahrenheit for about 10 minutes.

3.   Divide among plates and serve.

Enjoy the recipe!

The nutritional facts: calories 120, fat 3, fiber 1, carbs 3, protein 7

SESAME MUSTARD GREENS

Prep. time: 10 minutes

The cooking time: 11 minutes

The recipe servings: 4

2garlic cloves, minced

1 pound mustard greens, torn 1 tablespoon of olive oil

½ cup yellow onion, cut

Salt and dark pepper to the taste 3 tablespoons veggie stock

¼ teaspoon dull sesame oil

Guidelines:

1.   Heat up a dish that accommodates the air fryer cooker with the oil over medium heat, include onions, mix and dark colored them for 5 minutes.

2.   Add garlic, stock, greens, salt and pepper, mix, present in the air fryer cooker and cook at 350 Deg. Fahrenheit for about 6 minutes.

3.   Add sesame oil, hurl to cover, separate among plates and serve.

Enjoy the recipe!

The nutritional facts: calories 120, fat 3, fiber 1, carbs 3, protein 7

RADISH HASH

Prep. time: 10 minutes

The cooking time: 7 minutes

The recipe servings: 4

Fixings:

½ teaspoon onion powder 1 pound radishes, cut

½ teaspoon garlic powder

Salt and dark pepper to the taste 4 eggs

1/3 cup parmesan, ground

Guidelines:

1.   In a bowl, blend radishes in with salt, pepper, onion and garlic powder, eggs and parmesan and mix well.

2.   Transfer radishes to a container that accommodates the air fryer cooker and cook at 350 Deg. Fahrenheit for about 7 minutes.

3.   Divide hash on plates and serve.

Enjoy the recipe!

The nutritional facts: calories 80, fat 5, fiber 2, carbs 5, protein 7

DELIGHTFUL ZUCCHINI MIX

Prep. time: 10 minutes

The cooking time: 14 minutes

The recipe servings: 6

6 zucchinis, split and afterward cut Salt and dark pepper to the taste 1 tablespoon margarine

1   teaspoon oregano, dried

½ cup yellow onion, cleaved 3 garlic cloves, minced

2   ounces parmesan, ground

¾ cup overwhelming cream

Guidelines:

1.   Heat up a container that accommodates the air fryer cooker with the spread over medium high heat, include onion, mix and cook for 4 minutes.

2.   Add garlic, zucchinis, oregano, salt, pepper and overwhelming cream, hurl, present in the air fryer cooker and cook at 350 Deg. Fahrenheit for about 10 minutes.

3.   Add parmesan, mix, partition among plates and serve.

Enjoy the recipe!

The nutritional facts: calories 160, fat 4, fiber 2, carbs 8, protein 8

SWISS CHARD AND SAUSAGE

Prep. time: 10 minutes

The cooking time: 20 minutes

The recipe servings: 8

8 cups Swiss chard, cleaved

½ cup onion, cleaved 1 tablespoon of olive oil 1 garlic clove, minced

Salt and dark pepper to the taste 3 eggs

2 cups ricotta cheddar

1 cup mozzarella, destroyed A spot of nutmeg

¼ cup parmesan, ground

1 pound wiener, hacked

Guidelines:

1.   Heat up a skillet that accommodates the air fryer cooker with the oil over medium heat, include onions, garlic, Swiss chard, salt, pepper and nutmeg, mix, cook for 2 minutes and take off heat.

2.   In a bowl, whisk eggs with mozzarella, parmesan and ricotta, mix, pour over Swiss chard blend, hurl, present in the air fryer cooker and cook at 320 Deg. Fahrenheit for about 17 minutes.

3.   Divide among plates and serve.

Enjoy the recipe!

The nutritional facts: calories 332, fat 13, fiber 3, carbs 14, protein 23

SWISS CHARD SALAD

Prep. time: 10 minutes

The cooking time: 13 minutes

The recipe servings: 4

1 bundle Swiss chard, torn 2 tablespoons olive oil

1 little yellow onion, slashed A spot of red pepper chips

¼ cup pine nuts, toasted

¼ cup raisins

1 tablespoon balsamic vinegar Salt and dark pepper to the taste

Guidelines:

1.   Heat up a skillet that accommodates the air fryer cooker with the oil over medium heat, include chard and onions, mix and cook for 5 minutes.

2.   Add salt, pepper, pepper drops, raisins, pine nuts and vinegar, mix, present in the air fryer cooker and cook at 350 Deg. Fahrenheit for about 8 minutes.

3.   Divide among plates and serve.

Enjoy the recipe!

The nutritional facts: calories 120, fat 2, fiber 1, carbs 8, protein 8

SPANISH GREENS

Prep. time: 10 minutes

The cooking time: 8 minutes

The recipe servings: 4

Fixings:

1 apple, cored and slashed 1 yellow onion, cut

3 tablespoons olive oil

¼ cup raisins

6 garlic cloves, slashed

¼ cup pine nuts, toasted

¼ cup balsamic vinegar

5 cups blended spinach and chard Salt and dark pepper to the taste A spot of nutmeg

Guidelines:

1.   Heat up a skillet that accommodates the air fryer cooker with the oil over medium high heat, include onion, mix and cook for 3 minutes.

2.   Add apple, garlic, raisins, vinegar, blended spinach and chard, nutmeg, salt and pepper, mix, present in preheated air fryer and cook at 350 Deg. Fahrenheit for about 5 minutes.

3.   Divide between the plates, and sprinkle pine nuts on top and serve.

Enjoy the recipe!

The nutritional facts: calories 120, fat 1, fiber 2, carbs 3, protein 6

ENHANCED AIR FRIED TOMATOES

Prep. time: 10 minutes

The cooking time: 15

The recipe servings: 8

Fixings:

1   jalapeno pepper, slashed 4 garlic cloves, minced

2   pounds cherry tomatoes, divided Salt and dark pepper to the taste

¼ cup olive oil

½ teaspoon oregano, dried

¼ cup basil, slashed

½ cup parmesan, ground

Guidelines:

1.   In a bowl, blend tomatoes in with garlic, jalapeno, season with salt, pepper and oregano and sprinkle the oil, hurl to cover, present in the air fryer cooker and cook at 380 Deg. Fahrenheit for about 15 minutes.

2.   Transfer tomatoes to a bowl, include basil and parmesan, hurl and serve. Enjoy the recipe!

The nutritional facts: calories 140, fat 2, fiber 2, carbs 6, protein 8

ITALIAN EGGPLANT STEW

Prep. time: 10 minutes

The cooking time: 15 minutes

The recipe servings: 4

Fixings:

1   red onion, hacked

2   garlic cloves, hacked 1 bundle parsley, slashed

Salt and dark pepper to the taste 1 teaspoon oregano, dried

2 eggplants, cut into medium pieces 2 tablespoons olive oil

2 tablespoons tricks, slashed

1 bunch green olives, hollowed and cut 5 tomatoes, hacked

3 tablespoons herb vinegar

Guidelines:

1.   Heat up a dish that accommodates the air fryer cooker with the oil over medium heat, include eggplant, oregano, salt and pepper, mix and cook for 5 minutes.

2.   Add garlic, onion, parsley, tricks, olives, vinegar and tomatoes, mix, present in the air fryer cooker and cook at 360 Deg. Fahrenheit for about 15 minutes.

3.   Divide into bowls and serve.

Enjoy the recipe!

The nutritional facts: calories 170, fat 13, fiber 3, carbs 5, protein 7

RUTABAGA AND CHERRY TOMATOES MIX

Prep. time: 10 minutes The cooking time: 15 minutes The recipe servings: 4

Fixings:

1 tablespoon shallot, hacked 1 garlic clove, minced

¾ cup cashews, splashed for a few hours and depleted 2 tablespoons The nutritional factsal yeast

½ cup veggie stock

Salt and dark pepper to the taste 2 teaspoons lemon juice

For the pasta:

1   cup cherry tomatoes, divided 5 teaspoons olive oil

¼ teaspoon garlic powder

2   rutabagas, stripped and cut into thick noodles

Guidelines:

1.   Place tomatoes and rutabaga noodles into a container that accommodates the air fryer cooker, shower the oil over them, season with salt, dark pepper and garlic powder, hurl to cover and cook in the air fryer cooker at 350 Deg. Fahrenheit for about 15 minutes.

2.   Meanwhile, in a food processor, blend garlic in with shallots, cashews, veggie stock, The nutritional factsal yeast, lemon squeeze, a spot of ocean salt and dark pepper to the taste and mix well.

3.   Divide rutabaga pasta on plates, top with tomatoes, sprinkle the sauce over them and serve.

Enjoy the recipe!

The nutritional facts: calories 160, fat 2, fiber 5, carbs 10, protein 8

GARLIC TOMATOES

Prep. time: 10 minutes

The cooking time: 15 minutes

The recipe servings: 4

4 garlic cloves, squashed

1 pound blended cherry tomatoes 3 thyme springs, hacked

Salt and dark pepper to the taste

¼ cup olive oil

Guidelines:

1.   In a bowl, blend tomatoes in with salt, dark pepper, garlic, olive oil and thyme, hurl to cover, present in the air fryer cooker and cook at 360 Deg. Fahrenheit for about 15 minutes.

2.   Divide tomatoes blend on plates and serve.

Enjoy the recipe!

The nutritional facts: calories 100, fat 0, fiber 1, carbs 1, protein 6

TOMATO AND BASIL TART

Prep. time: 10 minutes

The cooking time: 14 minutes

The recipe servings: 2

1 bundle basil, hacked 4 eggs

1   garlic clove, minced

Salt and dark pepper to the taste

½ cup cherry tomatoes, divided

¼ cup cheddar, ground

Guidelines:

1.   In a bowl, blend eggs in with salt, dark pepper, cheddar and basil and whisk well.

2.   Pour this into a heating dish that accommodates the air fryer cooker, mastermind tomatoes on top, present in the fryer and cook at 320 Deg. Fahrenheit for about 14 minutes.

3.   Slice and serve immediately.

Enjoy the recipe!

The nutritional facts: calories 140, fat 1, fiber 1, carbs 2, protein 10

ZUCCHINI NOODLES DELIGHT

Prep. time: 10 minutes

The cooking time: 20 minutes

The recipe servings: 6

2tablespoons olive oil

2   zucchinis, cut with a spiralizer 16 ounces mushrooms, cut

¼ cup sun dried tomatoes, cleaved 1 teaspoon garlic, minced

½ cup cherry tomatoes, divided 2 cups tomatoes sauce

2 cups spinach, torn

Salt and dark pepper to the taste A bunch basil, cleaved

Guidelines:

1.   Put zucchini noodles in a bowl, season salt and dark pepper and leave them aside for 10 minutes.

2.   Heat up a container that accommodates the air fryer cooker with the oil over medium high heat, include garlic, mix and cook for 1 moment.

3.   Add mushrooms, sun dried tomatoes, cherry tomatoes, spinach, cayenne, sauce and zucchini noodles, mix, present in the air fryer cooker and cook at 320 Deg. Fahrenheit for about 10 minutes.

4.   Divide among plates and present with basil sprinkled on top.

Enjoy the recipe!

The nutritional facts: calories 120, fat 1, fiber 1, carbs 2, protein 9

BASIC TOMATOES AND BELL PEPPER SAUCE

Prep. time: 10 minutes

The cooking time: 15 minutes

The recipe servings: 4

2 red ringer peppers, slashed 2 garlic cloves, minced

1 pound cherry tomatoes, divided 1 teaspoon rosemary, dried

3 straight leaves

2 tablespoons olive oil

1 tablespoon balsamic vinegar Salt and dark pepper to the taste

Guidelines:

1.   In a bowl blend tomatoes in with garlic, salt, dark pepper, rosemary, straight leaves, half of the oil and half of the vinegar, hurl to cover, present in the air fryer cooker and meal them at 320 Deg. Fahrenheit for about 15 minutes.

2.   Meanwhile, in your food processor, blend ringer peppers with a spot of ocean salt, dark pepper, the remainder of the oil and the remainder of the vinegar and mix well indeed.

3.   Divide cooked tomatoes on plates, shower the chime peppers sauce over them and serve.

Enjoy the recipe!

The nutritional facts: calories 123, fat 1, fiber 1, carbs 8, protein 10

CHERRY TOMATOES SKEWERS

Prep. time: 10 minutes

The cooking time: 6 minutes

The recipe servings: 4

Fixings:

3 tablespoons balsamic vinegar 24 cherry tomatoes

1 tablespoons thyme, cleaved Salt and dark pepper to the taste

For the dressing:

2   tablespoons balsamic vinegar Salt and dark pepper to the taste 4 tablespoons olive oil

Guidelines:

1.   In a bowl, blend 2 tablespoons oil with 3 tablespoons vinegar, 3 garlic cloves, thyme, salt and dark pepper and whisk well.

2.   Add tomatoes, hurl to cover and leave aside for 30 minutes.

3.   Arrange 6 tomatoes on one stick and rehash with the remainder of the tomatoes.

4.   Introduce them in the air fryer cooker and cook at 360 Deg. Fahrenheit for about 6 minutes.

5.   In another bowl, blend 2 tablespoons vinegar in with salt, pepper and 4 tablespoons oil and whisk well.

6.   Arrange tomato sticks on plates and present with the dressing showered on top.

Enjoy

The nutritional facts: calories 140, fat 1, fiber 1, carbs 2, protein 7

FLAVORFUL PORTOBELLO MUSHROOMS

Prep. time: 10 minutes

The cooking time: 12 minutes

The recipe servings: 4

10 basil leaves

1 cup infant spinach

3 garlic cloves, slashed

1 cup almonds, generally slashed 1 tablespoon parsley

¼ cup olive oil

8 cherry tomatoes, divided

Salt and dark pepper to the taste

4 Portobello mushrooms, stems evacuated and slashed

Guidelines:

1.   In your food processor, blend basil in with spinach, garlic, almonds, parsley, oil, salt, dark pepper to the taste and mushroom stems and mix well.

2.   Stuff each mushroom with this blend, place them in the air fryer cooker and cook at 350 Deg. Fahrenheit for about 12 minutes.

3.   Divide mushrooms on plates and serve.

Enjoy the recipe!

The nutritional facts: calories 145, fat 3, fiber 2, carbs 6, protein 17

MEXICAN PEPPERS

Prep. time: 10 minutes

The cooking time: 25 minutes

The recipe servings: 4

4 ringer peppers, finishes cut off and seeds evacuated

½ cup tomato juice

2 tablespoons jostled jalapenos, hacked 4 chicken bosoms

1 cup tomatoes, hacked

¼ cup yellow onion, slashed

¼ cup green peppers, slashed 2 cups tomato sauce

Salt and dark pepper to the taste 2 teaspoons onion powder

½ teaspoon red pepper, squashed 1 teaspoon bean stew powder

½ teaspoons garlic powder 1 teaspoon cumin, ground

Guidelines:

1.   In a skillet that accommodates the air fryer cooker, blend chicken bosoms in with tomato juice, jalapenos, tomatoes, onion, green peppers, salt, pepper, onion powder, red pepper, stew powder, garlic powder, oregano and cumin, mix well, present in the air fryer cooker and cook at 350 Deg. Fahrenheit for about 15 minutes,

2.   Shred meat utilizing 2 forks, mix, stuff ringer peppers with this blend, place them in the air fryer cooker and cook at 320 Deg. Fahrenheit for about 10 minutes more.

3.   Divide stuffed peppers on plates and serve.

Enjoy the recipe!

The nutritional facts: calories 180, fat 4, fiber 3, carbs 7, protein 14

PEPPERS STUFFED WITH BEEF

Prep. time: 10 minutes

The cooking time: 55 minutes

The recipe servings: 4

1 pound hamburger, ground

1 teaspoon coriander, ground 1 onion, slashed

3 garlic cloves, minced & 2 tablespoonful of olive oil

1 tablespoon ginger, ground

½ teaspoon cumin, ground

½ teaspoon turmeric powder

1 tablespoon hot curry powder Salt and dark pepper to the taste 1 egg

4 ringer peppers, cut into equal parts and seeds evacuated 1/3 cup raisins

1/3 cup pecans, slashed

Guidelines:

1.   Heat up a skillet with the oil over medium high heat, include onion, mix and cook for 4 minutes.

2.   Add garlic and hamburger, mix and cook for 10 minutes.

3.   Add coriander, ginger, cumin, curry powder, salt, pepper, turmeric, pecans and raisins, mix take off heat and blend in with the egg.

4.   Stuff pepper parts with this blend, present them in the air fryer cooker and cook at 320 Deg. Fahrenheit for about 20 minutes.

5.   Divide among plates and serve.

Enjoy the recipe!

The nutritional facts: calories 170, fat 4, fiber 3, carbs 7, protein 12

STUFFED POBLANO PEPPERS

Prep. time: 10 minutes

The cooking time: 15 minutes

The recipe servings: 4

2 teaspoons garlic, minced 1 white onion, slashed

10 poblano peppers, finishes cut off and deseeded 1 tablespoon of olive oil

8 ounces mushrooms, slashed Salt and dark pepper to the taste

½ cup cilantro, slashed

Guidelines:

1.   Heat up a skillet with the oil over medium high heat, include onion and mushrooms, mix and cook for 5 minutes.

2.   Add garlic, cilantro, salt and dark pepper, mix and cook for 2 minutes.

3.   Divide this blend into poblanos, present them in the air fryer cooker and cook at 350 Deg. Fahrenheit for about 15 minutes.

4.   Divide among plates and serve.

Enjoy the recipe!

The nutritional facts: calories 150, fat 3, fiber 2, carbs 7, protein 10

STUFFED BABY PEPPERS

Prep. time: 10 minutes

The cooking time: 6 minutes

The recipe servings: 4

Fixings:

12 infant ringer peppers, cut into equal parts the long way

¼ teaspoon red pepper pieces, squashed

1 pound shrimp, cooked, stripped and deveined 6 tablespoons jolted basil pesto

Salt and dark pepper to the taste 1 tablespoon lemon juice

1   tablespoon of olive oil

A bunch parsley, hacked

Guidelines:

1.   In a bowl, blend shrimp in with pepper pieces, pesto, salt, dark pepper, lemon juice, oil and parsley, whisk well indeed and stuff chime pepper parts with this blend.

2.   Place them in the air fryer cooker and cook at 320 Deg. Fahrenheit for about 6 minutes,

3.   Arrange peppers on plates and serve.

Enjoy the recipe!

The nutritional facts: calories 130, fat 2, fiber 1, carbs 3, protein 15

EGGPLANT AND GARLIC SAUCE

Prep. time: 10 minutes

The cooking time: 10 minutes

The recipe servings: 4

2tablespoons olive oil 2 garlic cloves, minced

2   eggplants, split and cut 1 red stew pepper, slashed

1 green onion stalk, hacked 1 tablespoon ginger, ground 1 tablespoon soy sauce

1 tablespoon balsamic vinegar

Guidelines:

1.   Heat up a dish that accommodates the air fryer cooker with the oil over medium high heat, include eggplant cuts and cook for 2 minutes.

2.   Add stew pepper, garlic, green onions, ginger, soy sauce and vinegar, present in the air fryer cooker and cook at 320 Deg. Fahrenheit for about 7 minutes.

3.   Divide among plates and serve.

Enjoy the recipe!

The nutritional facts: calories 130, fat 2, fiber 4, carbs 7, protein 9

EGGPLANT HASH

Prep. time: 20 minutes

The cooking time: 10 minutes

The recipe servings: 4

1 eggplant, generally cleaved

½ cup olive oil

½ pound cherry tomatoes, divided 1 teaspoon Tabasco sauce

¼ cup basil, cleaved

¼ cup mint, cleaved

Salt and dark pepper to the taste

Guidelines:

1.   Heat up a container that accommodates the air fryer cooker with half of the oil over medium high heat, include eggplant pieces, cook for 3 minutes, flip, cook them for 3 minutes more and move to a bowl.

2.   Heat up a similar dish with the remainder of the oil over medium high heat, include tomatoes, mix and cook for 1-2 minutes.

3.   Return eggplant pieces to the skillet, include salt, dark pepper, basil, mint and Tabasco sauce, present in the air fryer cooker and cook at 320 Deg. Fahrenheit for about 6 minutes.

4.   Divide among plates and serve.

Enjoy the recipe!

The nutritional facts: calories 120, fat 1, fiber 4, carbs 8, protein 15

SWEET POTATOES MIX

Prep. time: 10 minutes

The cooking time: 15 minutes

The recipe servings: 4

3 sweet potatoes, cubed, 4 garlic cloves, minced

½ pound bacon, slashed Juice from 1 lime

Salt and dark pepper to the taste 2 tablespoons balsamic vinegar A bunch dill, slashed

2 green onions, slashed

A spot of cinnamon powder A touch of red pepper pieces

Guidelines:

1.   Arrange bacon and sweet potatoes in the air fryer cooker's container, include garlic and half of the oil, hurl well and cook at 350 degrees F and prepare for 15 minutes.

2.   Meanwhile, in a bowl, blend vinegar in with lime juice, olive oil, green onions, pepper drops, dill, salt, pepper and cinnamon and whisk.

3.   Transfer bacon and sweet potatoes to a plate of mixed greens bowl, include plate of mixed greens dressing, hurl well and serve immediately.

Enjoy the recipe!

The nutritional facts: calories 170, fat 3, fiber 2, carbs 5, protein 12

GREEK POTATO MIX

Prep. time: 10 minutes

The cooking time: 20 minutes

The recipe servings: 2

2 medium potatoes, cut into wedges 1 yellow onion, hacked

2 tablespoons spread

1 little carrot, generally hacked 1 and ½ tablespoon flour

1   bay leaf

½ cup chicken stock

2   tablespoons Greek yogurt

Salt and dark pepper to the taste

Guidelines:

1.   Heat up a dish that accommodates the air fryer cooker with the spread over medium high heat, include onion and carrot, mix and cook for 3-4 minutes.

2.   Add potatoes, flour, chicken stock, salt, pepper and sound leaf, mix, present in the air fryer cooker and cook at 320 Deg. Fahrenheit for about 16 minutes.

3.   Add Greek yogurt, hurl, separate among plates and serve. Enjoy the recipe!

The nutritional facts: calories 198, fat 3, fiber 2, carbs 6, protein 8

BROCCOLI HASH

Prep. time: 30 minutes

The cooking time: 8 minutes

The recipe servings: 2

Fixings:

10 ounces mushrooms, divided

1 broccoli head, florets isolated 1 garlic clove, minced

1 tablespoon balsamic vinegar 1 yellow onion, hacked

1 tablespoon of olive oil Salt and dark pepper 1 teaspoon basil, dried

1   avocado, stripped and pitted A spot of red pepper chips

Guidelines:

1.   In a bowl, blend mushrooms in with broccoli, onion, garlic and avocado.

2.   In another bowl, blend vinegar, oil, salt, pepper and basil and whisk well.

3.   Pour this over veggies, hurl to cover, leave aside for 30 minutes, move to the air fryer cooker's bin and cook at 350 Deg. Fahrenheit for about 8 minutes,

4.   Divide among plates and present with pepper pieces on top.

Enjoy the recipe!

The nutritional facts: calories 182, fat 3, fiber 3, carbs 5, protein 8

AIR FRIED ASPARAGUS

Prep. time: 10 minutes

The cooking time: 15 minutes

The recipe servings: 4

2   2pounds crisp asparagus, cut

¼ cup olive oil

Salt and dark pepper to the taste 1 teaspoon lemon pizzazz

4 garlic cloves, minced

½ teaspoon oregano, dried

¼ teaspoon red pepper pieces

4 ounces feta cheddar, disintegrated

2 tablespoons parsley, finely cleaved Juice from 1 lemon

Guidelines:

1.   In a bowl, blend oil in with lemon pizzazz, garlic, pepper chips and oregano and whisk.

2.   Add asparagus, cheddar, salt and pepper, hurl, move to the air fryer cooker's container and cook at 350 Deg. Fahrenheit for about 8 minutes.

Partition asparagus on plates, shower lemon squeeze and sprinkle parsley on top and serve.

Enjoy the recipe!

The nutritional facts: calories 162, fat 13, fiber 5, carbs 12, protein 8

STUFFED EGGPLANTS

Prep. time: 10 minutes

The cooking time: 30 minutes

The recipe servings: 4

4 little eggplants, split the long way Salt and dark pepper to the taste

10 tablespoons olive oil

2 and ½ pounds tomatoes, cut into equal parts and ground 1 green ringer pepper, hacked

1 yellow onion, cleaved

1 tablespoon garlic, minced

½ cup cauliflower, cleaved 1 teaspoon oregano, slashed

½ cup parsley, cleaved

3 ounces feta cheddar, disintegrated

Rules:

1.   Season eggplants with salt, pepper and 4 tablespoons oil, hurl, put them in the air fryer cooker and cook at 350 Deg. Fahrenheit for about 16 minutes.

2.   Meanwhile, heat up a container with 3 tablespoons oil over medium high heat, include onion, mix and cook for 5 minutes.

3.   Add chime pepper, garlic and cauliflower, mix, cook for 5 minutes, take off heat, include parsley, tomato, salt, pepper, oregano and cheddar and whisk everything.

4.   Stuff eggplants with the veggie blend, shower the remainder of the oil over them, put them in the air fryer cooker and cook at 350 Deg. Fahrenheit for about 6 minutes more.

5.   Divide among plates and serve immediately.

Enjoy the formula!

The nutritional facts: calories 240, fat 4, fiber, 2, carbs 19, protein 2

GREEN BEANS AND PARMESAN

Prep. time: 10 minutes

The cooking time: 8 minutes

The recipe servings: 4

Fixings:

12 ounces green beans

2 teaspoons of garlic, minced with 2 tablespoons olive oil

Salt and dark pepper to the taste 1 egg, whisked

1/3 cup parmesan, ground

Rules:

1.   In a bowl, blend oil in with salt, pepper, garlic and egg and whisk well.

2.   Add green beans to this blend, hurl well and sprinkle parmesan everywhere.

3.   Transfer green beans to the air fryer cooker and cook them at 390 Deg. Fahrenheit for about 8 minutes.

4.   Divide green beans on plates and serve them immediately.

Enjoy the formula!

The nutritional facts: calories 120, fat 8, fiber 2, carbs 7, protein 4

TASTY CREAMY GREEN BEANS

Prep. time: 10 minutes

The cooking time: 15 minutes

The recipe servings: 4

½ cup overwhelming cream

1   cup mozzarella, destroyed 2/3 cup parmesan, ground

Salt and dark pepper to the taste 2 pounds green beans

2   teaspoons lemon get-up-and-go, ground A spot of red pepper pieces

Rules:

1.   Put the beans in a dish that accommodates the air fryer cooker, include overwhelming cream, salt, pepper, lemon pizzazz, pepper pieces, mozzarella and parmesan, hurl, present in the air fryer cooker and cook at 350 Deg. Fahrenheit for about 15 minutes.

2.   Divide among plates and serve immediately. Enjoy the formula!

The nutritional facts: calories 231, fat 6, fiber 7, carbs 8, protein 5

GREEN BEANS AND TOMATOES

Prep. time: 10 minutes

The cooking time: 15 minutes

The recipe servings: 4

Fixings:

1pint cherry tomatoes 1 pound green beans

1   tablespoons olive oil

Salt and dark pepper to the taste

Rules:

1.   In a bowl, blend cherry tomatoes in with green beans, olive oil, salt and pepper, hurl, move to the air fryer cooker and cook at 400 Deg. Fahrenheit for about 15 minutes.

2.   Divide among plates and serve immediately. Enjoy the formula!

The nutritional facts: calories 162, fat 6, fiber 5, carbs 8, protein 9

SIMPLE GREEN BEANS AND POTATOES

Prep. time: 10 minutes

The cooking time: 15 minutes

The recipe servings: 5

2 pounds green beans 6 new potatoes, split

Salt and dark pepper to the taste A shower of olive oil

6 bacon cuts, cooked and hacked

Rules:

1.   In a bowl, blend green beans in with potatoes, salt, pepper and oil, hurl, move to the air fryer cooker and cook at 390 Deg. Fahrenheit for about 15 minutes.

2.   Divide among plates and present with bacon sprinkled on top. Enjoy the formula!

The nutritional facts: calories 374, fat 15, fiber 12, carbs 28, protein 12

ENHANCED GREEN BEANS

Prep. time: 10 minutes

The cooking time: 15minutes

The recipe servings: 4

Fixings:

1pound red potatoes, cut into wedges 1 pound green beans

1   garlic cloves, minced 2 tablespoons olive oil

Salt and dark pepper to the taste

½ teaspoon oregano, dried

Rules:

1.   In a skillet that accommodates the air fryer cooker, consolidate potatoes with green beans, garlic, oil, salt, pepper and oregano, hurl, present in the air fryer cooker and cook at 380 Deg. Fahrenheit for about 15 minutes.

2.   Divide among plates and serve. Enjoy the formula!

The nutritional facts: calories 211, fat 6, fiber 7, carbs 8, protein 5

POTATOES AND TOMATOES MIX

Prep. time: 10 minutes

The cooking time: 16 minutes

The recipe servings: 4

Fixings:

1 and ½ pounds red potatoes, quartered 2 tablespoons olive oil

1 16 ounces cherry tomatoes

1 teaspoon sweet paprika

1 tablespoons rosemary, cleaved Salt and dark pepper to the taste 3 garlic cloves, minced

Rules:

1.   In a bowl, blend potatoes in with tomatoes, oil, paprika, rosemary, garlic, salt and pepper, hurl, move to the air fryer cooker and cook at 380 Deg. Fahrenheit for about 16 minutes.

2.   Divide among plates and serve. Enjoy the formula!

The nutritional facts: calories 192, fat 4, fiber 4, carbs 30, protein 3

BALSAMIC POTATOES

Prep. time: 10 minutes The cooking time: 20 minutes The recipe servings: 4

Fixings:

1   and ½ pounds infant potatoes, split 2 garlic cloves, slashed

2   red onions, cleaved

9 ounces cherry tomatoes 3 tablespoons olive oil

1   and ½ tablespoons balsamic vinegar 2 thyme springs, cleaved

Salt and dark pepper to the taste

Rules:

1.   In your food processor, blend garlic in with onions, oil, vinegar, thyme, salt and pepper and heartbeat truly well.

2.   In a bowl, blend potatoes in with tomatoes and balsamic marinade, hurl well, move to the air fryer cooker and cook at 380 Deg. Fahrenheit for about 20 minutes.

3.   Divide among plates and serve. Enjoy the formula!

The nutritional facts: calories 301, fat 6, fiber 8, carbs 18, protein 6

POTATOES AND SPECIAL TOMATO SAUCE

Prep. time: 10 minutes The cooking time: 16 minutes The recipe servings: 4

Fixings:

2   pounds potatoes, cubed 4 garlic cloves, minced

1   yellow onion, hacked 1 cup tomato sauce

2   tablespoons basil, hacked 2 tablespoons olive oil

½ teaspoon oregano, dried

½ teaspoon parsley, dried

Rules:

1.   Heat up a dish that accommodates the air fryer cooker with the oil over medium heat, include onion, mix and cook for 1-2 minutes.

2.   Add garlic, potatoes, parsley, tomato sauce and oregano, mix, present in the air fryer cooker and cook at 370 degrees F and cook for 16 minutes.

3.   Add basil, hurl everything, separate among plates and serve. Enjoy the formula!

The nutritional facts: calories 211, fat 6, fiber 8, carbs 14, protein 6

AIR FRYER DESSERT RECIPES

DELICIOUS BANANA CAKE

Prep. time: 10 minutes The cooking time: 30 minutes The recipe servings: 4

Fixings:

1 tablespoon spread, delicate 1 egg

1/3 cup dark colored sugar 2 tablespoons HONNEY

1 banana, stripped and crushed 1 cup white flour

1 teaspoon preparing powder

½ teaspoon cinnamon powder Cooking splash

Rules:

1.   Spray a cake dish with some cooking splash and leave aside.

2.   In a bowl, blend margarine in with sugar, banana, HONNEY, egg, cinnamon, heating powder and flour and whisk

3.   Pour this into a cake skillet lubed with cooking splash, present in the air fryer cooker and cook at 350 Deg. Fahrenheit for about 30 minutes.

4.   Leave cake to chill off, cut and serve.

Enjoy the formula!

The nutritional facts: calories 232, fat 4, fiber 1, carbs 34, protein 4

BASIC CHEESECAKE

Prep. time: 10 minutes

The cooking time: 15 minutes

The recipe servings: 15

Fixings:

1 pound cream cheddar

½ teaspoon vanilla concentrate 2 eggs

4 tablespoons sugar

1 cup graham saltines, disintegrated 2 tablespoons spread

Rules:

1.   In a bowl, blend saltines in with spread.

2.	Press wafers blend on the base of a lined cake dish, present in the air fryer cooker and cook at 350 Deg. Fahrenheit for about 4 minutes.

3.	Meanwhile, in a bowl, blend sugar in with cream cheddar, eggs and vanilla and whisk well.

4.	Spread filling over saltines covering and cook your cheesecake in the air fryer cooker at 310 Deg. Fahrenheit for about 15 minutes.

5.	Leave cake in the ice chest for 3 hours, cut and serve.

Enjoy the formula!

The nutritional facts: calories 245, fat 12, fiber 1, carbs 20, protein 3

BREAD PUDDING

Prep. toime: 10 minutes

The cooking time: 60 minutes

The recipe servings: 4

Fixings:

6 coated doughnuts, disintegrated 1 cup fruits

4 egg yolks

1 and ½ cups whipping cream

½ cup raisins

¼ cup sugar

½ cup chocolate chips.

Rules:

1.   In a bowl, blend fruits in with egg yolks and whipping cream and mix well.

2.   In another bowl, blend raisins in with sugar, chocolate chips and doughnuts and mix.

3.   Combine the 2 blends, move everything to a lubed skillet that accommodates the air fryer cooker and cook at 310 Deg. Fahrenheit for about 60 minutes.

4.   Chill pudding before cutting and serving it.

Enjoy the formula!

The nutritional facts: calories 302, fat 8, fiber 2, carbs 23, protein 10

BREAD DOUGH AND AMARETTO DESSERT

Prep. time: 10 MINUTES

The cooking time: 12 minutes

The recipe servings: 12

Fixings:

1 pound bread mixture 1 cup sugar

½ cup margarine, liquefied 1 cup substantial cream

12 ounces chocolate chips

2 tablespoons amaretto alcohol

Rules:

1.   Roll mixture, cut into 20 cuts and afterward cut each cut in equal parts.

2.   Brush mixture pieces with margarine, sprinkle sugar, place them in the air fryer cooker's container after you've brushed it some spread, cook them at 350 Deg. Fahrenheit for about 5 minutes, flip them, cook for 3 minutes more and move to a platter.

3.   Heat up a skillet with the substantial cream over medium heat, include chocolate chips and mix until they soften.

4.   Add alcohol, mix once more, move to a bowl and serve bread scoops with this sauce.

Enjoy the formula!

The nutritional facts: calories 200, fat 1, fiber 0, carbs 6, protein 6

CINNAMON ROLLS AND CREAM CHEESE DIP

Prep. time: 2 hours The cooking time: 15 minutes The recipe servings: 8

Fixings:

1 pound bread batter

¾ cup dark colored sugar

1   and ½ tablespoons cinnamon, ground

¼ cup spread, softened

For the cream cheddar plunge:

2   tablespoons spread

4 ounces cream cheddar 1 and ¼ cups sugar

½ teaspoon vanilla

Rules:

1.   Roll batter on a floured working surface, shape a square shape and brush with ¼ cup margarine.

2.   In a bowl, blend cinnamon in with sugar, mix, sprinkle this over batter, fold mixture into a log, seal well and cut into 8 pieces.

3.   Leave moves to ascend for 2 hours, place them in the air fryer cooker's bin, cook at 350 Deg. Fahrenheit for about 5 minutes, flip them, cook for 4 minutes more and move to a platter.

4.   In a bowl, blend cream cheddar with spread, sugar and vanilla and whisk truly well.

5.   Serve your cinnamon moves with this cream cheddar plunge.

Enjoy the formula!

The nutritional facts: calories 200, fat 1, fiber 0, carbs 5, protein 6

PUMPKIN PIE

Prep. time: 10 minutes The cooking time: 15 minutes The recipe servings: 9

Fixings:

1   tablespoon sugar

2   tablespoons flour

1   tablespoon margarine

2   tablespoons water

For the pumpkin pie filling:

3.5 ounces pumpkin substance, slashed 1 teaspoon blended zest

1 teaspoon nutmeg

3 ounces water

1 egg, whisked

1 tablespoon sugar

Rules:

1.   Put 3 ounces water in a pot, heat to the point of boiling over medium high heat, include pumpkin, egg, 1 tablespoon sugar, zest and nutmeg, mix, bubble for 20 minutes, take off heat and mix utilizing a drenching blender.

2.   In a bowl, blend flour in with margarine, 1 tablespoon sugar and 2 tablespoons water and massage your mixture well.

3.   Grease a pie skillet that accommodates the air fryer cooker with margarine, press mixture into the dish, load up with pumpkin pie filling, place in the air fryer cooker's bushel and cook at 360 Deg. Fahrenheit for about 15 minutes.

4.   Slice and serve warm.

Enjoy the formula!

The nutritional facts: calories 200, fat 5, fiber 2, carbs 5, protein 6

WRAPPED PEARS

Prep. time: 10 minutes The cooking time: 15 minutes The recipe servings: 4

Fixings:

4 puff baked good sheets

14 ounces vanilla custard 2 pears, divided

1 egg, whisked

½ teaspoon cinnamon powder 2 tablespoons sugar

Rules:

1.   Place puff baked good cuts on a working surface, include spoonfuls of vanilla custard in the focal point of each, top with pear parts and wrap.

2.   Brush pears with egg, sprinkle sugar and cinnamon, place them in the air fryer cooker's container and cook at 320 Deg. Fahrenheit for about 15 minutes.

3.   Divide bundles on plates and serve.

Enjoy the formula!

The nutritional facts: calories 200, fat 2, fiber 1, carbs 14, protein 3

STRAWBERRY DONUTS

Prep. time: 10 minutes The cooking time: 15 minutes The recipe servings: 4

Fixings:

8 ounces flour

1 tablespoon darker sugar 1 tablespoon white sugar 1 egg

2 and ½ tablespoons margarine 4 ounces entire milk

1 teaspoon heating powder

For the strawberry icing:

2 tablespoons margarine

3.5 ounces icing sugar

½ teaspoon pink shading

¼ cup strawberries, slashed 1 tablespoon whipped cream

Rules:

1.   In a bowl, blend margarine, 1 tablespoon darker sugar, 1 tablespoon white sugar and flour and mix.

2.   In a subsequent bowl, blend egg in with 1 and ½ tablespoons margarine and milk and mix well.

3.   Combine the 2 blends, mix, shape doughnuts from this blend, place them in the air fryer cooker's bushel and cook at 360 Deg. Fahrenheit for about 15 minutes.

4.   Put 1 tablespoon spread, icing sugar, food shading, whipped cream and strawberry puree and whisk well.

5.   Arrange doughnuts on a platter and present with strawberry good to beat all.

Enjoy the formula!

The nutritional facts: calories 250, fat 12, fiber 1, carbs 32, protein 4

AIR FRIED BANANAS

Prep. time: 10 minutes The cooking time: 15 minutes The recipe servings: 4

Fixings:

3 tablespoons spread

2 eggs

8 bananas, stripped and split

½ cup corn flour

3 tablespoons cinnamon sugar 1 cup panko

Rules:

1.   Heat up a dish with the spread over medium high heat, include panko, mix and cook for 4 minutes and afterward move to a bowl.

2.   Roll each in flour, eggs and panko blend, orchestrate them in the air fryer cooker's bushel, and cook at 280 Deg. Fahrenheit for about 10 minutes.

3.   Serve immediately.

Enjoy the formula!

The nutritional facts: calories 164, fat 1, fiber 4, carbs 32, protein 4

COCOA CAKE

Prep. time: 10 minutes

The cooking time: 17 minutes

The recipe servings: 6

Fixings:

3.5 ounces spread, dissolved 3 eggs

3 ounces sugar

1 teaspoon cocoa powder 3 ounces flour

½ teaspoon lemon juice

Rules:

1. In a bowl, blend 1 tablespoon margarine with cocoa powder and whisk.

2. In another bowl, blend the remainder of the spread in with sugar, eggs, flour and lemon juice, whisk well and empty half into a cake container that accommodates the air fryer cooker.

3. Add portion of the cocoa blend, spread, include the remainder of the margarine layer and top with the remainder of cocoa.

4. Introduce in the air fryer cooker and cook at 360 Deg. Fahrenheit for about 17 minutes.

5. Cool cake down before cutting and serving.

Enjoy the formula!

The nutritional facts: calories 340, fat 11, fiber 3, carbs 25, protein 5

CHOCOLATE CAKE

Prep. time: 10 minutes

The cooking time: 30 minutes

The recipe servings: 12

Fixings:

¾ cup white flour

¾ cup entire wheat flour 1 teaspoon preparing pop

¾ teaspoon pumpkin pie flavor

¾ cup sugar

1 banana, squashed

½ teaspoon preparing powder 2 tablespoons canola oil

½ cup Greek yogurt

8 ounces canned pumpkin puree Cooking splash

1 egg

½ teaspoon vanilla concentrate 2/3 cup chocolate chips

Rules:

1.   In a bowl, blend white flour in with entire wheat flour, salt, preparing pop and powder and pumpkin flavor and mix.

2.   In another bowl, blend sugar in with oil, banana, yogurt, pumpkin puree, vanilla and egg and mix utilizing a blender.

3.   Combine the 2 blends, include chocolate chips, mix, empty this into a lubed Bundt container that accommodates the air fryer cooker.

4.   Introduce in the air fryer cooker and cook at 330 Deg. Fahrenheit for about 30 minutes.

5.   Leave the cake to chill off, before cutting and serving it.

Enjoy the formula!

The nutritional facts: calories 232, fat 7, fiber 7, carbs 29, protein 4

APPLE BREAD

Prep. time: 10 minutes

The cooking time: 40 minutes

The recipe servings: 6

Fixings:

3 cups apples, cored and cubed 1 cup sugar

1   tablespoon vanilla

2   eggs

1 tablespoon crusty fruit-filled treat flavor 2 cups white flour

1 tablespoon heating powder 1 stick spread

1 cup water

Rules:

1.   In a bowl blend egg in with 1 margarine stick, crusty fruit-filled treat flavor and sugar and mix utilizing your blender.

2.   Add apples and mix again well.

3.   In another bowl, blend heating powder in with flour and mix.

4.   Combine the 2 blends, mix and fill a spring structure skillet.

5.   Put spring structure dish in the air fryer cooker and cook at 320 Deg. Fahrenheit for about 40 minutes

6.   Slice and serve.

Enjoy the formula!

The nutritional facts: calories 192, fat 6, fiber 7, carbs 14, protein 7

BANANA BREAD

Prep. time: 10 minutes

The cooking time: 40 minutes

The recipe servings: 6

Fixings:

¾ cup sugar 1/3 cup spread

1   teaspoon vanilla concentrate 1 egg

2   bananas, crushed

1 teaspoon preparing powder 1 and ½ cups flour

½ teaspoons preparing soft drink 1/3 cup milk

1 and ½ teaspoons cream of tartar Cooking splash

Rules:

1.   In a bowl, blend milk in with cream of tartar, sugar, spread, egg, vanilla and bananas and mix everything.

2.   In another bowl, blend flour in with preparing powder and heating pop.

3.   Combine the 2 blends, mix well, empty this into a cake container lubed with some cooking splash, present in the air fryer cooker and cook at 320 Deg. Fahrenheit for about 40 minutes.

4.   Take bread out, leave aside to chill off, cut and serve it.

Enjoy the formula!

The nutritional facts: calories 292, fat 7, fiber 8, carbs 28, protein 4

MINI LAVA CAKES

Prep. time: 10 minutes

The cooking time: 20 minutes

The recipe servings: 3

Fixings:

1 egg

4 tablespoons sugar

2 tablespoons olive oil 4 tablespoons milk

4 tablespoons flour

1   tablespoon cocoa powder

½ teaspoon heating powder

½ teaspoon orange pizzazz

Rules:

1.   In a bowl, blend egg in with sugar, oil, milk, flour, salt, cocoa powder, heating powder and orange pizzazz, mix quite well and empty this into lubed ramekins.

2.   Add ramekins to the air fryer cooker and cook at 320 Deg. Fahrenheit for about 20 minutes.

3.   Serve magma cakes warm.

Enjoy the formula!

The nutritional facts: calories 201, fat 7, fiber 8, carbs 23, protein 4

FRESH APPLES

Prep. time: 10 minutes The cooking time: 10 minutes The recipe servings: 4

Fixings:

2   teaspoons cinnamon powder

5 apples, cored and cut into lumps

½ teaspoon nutmeg powder 1 tablespoon maple syrup

½ cup water

4   tablespoons margarine

¼ cup flour

¾ cup antiquated moved oats

¼ cup dark colored sugar

Rules:

1.   Put the apples in a dish that accommodates the air fryer cooker, include cinnamon, nutmeg, maple syrup and water.

2.   In a bowl, blend spread in with oats, sugar, salt and flour, mix, drop spoonfuls of this blend on apples, present in the air fryer cooker and cook at 350 Deg. Fahrenheit for about 10 minutes.

3.   Serve warm.

Enjoy the formula!

The nutritional facts: calories 200, fat 6, fiber 8, carbs 29, protein 12

CARROT CAKE

Prep. time: 10 minutes The cooking time: 45 minutes The recipe servings: 6

Fixings:

5   ounces flour

¾ teaspoon heating powder

½ teaspoon heating pop

½ teaspoon cinnamon powder

¼ teaspoon nutmeg, ground

½ teaspoon allspice 1 egg

3   tablespoons yogurt

½ cup sugar

¼ cup pineapple juice

4   tablespoons sunflower oil 1/3 cup carrots, ground

1/3 cup walnuts, toasted and slashed 1/3 cup coconut chips, destroyed Cooking shower

Rules:

1.　　　In a bowl, blend flour in with preparing pop and powder, salt, allspice, cinnamon and nutmeg and mix.

2.　　　In another bowl, blend egg in with yogurt, sugar, pineapple juice, oil, carrots, walnuts and coconut drops and mix well.

3.　　　Combine the two blends and mix well, empty this into a spring structure container that accommodates the air fryer cooker which you've lubed with some cooking shower, move to the air fryer cooker and cook on 320 Deg. Fahrenheit for about 45 minutes.

4.　　　Leave cake to chill off, at that point cut and serve it. Enjoy the formula!

The nutritional facts: calories 200, fat 6, fiber 20, carbs 22, protein 4

GINGER CHEESECAKE

Prep. time: 2 HOURS and 10 minutes

The cooking time: 20 minutes

Fixings:

2 teaspoons margarine, liquefied

½ cup ginger cookies, disintegrated 16 ounces cream cheddar, delicate

2 eggs

½ cup sugar

1 teaspoon rum

½ teaspoon vanilla concentrate

½ teaspoon nutmeg, ground

Rules:

1.   Grease a skillet with the margarine and spread cookie morsels on the base.

2.   In a bowl, beat cream cheddar with nutmeg, vanilla, rum and eggs, whisk well and spread over the cookie morsels.

3.   Introduce in the air fryer cooker and cook at 340 Deg. Fahrenheit for about 20 minutes.

4.   Leave cheesecake to chill off and keep in the ice chest for 2 hours before cutting and serving it.

Enjoy the formula!

The nutritional facts: calories 412, fat 12, fiber 6, carbs 20, protein 6

STRAWBERRY PIE

Prep. time: 10 minutes

The cooking time: 20 minutes

The recipe servings:12

Fixings:

For the covering:

1 cup coconut, destroyed 1 cup sunflower seeds

¼ cup spread

For the filling:

1 teaspoon gelatin

8 ounces cream cheddar 4 ounces strawberries

2 tablespoons water

½ tablespoon lemon juice

¼ teaspoon stevia

½ cup overwhelming cream

8 ounces strawberries, hacked for serving

Rules:

1.   In your food processor, blend sunflower seeds with coconut, a touch of salt and spread, heartbeat and press this on the base of a cake skillet that accommodates the air fryer cooker.

2.   Heat up a skillet with the water over medium heat, include gelatin, mix until it breaks up, leave aside to chill off, add this to your food processor, blend in with 4 ounces strawberries, cream cheddar, lemon juice and stevia and mix well.

3.   Add overwhelming cream, mix well and spread this over outside.

4.   Top with 8 ounces strawberries, present in the air fryer cooker and cook at 330 Deg. Fahrenheit for about 15 minutes.

5.   Keep in the refrigerator until you serve it.

Enjoy the formula!

The nutritional facts: calories 234, fat 23, fiber 2, carbs 6, protein 7

ESPRESSO CHEESECAKES

Prep. time: 10 minutes The cooking time: 20 minutes The recipe servings: 6

Fixings:

For the cheesecakes:

2 tablespoons spread

8 ounces cream cheddar 3 tablespoons espresso

3 eggs

1/3 cup sugar

1 tablespoon caramel syrup

For the icing:

3 tablespoons caramel syrup 3 tablespoons spread

8 ounces mascarpone cheddar, delicate 2 tablespoons sugar

Rules:

1.   In your blender, blend cream cheddar with eggs, 2 tablespoons spread, espresso, 1 tablespoon caramel syrup and 1/3 cup sugar and heartbeat quite well, spoon into a cupcakes dish that accommodates the air fryer cooker, present in the fryer and cook at 320 degrees F and heat for 20 minutes.

2.   Leave aside to chill off and afterward keep in the cooler for 3 hours.

3.   Meanwhile, in a bowl, blend 3 tablespoons spread with 3 tablespoons caramel syrup, 2 tablespoons sugar and mascarpone, mix well, spoon this over cheesecakes and serve them.

Enjoy the formula!

The nutritional facts: calories 254, fat 23, fiber 0, carbs 21, protein 5

COCOA COOKIES

Prep. time: 10 minutes

The cooking time: 14 minutes

The recipe servings: 12

Fixings:

6 ounces coconut oil, liquefied 6 eggs

3 ounces cocoa powder 2 teaspoons vanilla

½ teaspoon preparing powder 4 ounces cream cheddar

5 tablespoons sugar

Rules:

1.   In a blender, blend eggs in with coconut oil, cocoa powder, preparing powder, vanilla, cream cheddar and swerve and mix utilizing a blender.

2.   Pour this into a lined heating dish that accommodates the air fryer cooker, present in the fryer at 320 degrees F and prepare for 14 minutes.

3.   Slice cookie sheet into square shapes and serve.

Enjoy the formula!

The nutritional facts: calories 178, fat 14, fiber 2, carbs 3, protein 5

UNIQUE BROWNIES

Prep. time: 10 minutes

The cooking time: 17 minutes

The recipe servings: 4

Fixings:

1 egg

1/3 cup of cocoa powder and 1/3 cup of sugar

7 tablespoons spread

½ teaspoon vanilla concentrate

¼ cup white flour

¼ cup pecans, hacked

½ teaspoon preparing powder 1 tablespoon nutty spread

Rules:

1.   Heat up a dish with 6 tablespoons spread and the sugar over medium heat, mix, cook for 5 minutes, move this to a bowl, include salt, vanilla concentrate, cocoa powder, egg, preparing powder, pecans and flour, mix the entire thing truly well and fill a skillet that accommodates the air fryer cooker.

2.   In a bowl, blend 1 tablespoon spread with nutty spread, heat up in your microwave for a couple of moments, mix well and sprinkle this over brownies blend.

3.   Introduce in the air fryer cooker and prepare at 320 degrees F and heat for 17 minutes.

4.   Leave brownies to chill off, cut and serve.

Enjoy the formula!

The nutritional facts: calories 223, fat 32, fiber 1, carbs 3, protein 6

BLUEBERRY SCONES

Prep. time: 10 minutes The cooking time: 10 minutes The recipe servings: 10

Fixings:

1   cup white flour 1 cup blueberries

2   eggs

½ cup overwhelming cream

½ cup spread

5 tablespoons sugar

2 teaspoons vanilla concentrate 2 teaspoons preparing powder

Rules:

1.   In a bowl, blend flour, salt, preparing powder and blueberries and mix.

2.   In another bowl, blend overwhelming cream in with spread, vanilla concentrate, sugar and eggs and mix well.

3.   Combine the 2 blends, ply until you acquire your batter, shape 10 triangles from this blend, place them on a lined preparing sheet that accommodates the air fryer cooker and cook them at 320 Deg. Fahrenheit for about 10 minutes.

4.   Serve them cold.

Enjoy the formula!

The nutritional facts: calories 130, fat 2, fiber 2, carbs 4, protein 3

CHOCOLATE COOKIES

Prep. time: 10 minutes

The cooking time: 25 minutes

The recipe servings:12

Fixings:

1 teaspoon vanilla concentrate

½ cup spread 1 egg

4 tablespoons sugar

2 cups flour

½ cup unsweetened chocolate chips

Rules:

1.   Heat up a container with the spread over medium heat, mix and cook for 1 moment.

2.   In a bowl, blend egg in with vanilla concentrate and sugar and mix well.

3.   Add liquefied margarine, flour and half of the chocolate chips and mix everything.

4. Transfer this to a container that accommodates the air fryer cooker, spread the remainder of the chocolate chips on top, present in the fryer at 330 degrees F and prepare for 25 minutes.

5. Slice when it's cold and serve.

Enjoy the recipe!

The nutritional facts: calories 230, fat 12, fiber 2, carbs 4, protein 5

DELECTABLE ORANGE CAKE

Prep. time: 10 minutes

The cooking time: 32 minutes

The recipe servings:12

Fixings:

6 eggs

1 orange, stripped and cut into quarters 1 teaspoon vanilla concentrate

1   teaspoon preparing powder 9 ounces flour

2   ounces sugar+ 2 tablespoons 2 tablespoons orange get-up-and-go

4 ounces cream cheddar 4 ounces yogurt

Rules:

1. In your food processor, beat orange quite well.

2. Add flour, 2 tablespoons sugar, eggs, preparing powder, vanilla concentrate and heartbeat well once more.

3. Transfer this into 2 spring structure container, present each in your fryer and cook at 330 Deg. Fahrenheit for about 16 minutes.

4. Meanwhile, in a bowl, blend cream cheddar with orange get-up-and-go, yogurt and the remainder of the sugar and mix well.

5. Place one cake layer on a plate, include half of the cream cheddar blend, include the other cake layer and top with the remainder of the cream cheddar blend.

6. Spread it well, cut and serve.

Enjoy the recipe!

The nutritional facts: calories 200, fat 13, fiber 2, carbs 9, protein 8

MACAROONS

Prep. time: 10 minutes

The cooking time: 8 minutes

The recipe servings: 20

Fixings:

2 tablespoons sugar

4 egg whites

2 cup coconut, destroyed 1 teaspoon vanilla concentrate

Rules:

1.   In a bowl, blend egg whites with stevia and beat utilizing your blender.

2.   Add coconut and vanilla concentrate, whisk once more, shape little balls out of this blend, present them in the air fryer cooker and cook at 340 Deg. Fahrenheit for about 8 minutes.

3.   Serve macaroons cold.

Enjoy the recipe!

The nutritional facts: calories 55, fat 6, fiber 1, carbs 2, protein 1

LIME CHEESECAKE

Prep. time: 4 hours and 10 minutes

The cooking time: 4 minutes

The recipe servings: 10

Fixings:

2 tablespoons margarine, softened 2 teaspoons sugar

4 ounces flour

¼ cup coconut, destroyed

For the filling:

1   pound cream cheddar Zest from 1 lime, ground Juice structure 1 lime

2   cups hot water

2 sachets lime jam

Rules:

1.   In a bowl, blend coconut in with flour, spread and sugar, mix well and press this on the base of a container that accommodates the air fryer cooker.

2.   Meanwhile, put the hot water in a bowl, include jam sachets and mix until it breaks up.

3.   Put cream cheddar in a bowl, include jam, lime squeeze and get-up-and-go and whisk truly well.

4.	Add this over the outside, spread, present in the air fryer and cook at 300 Deg. Fahrenheit for about 4 minutes.

5.	Keep in the ice chest for 4 hours before serving.

Enjoy the recipe!

The nutritional facts: calories 260, fat 23, fiber 2, carbs 5, protein 7

SIMPLE GRANOLA

Prep. time: 10 minutes The cooking time: 35 minutes The recipe servings: 4

Fixings:

1	cup coconut, destroyed

½ cup almonds

½ cup walnuts, cleaved 2 tablespoons sugar

½ cup pumpkin seeds

½ cup sunflower seeds

2	tablespoons sunflower oil 1 teaspoon nutmeg, ground

1 teaspoon crusty fruit-filled treat zest blend

Rules:

1.   In a bowl, blend almonds and walnuts in with pumpkin seeds, sunflower seeds, coconut, nutmeg and crusty fruit-filled treat flavor blend and mix well.

2.   Heat up a dish with the oil over medium heat, include sugar and mix well.

3.   Pour this over nuts and coconut blend and mix well.

4.   Spread this on a lined preparing sheet that accommodates the air fryer cooker, present in the air fryer cooker and cook at 300 degrees F and heat for 25 minutes.

5.   Leave your granola to chill off, cut and serve.

Enjoy the recipe!

The nutritional facts: calories 322, fat 7, fiber 8, carbs 12, protein 7

STRAWBERRY COBBLER

Prep. time: 10 minutes The cooking time: 25 minutes The recipe servings: 6

Fixings:

¾ cup sugar

6 cups strawberries, split 1/8 teaspoon heating powder 1 tablespoon lemon juice

½ cup flour

A spot of heating pop

½ cup water

3 and ½ tablespoon of olive oil Cooking shower

Rules:

1.   In a bowl, blend strawberries in with half of sugar, sprinkle some flour, include lemon squeeze, whisk and fill the heating dish that accommodates the air fryer cooker and lubed with cooking splash

2.   In another bowl, blend flour in with the remainder of the sugar, preparing powder and pop and mix well.

3.   Add the olive oil and blend until the entire thing with your hands.

4.   Add ½ cup water and spread over strawberries.

5.   Introduce in the fryer at 355 degrees F and prepare for 25 minutes.

6.   Leave shoemaker aside to chill off, cut and serve. Enjoy

The nutritional facts: calories 221, fat 3, fiber 3, carbs 6, protein 9

DARK TEA CAKE

Prep. time: 10 minutes The cooking time: 35 minutes The recipe servings: 12

Fixings:

6 tablespoons dark tea powder 2 cups milk

½ cup spread 2 cups sugar

4 eggs

2   teaspoons vanilla concentrate

½ cup olive oil

3   and ½ cups flour

1 teaspoon heating pop

3 teaspoons heating powder

For the cream:

6 tablespoons HONNEY

4 cups sugar

1 cup margarine, delicate

Rules:

1.   Put the milk in a pot, heat up over medium heat, include tea, mix well, take off heat and leave aside to chill off.

2.   In a bowl, blend ½ cup margarine with 2 cups sugar, eggs, vegetable oil, vanilla concentrate, preparing powder, heating pop and 3 and ½ cups flour and mix everything truly well.

3.   Pour this into 2 lubed round container, present each in the fryer at 330 degrees F and prepare for 25 minutes.

4.   In a bowl, blend 1 cup spread with HONNEY and 4 cups sugar and mix truly well.

5.   Arrange one cake on a platter, spread the cream all finished, top with the other cake and keep in the cooler until you serve it.

Enjoy the recipe!

The nutritional facts: calories 200, fat 4, fiber 4, carbs 6, protein 2

PLUM CAKE

Prep. time: 1 hour and 20 minutes

The cooking time: 36 minutes

The recipe servings: 8

Fixings:

7 ounces flour

1 bundle dried yeast 1 ounce margarine, delicate

1 egg, whisked

5 tablespoons sugar 3 ounces warm milk

1 and ¾ pounds plums, hollowed and cut into quarters Zest from 1 lemon, ground

1 ounce almond drops

Rules:

1.   In a bowl, blend yeast in with margarine, flour and 3 tablespoons sugar and mix well.

2.   Add milk and egg and rush for 4 minutes until your acquire a mixture.

3.   Arrange the batter in a spring structure skillet that accommodates the air fryer cooker and which you've lubed with some margarine, spread and leave aside for 60 minutes.

4.   Arrange plumps on the margarine, sprinkle the remainder of the sugar, present in the air fryer cooker at 350 degrees F, heat for 36 minutes, chill off, sprinkle almond chips and lemon get-up-and-go on top, cut and serve.

Enjoy the recipe!

The nutritional facts: calories 192, fat 4, fiber 2, carbs 6, protein 7

LENTILS COOKIES

Prep. time: 10 minutes The cooking time: 25 minutes The recipe servings: 36

Fixings:

1 cup water

1 cup canned lentils, depleted and pounded 1 cup white flour

1 teaspoon cinnamon powder 1 cup entire wheat flour

1   teaspoon heating powder

½ teaspoon nutmeg, ground 1 cup margarine, delicate

½ cup darker sugar

½ cup white sugar 1 egg

2   teaspoons almond separate 1 cup raisins

1 cup moved oats

1 cup coconut, unsweetened and destroyed

Rules:

1.

2.   In a bowl, blend white and entire wheat flour with salt, cinnamon, preparing powder and nutmeg and mix.

3.   In a bowl, blend spread in with white and dark colored sugar and mix utilizing your kitchen blender for 2 minutes.

4.   Add egg, almond remove, lentils blend, flour blend, oats, raisins and coconut and mix everything great.

5.   Scoop tablespoons of batter on a lined heating sheet that accommodates the air fryer cooker, present them in the fryer and cook at 350 Deg. Fahrenheit for about 15 minutes.

6.   Arrange cookies on a serving platter and serve Enjoy the recipe!

The nutritional facts: calories 154, fat 2, fiber 2, carbs 4, protein 7

LENTILS AND DATES BROWNIES

Prep. time: 10 minutes

The cooking time: 15 minutes

The recipe servings: 8

Fixings:

28 ounces canned lentils, washed and depleted 12 dates

1 tablespoon HONNEY

1 banana, stripped and hacked

½ teaspoon preparing pop

4 tablespoons almond spread 2 tablespoons cocoa powder

Guidelines:

1.   In your food processor, blend lentils in with spread, banana, cocoa, heating pop and HONNEY and mix truly well.

2.   Add dates, beat a couple of more occasions, empty this into a lubed skillet that accommodates the air fryer cooker, spread equally, present in the fryer at 360 degrees F and prepare for 15 minutes.

3.   Take brownies blend out of the oven, cut, organize on a platter and serve. Enjoy the recipe!

The nutritional facts: calories 162, fat 4, fiber 2, carbs 3, protein 4

MAPLE CUPCAKES

Prep. time: 10 minutes

The cooking time: 20 minutes

The recipe servings: 4

Fixings:

4 tablespoons margarine

4 eggs

½ cup unadulterated fruit purée

2 teaspoons cinnamon powder 1 teaspoon vanilla concentrate

½ apple, cored and cleaved 4 teaspoons maple syrup

¾ cup white flour

½ teaspoon heating powder

Guidelines:

1. Heat up a container with the margarine over medium heat, include fruit purée, vanilla, eggs and maple syrup, mix, take off heat and leave aside to chill off.

2. Add flour, cinnamon, heating powder and apples, whisk, pour in a cupcake skillet, present in the air fryer cooker at 350 degrees F and prepare for 20 minutes.

3. Leave cupcakes them to chill off, move to a platter and serve them. Enjoy the recipe!

The nutritional facts: calories 150, fat 3, fiber 1, carbs 5, protein 4

RHUBARB PIE

Prep. time: 30 minutes

The cooking time: 45 minutes

The recipe servings: 6

Fixings:

1 and ¼ cups almond flour 8 tablespoons margarine

5 tablespoons cold water 1 teaspoon sugar

For the filling:

3 cups rhubarb, slashed 3 tablespoons flour

1   and ½ cups sugar 2 eggs

½ teaspoon nutmeg, ground 1 tablespoon margarine

2   tablespoons low fat milk

Guidelines:

1.   In a bowl, blend 1 and ¼ cups flour with 1 teaspoon sugar, 8 tablespoons margarine and cold water, mix and work until you acquire a batter.

2.   Transfer batter to a floured working surface, shape a circle, level, envelop by plastic, keep in the refrigerator for around 30 minutes, roll and push on the base of a pie container that accommodates the air fryer cooker.

3.   In a bowl, blend rhubarb in with 1 and ½ cups sugar, nutmeg, 3 tablespoons flour and whisk.

4.   In another bowl, whisk eggs with milk, add to rhubarb blend, empty the entire blend into the pie outside, present in the air fryer cooker and cook at 390 Deg. Fahrenheit for about 45 minutes.

5.   Cut and serve it cold. Enjoy the recipe!

The nutritional facts: calories 200, fat 2, fiber 1, carbs 6, protein 3

LEMON TART

Prep. time:1 HOUR

The cooking time: 35 minutes

The recipe servings: 6

Fixings:

For the outside:

2   tablespoons sugar 2 cups white flour A touch of salt

3   tablespoons ice water 12 tablespoons cold spread

For the filling:

2 eggs, whisked

1 and ¼ cup sugar

10 tablespoons softened and chilled spread Juice from 2 lemons

Pizzazz from 2 lemons, ground

Guidelines:

1.   In a bowl, blend 2 cups flour with a spot of salt and 2 tablespoons sugar and whisk.

2.   Add 12 tablespoons spread and the water, ply until you get a batter, shape a ball, enclose by foil and keep in the ice chest for 60 minutes.

3.   Transfer mixture to a floured surface, straighten it, organize on the base of a tart dish, prick with a fork, keep in the ice chest for 20 minutes, present in the air fryer cooker at 360 degrees F and heat for 15 minutes.

4.   In a bowl, blend 1 and ¼ cup sugar with eggs, 10 tablespoons spread, lemon juice and lemon get-up-and-go and whisk well overall.

5.   Pour this into pie outside layer, spread equitably, present in the fryer and cook at 360 Deg. Fahrenheit for about 20 minutes.

6.   Cut and serve it. Enjoy the recipe!

The nutritional facts: calories 182, fat 4, fiber 1, carbs 2, protein 3

MANDARIN PUDDDING

Prep. time: 20 minutes

The cooking time: 40 minutes

The recipe servings: 8

Fixings:

1mandarin, stripped and cut Juice from 2 mandarins

1   tablespoons darker sugar 4 ounces margarine, delicate

2 eggs, whisked

¾ cup sugar

¾ cup white flour

¾ cup almonds, ground Honey for serving

Guidelines:

1.   Grease a portion skillet with some margarine, sprinkle dark colored sugar on the base and mastermind mandarin cuts.

2.   In a bowl, blend spread in with sugar, eggs, almonds, flour and mandarin juice, mix, spoon this over mandarin cuts, place container in the air fryer cooker and cook at 360 Deg. Fahrenheit for about 40 minutes.

3.   Transfer pudding to a plate and present with HONNEY on top. Enjoy the recipe!

The nutritional facts: calories 162, fat 3, fiber 2, carbs 3, protein 6

STRAWBERRY SHORTCAKES

Prep. time: 20 minutes

The cooking time: 45 minutes

The recipe servings: 6

Fixings:

Cooking splash

¼ cup sugar+ 4 tablespoons 1 and ½ cup flour

1 teaspoon preparing powder

¼ teaspoon preparing soft drink 1/3 cup spread

1 cup buttermilk

1   egg, whisked

2   cups strawberries, cut 1 tablespoon rum

1 tablespoon mint, cleaved 1 teaspoon lime get-up-and-go, ground

½ cup whipping cream

Guidelines:

1.   In a bowl, blend flour in with ¼ cup sugar, preparing powder and heating pop and mix.

2.   In another bowl, blend buttermilk in with egg, mix, add to flour blend and whisk.

3.   Spoon this mixture into 6 containers lubed with cooking shower, spread with tin foil, mastermind them in the air fryer cooker cook at 360 Deg. Fahrenheit for about 45 minutes.

4.   Meanwhile, in a bowl, blend strawberries in with 3 tablespoons sugar, rum, mint and lime pizzazz, mix and leave aside in a virus place.

5.   In another bowl, blend whipping cream in with 1 tablespoon sugar and mix.

6.   Take containers out, separate strawberry blend and whipped cream on top and serve. Enjoy the recipe!

The nutritional facts: calories 164, fat 2, fiber 3, carbs 5, protein 2

WIPE CAKE

Prep. time: 10 minutes The cooking time: 20 minutes The recipe servings: 12

Fixings:

3 cups flour

3 teaspoons preparing powder

½ cup cornstarch

1 teaspoon preparing soft drink 1 cup olive oil

1 and ½ cup milk

1   and 2/3 cup sugar 2 cups water

¼ cup lemon juice

2   teaspoons vanilla concentrate

Guidelines:

1.   In a bowl, blend flour in with cornstarch, heating powder, preparing pop and sugar and whisk well.

2.   In another bowl, blend oil in with milk, water, vanilla and lemon squeeze and whisk.

3.   Combine the two blends, mix, pour in a lubed preparing dish that accommodates the air fryer cooker, present in the fryer and cook at 350 Deg. Fahrenheit for about 20 minutes.

4.   Leave cake to chill off, cut and serve. Enjoy the recipe!

The nutritional facts: calories 246, fat 3, fiber 1, carbs 6, protein 2

RICOTTA AND LEMON CAKE

The cooking time: 1 hour and 10 minutes

The recipe servings: 4

Fixings:

8 eggs, whisked

3 pounds ricotta cheddar

½ pound sugar

Get-up-and-go from 1 lemon, ground Zest from 1 orange, ground Butter for the container

Guidelines:

1.   In a bowl, blend eggs in with sugar, cheddar, lemon and orange get-up-and-go and mix quite well.

2.   Grease a heating container that accommodates the air fryer cooker with some hitter, spread ricotta blend, present in the fryer at 390 degrees F and prepare for 30 minutes.

3.   Reduce heat at 380 degrees F and prepare for 40 additional minutes.

4.   Take out of the oven, leave cake to chill off and serve! Enjoy the recipe!

The nutritional facts: calories 110, fat 3, fiber 2, carbs 3, protein 4

TANGERINE CAKE

Prep. time: 10 minutes

The cooking time: 20 minutes

The recipe servings: 8

Fixings:

¾ cup sugar 2 cups flour

¼ cup olive oil

½ cup milk

1   teaspoon juice vinegar

½ teaspoon vanilla concentrate Juice and get-up-and-go from 2 lemons Juice and get-up-and-go from 1 tangerine

Tangerine sections, for serving

Guidelines:

1.   In a bowl, blend flour in with sugar and mix.

2.   In another bowl, blend oil in with milk, vinegar, vanilla concentrate, lemon squeeze and pizzazz and tangerine get-up-and-go and whisk quite well.

3.   Add flour, mix well, empty this into a cake skillet that accommodates the air fryer cooker, present in the fryer and cook at 360 Deg. Fahrenheit for about 20 minutes.

4.   Serve immediately with tangerine sections on top. Enjoy the recipe!

The nutritional facts: calories 190, fat 1, fiber 1, carbs 4, protein 4

BLUEBERRY PUDDING

Prep. time: 10 minutes

The cooking time: 25 minutes

The recipe servings: 6

Fixings:

2cups flour

2 cups moved oats 8 cups blueberries

1 stick margarine, dissolved

1 cup pecans, slashed

3 tablespoons maple syrup

2 tablespoons rosemary, slashed

Guidelines:

1.   Spread blueberries in a lubed heating dish and leave aside.

2.   In your food processor, blend moved oats in with flour, pecans, margarine, maple syrup and rosemary, mix well, layer this over blueberries, present everything in the air fryer cooker and cook at 350 degrees for 25 minutes.

3.   Leave treat to chill off, cut and serve. Enjoy the recipe!

The nutritional facts: calories 150, fat 3, fiber 2, carbs 7, protein 4

COCOA AND ALMONDS BARS

Prep. time: 30 minutes

The cooking time: 4 minutes

The recipe servings: 6

Fixings:

¼ cup cocoa nibs

1 cup almonds, drenched and depleted 2 tablespoons cocoa powder

¼ cup hemp seeds

¼ cup goji berries

¼ cup coconut, destroyed 8 dates, hollowed and drenched

Guidelines:

1.   Put almonds in your food processor, mix, include hemp seeds, cocoa nibs, cocoa powder, goji, coconut and mix quite well.

2.   Add dates, mix well once more, spread on a lined heating sheet that accommodates the air fryer cooker and cook at 320 Deg. Fahrenheit for about 4 minutes.

3.   Cut into two halves and keep in the cooler for 30 minutes before serving.

Enjoy the recipe!

The nutritional facts: calories 140, fat 6, fiber 3, carbs 7, protein 19

CHOCOLATE AND POMEGRANATE BARS

Prep. time: 2 hours The cooking time: 10 minutes The recipe servings: 6

Fixings:

½ cup milk

1 teaspoon vanilla concentrate

1 and ½ cups dim chocolate, cleaved

½ cup almonds, slashed

½ cup pomegranate seeds

Guidelines:

1.   Heat up a skillet with the milk over medium low heat, include chocolate, mix for 5 minutes, take off heat include vanilla concentrate, half of the pomegranate seeds and half of the nuts and mix.

2.   Pour this into a lined heating container, spread, sprinkle a touch of salt, the remainder of the pomegranate arils and nuts, present in the air fryer cooker and cook at 300 Deg. Fahrenheit for about 4 minutes.

2.   Pour this into a lined baking pan, spread, sprinkle a pinch of salt, the rest of the pomegranate arils and nuts, introduce in the air fryer cooker and cook at 300 Deg. Fahrenheit for about 4 minutes.

3.   Keep in the fridge for 2 hours before serving. Enjoy the recipe!

The nutritional facts: calories 68, fat 1, fiber 4, carbs 6, protein 1

TOMATO CAKE

Prep. time: 10 minutes The cooking time: 30 minutes The recipe servings: 4

Fixings:

1 and ½ cups flour

1 teaspoon cinnamon powder 1 teaspoon preparing powder

1 teaspoon preparing pop

¾ cup maple syrup

1   cup tomatoes hacked

½ cup olive oil

2   tablespoon apple juice vinegar

Guidelines:

1.   In a bowl, blend flour in with preparing powder, heating pop, cinnamon and maple syrup and mix well.

2.   In another bowl, blend tomatoes in with olive oil and vinegar and mix well.

3.   Combine the 2 blends, mix well, fill a lubed round skillet that accommodates the air fryer cooker, present in the fryer and cook at 360 Deg. Fahrenheit for about 30 minutes.

4.   Leave cake to chill off, cut and serve.

Enjoy the recipe!

The nutritional facts: calories 153, fat 2, fiber 1, carbs 25, protein 4

BERIES MIX

Prep. time: 5 minutes The cooking time: 6 minutes The recipe servings: 4

Fixings:

2 tablespoons lemon juice

1 and ½ tablespoons maple syrup

1 and ½ tablespoons champagne vinegar 1 tablespoon of olive oil

1 pound strawberries, split 1 and ½ cups blueberries

¼ cup basil leaves, torn

Guidelines:

1.   In a dish that accommodates the air fryer cooker, blend lemon squeeze in with maple syrup and vinegar, heat to the point of boiling over medium high heat, include oil, blueberries and strawberries, mix, present in the air fryer cooker and cook at 310 Deg. Fahrenheit for about 6 minutes.

2.   Sprinkle basil on top and serve!

Enjoy the recipe!

The nutritional facts: calories 163, fat 4, fiber 4, carbs 10, protein 2.1

ENERGY FRUIT PUDDING

Prep. time: 10 minutes

The cooking time: 40 minutes

The recipe servings: 6

Fixings:

1 cup Paleo energy natural product curd 4 enthusiasm organic products, mash and seeds 3 and ½ ounces maple syrup

3 eggs

2   ounces ghee, dissolved

3   and ½ ounces almond milk

½ cup almond flour

½ teaspoon preparing powder

Guidelines:

1.   In a bowl, blend the half of the natural product curd with energy organic product seeds and mash, mix and gap into 6 heat verification ramekins.

2.   In a bowl, whisked eggs with maple syrup, ghee, the remainder of the curd, preparing powder, milk and flour and mix well.

3.   Divide this into the ramekins also, present in the fryer and cook at 200 Deg. Fahrenheit for about 40 minutes.

4.   Leave puddings to chill off and serve!

Enjoy the recipe!

The nutritional facts: calories 430, fat 22, fiber 3, carbs 7, protein 8

AIR FRIED APPLES

Prep. time: 10 minutes

The cooking time: 17 minutes

The recipe servings: 4

Fixings:

4big apples, cored A bunch raisins

1   tablespoon cinnamon, ground Raw HONNEY to the taste

Guidelines:

1.   Fill every apple with raisins, sprinkle cinnamon, shower HONNEY, put them in the air fryer cooker and cook at 367 Deg. Fahrenheit for about 17 minutes.

2.   Leave them to chill off and serve.

Enjoy the recipe!

The nutritional facts: calories 220, fat 3, fiber 4, carbs 6, protein 10

PUMPKIN COOKIES

Prep. time: 10 minutes

The cooking time: 15minutes

The recipe servings: 24

Fixings:

2 ½ cups flour

½ teaspoon heating pop

1   tablespoon flax seed, ground 3 tablespoons water

½ cup pumpkin substance, pounded

¼ cup HONNEY

2   tablespoons margarine

1   teaspoon vanilla concentrate

½ cup dim chocolate chips

Guidelines:

1.   In a bowl, blend flax seed with water, mix and leave aside for a couple of moments.

2.   In another bowl, blend flour in with salt and preparing pop.

3.   In a third bowl, blend HONNEY in with pumpkin puree, spread, vanilla concentrate and flaxseed.

4.   Combine flour with HONNEY blend and chocolate chips and mix.

5.   Scoop 1 tablespoon of cookie mixture on a lined heating sheet that accommodates the air fryer cooker, rehash with the remainder of the batter, present them in the air fryer cooker and cook at 350 Deg. Fahrenheit for about 15 minutes.

6.   Leave cookies to chill off and serve.

Enjoy the recipe!

The nutritional facts: calories 140, fat 2, fiber 2, carbs 7, protein 10

FIGS AND COCNUT BUTTER MIX

Prep. time: 6 minutes The cooking time: 4 minutes The recipe servings: 3

Fixings:

2   tablespoons coconut margarine 12 figs, divided

¼ cup sugar

1 cup almonds, toasted and cleaved

Guidelines:

1.   Put spread in a container that accommodates the air fryer cooker and dissolve over medium high heat.

2.   Add figs, sugar and almonds, hurl, present in the air fryer cooker and cook at 300 Deg. Fahrenheit for about 4 minutes.

3.   Divide into bowls and serve cold.

Enjoy the recipe!

The nutritional facts: calories 170, fat 4, fiber 5, carbs 7, protein 9

LEMON BARS

Prep. time: 10 minutes

The cooking time: 25 minutes

The recipe servings: 6

Fixings:

4 eggs

2 and ¼ cups flour Juice from 2 lemons 1 cup spread, delicate

2 cups sugar

Guidelines:

1.   In a bowl, blend spread in with ½ cup sugar and 2 cups flour, mix well, push on the base of a container that accommodates the air fryer cooker, present in the fryer and cook at 350 Deg. Fahrenheit for about 10 minutes.

2.	In another bowl, blend the remainder of the sugar in with the remainder of the flour, eggs and lemon juice, whisk well and spread over outside.

3.	Introduce in the fryer at 350 Deg. Fahrenheit for about 15 minutes more, leave aside to chill off, cut bars and serve them.

Enjoy the recipe!

The nutritional facts: calories 125, fat 4, fiber 4, carbs 16, protein 2

PEARS AND ESPRESSO CREAM

Prep. time: 10 minutes

The cooking time: 30 minutes

The recipe servings: 4

Fixings:

4 pears, divided and cored 2 tablespoons lemon juice 1 tablespoon sugar

2 tablespoons water

2 tablespoons spread

For the cream:

1	cup whipping cream 1 cup mascarpone

1/3 cup sugar

2   tablespoons coffee, cold

Guidelines:

1.   In a bowl, blend pears parts with lemon juice, 1 tablespoons sugar, spread and water, hurl well, move them to the air fryer cooker and cook at 360 Deg. Fahrenheit for about 30 minutes.

2.   Meanwhile, in a bowl, blend whipping cream in with mascarpone, 1/3 cup sugar and coffee, whisk truly well and keep in the ice chest until pears are finished.

3.   Divide pears on plates, top with coffee cream and serve them. Enjoy the recipe!

The nutritional facts: calories 211, fat 5, fiber 7, carbs 8, protein 7

POPPYSEED CAKE

Prep. time: 10 minutes

The cooking time: 30 minutes

The recipe servings: 6

Fixings:

1 and ¼ cups flour

1 teaspoon heating powder

¾ cup sugar

1 tablespoon orange pizzazz, ground 2 teaspoons lime get-up-and-go, ground

½ cup margarine, delicate 2 eggs, whisked

½ teaspoon vanilla concentrate 2 tablespoons poppy seeds 1 cup milk

For the cream:

1 cup sugar

½ cup enthusiasm organic product puree

3 tablespoons margarine, softened 4 egg yolks

Guidelines:

1.   In a bowl, blend flour in with heating powder, ¾ cup sugar, orange pizzazz and lime get-up-and-go and mix.

2.   Add ½ cup spread, eggs, poppy seeds, vanilla and milk, mix utilizing your blender, fill a cake dish that accommodates the air fryer cooker and cook at 350 Deg. Fahrenheit for about around 30 minutes.

3.   Meanwhile, heat up a dish with 3 tablespoons spread over medium heat, include sugar and mix until it breaks down.

4.   Take off heat, include energy natural product puree and egg yolks step by step and whisk truly well.

5.   Take cake out of the fryer, chill it off a piece and cut into equal parts on a level plane.

6.   Spread ¼ of energy natural product cream more than one half, top with the other cake half

also, spread ¼ of the cream on top.

7.   Serve virus. Enjoy the recipe!

The nutritional facts: calories 211, fat 6, fiber 7, carbs 12, protein 6

SWEET SQUARES

Prep. time: 10 minutes

The cooking time: 30 minutes

The recipe servings: 6

Fixings:

1cup flour

½ cup spread, delicate 1 cup sugar

¼ cup powdered sugar

1 teaspoons lemon strip, ground 2 tablespoons lemon juice

2 eggs, whisked

½ teaspoon preparing powder

Guidelines:

1. In a bowl, blend flour in with powdered sugar and spread, mix well, push on the base of a dish that accommodates the air fryer cooker, present in the fryer and heat at 350 Deg. Fahrenheit for about 14 minutes.

2. In another bowl, blend sugar in with lemon juice, lemon strip, eggs and heating powder, mix utilizing your blender and spread over prepared hull.

3. Bake for 15 minutes more, leave aside to chill off, cut into medium squares and serve cold.

Enjoy the recipe!

The nutritional facts: calories 100, fat 4, fiber 1, carbs 12, protein 1

PLUM BARS

Prep. time: 10 minutes

The cooking time: 16 minutes

The recipe servings: 8

Fixings:

2 cups dried plums 6 tablespoons water 2 cup moved oats

1 cup dark colored sugar

½ teaspoon preparing pop

1 teaspoon cinnamon powder 2 tablespoons spread, liquefied 1 egg, whisked

Cooking splash

Guidelines:

1.   In your food processor, blend plums with water and mix until you get a clingy spread.

2.   In a bowl, blend oats in with cinnamon, preparing pop, sugar, egg and margarine and whisk truly well.

3.   Press portion of the oats blend in a preparing dish that accommodates the air fryer cooker showered with cooking oil, spread plums blend and top with the other portion of the oats blend.

4.   Introduce in the air fryer cooker and cook at 350 Deg. Fahrenheit for about 16 minutes.

5.   Leave blend aside to chill off, cut into medium bars and serve. Enjoy the recipe!

The nutritional facts: calories 111, fat 5, fiber 6, carbs 12, protein 6

PLUM AND CURRENT TART

Prep. time: 10 minutes

The cooking time: 35 minutes

The recipe servings: 6

Fixings:

For the disintegrate:

¼ cup almond flour

¼ cup millet flour

1 cup dark colored rice flour

½ cup genuine sweetener

10 tablespoons margarine, delicate 3 tablespoons milk

For the filling:

1   pound little plums, pitted and divided 1 cup white currants

2   tablespoons cornstarch

3   tablespoons sugar

½ teaspoon vanilla concentrate

½ teaspoon cinnamon powder

¼ teaspoon ginger powder 1 teaspoon lime juice

Guidelines:

1.   In a bowl, blend darker rice flour with ½ cup sugar, millet flour, almond flour, spread and milk and mix until you get a sand like mixture.

2.   Reserve ¼ of the mixture, press the remainder of the batter into a tart container that accommodates the air fryer cooker and keep in the refrigerator for 30 minutes.

3.   Meanwhile, in a bowl, blend plums with currants, 3 tablespoons sugar, cornstarch, vanilla concentrate, cinnamon, ginger and lime squeeze and mix well.

4.   Pour this over tart outside layer, disintegrate reserved mixture on top, present in the air fryer cooker and cook at 350 Deg. Fahrenheit for about 35 minutes.

5.   Leave tart to chill off, cut and serve. Enjoy the recipe!

The nutritional facts: calories 200, fat 5, fiber 4, carbs 8, protein 6

DELICIOUS ORANGE COOKIES

Prep. time: 10 minutes

The cooking time: 12 minutes

The recipe servings: 8

Fixings:

2 cups flour

1 teaspoon heating powder

½ cup margarine, delicate

¾ cup sugar

1 egg, whisked

1 teaspoon vanilla concentrate

1 tablespoon orange pizzazz, ground

For the filling:

4 ounces cream cheddar, delicate

½ cup margarine

2 cups powdered sugar

Guidelines:

1.	In a bowl, blend cream cheddar with ½ cup spread and 2 cups powdered sugar, mix well utilizing your blender and leave aside until further notice.

2.	In another bowl, blend flour in with heating powder.

3.	In a third bowl, blend ½ cup spread with ¾ cup sugar, egg, vanilla concentrate and orange pizzazz and whisk well.

4.	Combine flour with orange blend, mix well and scoop 1 tablespoon of the blend on a lined heating sheet that accommodates the air fryer cooker.

5.	Repeat with the remainder of the orange player, present in the fryer and cook at 340 Deg. Fahrenheit for about 12 minutes.

6.	Leave cookies to chill off, spread cream filling on half of them top with different cookies and serve.

Enjoy the recipe!

The nutritional facts: calories 124, fat 5, fiber 6, carbs 8, protein 4

CAHEW BARS

Prep. time: 10 minutes

The cooking time: 15 minutes

The recipe servings: 6

Fixings:

1/3 cup HONNEY

¼ cup almond meal

1 tablespoon almond spread

1 and ½ cups cashews, hacked 4 dates, slashed

¾ cup coconut, destroyed 1 tablespoon chia seeds

Guidelines:

1.   In a bowl, blend HONNEY in with almond meal and almond spread and mix well.

2.   Add cashews, coconut, dates and chia seeds and mix well once more.

3.   Spread this on a lined heating sheet that accommodates the air fryer cooker and press well.

4.   Introduce in the fryer and cook at 300 Deg. Fahrenheit for about 15 minutes.

5.   Leave blend to chill off, cut into medium bars and serve. Enjoy the recipe!

The nutritional facts: calories 121, fat 4, fiber 7, carbs 5, protein 6

DARK COLORED BUTTER COOKIES

Prep. time: 10 minutes The cooking time: 10 minutes The recipe servings: 6

Fixings:

1 and ½ cups spread 2 cups dark colored sugar 2 eggs, whisked

3 cups flour

2/3 cup walnuts, hacked

2 teaspoons vanilla concentrate 1 teaspoon preparing pop

½ teaspoon preparing powder

Guidelines:

1.   Heat up a dish with the spread over medium heat, mix until it liquefies, include dark colored sugar and mix until this disintegrates.

2.   In a bowl, blend flour in with walnuts, vanilla concentrate, preparing pop, heating powder and eggs and mix well.

3.	Add dark colored margarine, mix well and organize spoonfuls of this blend on a lined heating sheet that accommodates the air fryer cooker.

4.	Introduce in the fryer and cook at 340 Deg. Fahrenheit for about 10 minutes.

5.	Leave cookies to chill off and serve. Enjoy the recipe!

The nutritional facts: calories 144, fat 5, fiber 6, carbs 19, protein 2

SWEET POTATO CHEESECAKE

Prep. time: 10 minutes

The cooking time: 5 minutes

The recipe servings: 4

Fixings:

4 tablespoons spread, softened 6 ounces mascarpone, delicate 8 ounces cream cheddar, delicate

2/3 cup graham wafers, disintegrated

¾ cup milk

1 teaspoon vanilla concentrate 2/3 cup sweet potato puree

¼ teaspoons cinnamon powder

Guidelines:

1.   In a bowl, blend spread in with disintegrated saltines, mix well, push on the base of a cake dish that accommodates the air fryer cooker and keep in the ice chest for the time being.

2.   In another bowl, blend cream cheddar with mascarpone, sweet potato puree, milk, cinnamon and vanilla and whisk truly well.

3.   Spread this over covering, present in the air fryer cooker, cook at 300 Deg. Fahrenheit for about 4 minutes and keep in the cooler for a couple of hours before serving.

Enjoy the recipe!

The nutritional facts: calories 172, fat 4, fiber 6, carbs 8, protein 3

The cooking time: 35 minutes

The recipe servings: 4

Fixings:

1   pie mixture

2   and ¼ pounds peaches, hollowed and cleaved 2 tablespoons cornstarch

½ cup sugar

2 tablespoons flour

A spot of nutmeg, ground 1 tablespoon dim rum

1   tablespoon lemon juice

2   tablespoons spread, dissolved

Guidelines:

1.   Roll pie batter into a pie dish that accommodates the air fryer cooker and press well.

2.   In a bowl, blend peaches in with cornstarch, sugar, flour, nutmeg, rum, lemon squeeze and margarine and mix well.

3.   Pour and spread this into pie container, present in the air fryer cooker and cook at 350 Deg. Fahrenheit for about 35 minutes.

4.   Serve warm or cold. Enjoy the recipe!

The nutritional facts: calories 231, fat 6, fiber 7, carbs 9, protein 5

VEGAN STARTERS AND MAINS

Fixings:

Masala galette

2 tbsp. garam masala

2   medium potatoes bubbled and pounded 1 ½ cup coarsely squashed peanuts

3   tsp. ginger finely slashed

1-2 tbsp. crisp coriander leaves

2 or 3 green chilies finely slashed 1 ½ tbsp. lemon juice

Salt and pepper to taste

Technique:

Mix the fixings in an unblemished bowl.

Shape this mix into round and level galettes.

Wet the galettes possibly with water. Coat each galette with the squashed peanuts.

Pre heat the Air-Fryer at 160 deg. Fahrenheit for 5 about minutes. Recognize the galettes in the fry bushel and let them cook for an extra 25 minutes at a comparable temperature. Keep giving them to get auniform cook. Serve either with mint chutney or ketchup.

POTATO SAMOSA

Fixings: For wrappers:

2 tbsp. unsalted spread

1 ½ cup generally useful flour A spot of salt to taste

Include as a lot of water as required to make the batter solid and firm

For filling:

2-3 major potatoes bubbled and pounded

¼ cup bubbled peas

1 tsp. of powdered ginger

1 to 2 green chilies that are finely slashed or crushed

½ tsp. cumin

1   tsp. coarsely squashed coriander 1 dry red bean stew broken into pieces A limited quantity of salt (to taste)

½ tsp. dried mango powder

½ tsp. red bean stew power. 1-2 tbsp. coriander.

Technique:

Blend the mixture for the external covering and make it hardened and smooth. Leave it to rest in a holder while making the filling.

Cook the fixings in a dish and mix them well to make a thick glue. Turn the glue out.

Fold the batter into balls and straighten them. Cut them in equal parts and include the filling. Use water to assist you with collapsing the edges to make the state of a cone.

Pre-heat the air-fyer for about 5 to 6 minutes at 300 Fahrenheit. See all the samosas in the fry canister and close the holder sensibly. Keep the air-fryer at 200 Deg. for another 20 to 25 minutes. Around the midpoint, open the vault and turn the samosas over for uniform cooking. Then, fry at 250 Deg. for around 10 minutes in order to give them the perfect astonishing weak tinted covering. Serve hot. Proposed sides are tamarind or mint chutney.

VEGETABLE KEBAB

Fixing:

2cups blended vegetables 3 onions hacked

5 green chilies-generally hacked 1 ½ tbsp. ginger glue

1 ½ tsp. garlic glue 1 ½ tsp. salt

3 tsp. lemon juice

2 tsp. garam masala

4 tbsp. hacked coriander 3 tbsp. cream

3 tbsp. hacked capsicum 3 eggs

2 ½ tbsp. white sesame seeds

Strategy:

Crush the fixings with the exception of the egg and structure a smooth glue. Coat the vegetables in the glue.

Dunk the covered vegetables in the egg blend and afterward move to the sesame seeds and coat the vegetables well. Detect the vegetables on a stick.

Pre heat the air-fryer at 160 Deg Fahrenheit for around 5 minutes. Detect the sticks in the container and let them cook for an extra 25 minutes at a comparable temperature.

SAGO GALETTE

Fixing:

2 cup sago drenched

1   ½ cup coarsely squashed peanuts 3 tsp. ginger finely cleaved

1-2 tbsp. new coriander leaves

2   or 3 green chilies finely slashed 1 ½ tbsp. lemon juice

Salt and pepper to taste

Technique:

Wash the doused sago and blend it in with the remainder of the fixings in a perfect bowl.

Structure this mix into round and level galettes.

Wet the galettes to some degree with water. Coat each galette with the squashed peanuts.

Pre heat the air-fryer at 160 Deg,. Fahrenheit for 5 minutes. Detect the galettes in the fry case and let them cook for an extra 25 minutes at a comparable temperature. Keep giving them to get auniform cook. Serve either with mint chutney or ketchup.

STUFFED CAPSICUM BASKETS

Fixings: For bushels:

3-4 long capsicum

½ tsp. salt

½ tsp. pepper powder

For filling:

1   medium onion finely hacked 1 green stew finely cleaved

2   or 3 huge potatoes bubbled and pounded 1 ½ tbsp. slashed coriander leaves

1 tsp. fenugreek

1 tsp. dried mango powder 1 tsp. cumin powder

Salt and pepper to taste

For fixing:

3 tbsp. ground cheddar 1 tsp. red bean stew drops

½ tsp. oregano

½ tsp. basil

½ tsp. parsley

Strategy:

Take all the fixings under the heading "Filling" and combine them in a bowl.

Expel the stem of the capsicum. Remove the tops. Expel the seeds also. Sprinkle some salt and pepper inside the capsicums. Leave them aside for a long time.

By and by round the exhausted out capsicums with the filling organized at this point leave a little space at the top. Sprinkle ground cheddar and moreover incorporate the enhancing.

Preheat the Air-fryer at 140 degrees Fahrenheit for 5 minutes. Put the capsicums in the fry canister and close it. Let them cook at a comparable temperature for an extra 20 minutes. Turn them over in the center of to hinder over cooking.

HEATED MACARONI PASTA

Fixings:

1 cup pasta

7 cups of bubbling water 1 ½ tbsp. olive oil

A spot of salt

For hurling pasta:

1   ½ tbsp. olive oil

½ cup carrot little pieces Salt and pepper to taste

½ tsp. oregano

½ tsp. basil

For white sauce:

2   tbsp. olive oil

2 tbsp. universally handy flour 2 cups of milk

1 tsp. of dried oregano

½ tsp. of dried basil

½ tablespoon of the dried parsley Salt and pepper to taste Method:

Heat up the pasta and sifter it when done. You should hurl the pasta in the fixings referenced above and put in a safe spot.

For the sauce, add the fixings to a skillet and heat the fixings to the point of boiling. Mix the sauce and keep on stewing to make a thicker sauce. Add the pasta to the sauce and move this into a glass bowl embellished with cheddar. Pre-heat the Air-fryer at 160 degrees for 5 minutes. Spot the bowl in the crate and close it. Let it keep on cooking at a similar temperature for 10 minutes more. Continue blending the pasta in the middle.

MACARONI SAMOSA

Fixings: For wrappers: 1 cup generally useful flour 2 tbsp. unsalted margarine A touch of salt to taste

Take the measure of water sufficiently adequate to make a firm batter

For filling:

3 cups bubbled macaroni 2 onion cut

2 capsicum cut

2 carrot cut

2 cabbage cut 2 tbsp. soya sauce 2 tsp. vinegar

2 tbsp. ginger finely slashed 2 tbsp. garlic finely hacked

2 tbsp. green chilies finely slashed 2 tbsp. ginger-garlic glue

Add some salt and pepper to taste 2 tbsp. olive oil

½ tsp. ajinomoto

Technique:

Blend the batter for the external covering and make it firm and smooth. Leave it to rest in a compartment while making the filling.

Cook the fixings in a container and mix them well to make a thick glue. Turn the glue out.

Fold the batter into balls and smooth them. Cut them in equal parts and include the filling. Use water to assist you with collapsing the edges to make the state of a cone.

Pre-heat the Air Fryer for about 5-6 minutes at 300 Fahrenheit. Spot all the samosas in the fry bushel and close the bin appropriately. Keep the air-fryer cooker at 200 De for another 20 to 25 minutes. Around the midpoint, open the container and turn the samosas over for uniform cooking. After this, fry at 250 deg. F for about 10 minutes so as to give them the ideal brilliant darker shading. Serve hot. Prescribed sides are tamarind or mint chutney.

Fixings: Refried beans:

BURRITOS

½ cup red kidney beans (splashed medium-term)

½ little onion hacked 1 tbsp. olive oil

2 tbsp. of tomato puree

¼ tsp. of red stew powder 1 tsp. of salt to taste

4-5 flour tortillas

Vegetable Filling:

1 tbsp. Olive oil

1 medium onion finely cut 3 chips garlic squashed

½ cup French beans (Slice them longwise into thin and long cuts)

½ cup mushrooms daintily cut

1 cup curds slice in to long and somewhat thick fingers

½ cup destroyed cabbage 1 tbsp. coriander, cleaved 1 tbsp. vinegar

1 tsp. white wine

A spot of salt to taste

½ tsp. red bean stew chips

1 tsp. crisply ground peppercorns

½ cup salted jalapenos (Chop them up finely) 2 carrots (Cut in to long thin cuts)

Serving of mixed greens:

1-2 lettuce leaves destroyed.

1 or 2 spring onions slashed finely. Additionally cut the greens.

Take one tomato. Evacuate the seeds and hack it into little pieces. 1 green bean stew slashed.

1 cup of cheddar ground.

Strategy:

Cook the beans alongside the onion and garlic and pound them finely.

Presently, make the sauce you will requirement for the burrito. Guarantee that you make a marginally thick sauce.

For the filling, you should cook the fixings well in a dish and guarantee that the vegetables have seared outwardly.

To make the serving of mixed greens, hurl the fixings together.

Spot the tortilla and include a layer of sauce, trailed by the beans and the filling at the middle. Before you move it, you should put the plate of mixed greens on the filling.

Pre-heat the Air-fryer for 5 minutes at 200 Fahrenheit. Open the fry container and keep the burritos inside. Close the bin appropriately. Let the Air Fryer stay at 200 Fahrenheit for an additional 15 minutes or thereabouts. Part of the way through, evacuate the container and turn all the burritos over so as to get a uniform cook.

Fixings:

Cheddar and Bean Enchiladas

Flour tortillas (the same number of as required)

Red sauce:

4 tbsp. of olive oil

1 ½ tsp. of garlic that has been slashed 1 ½ cups of readymade tomato puree

3 medium tomatoes. Puree them in a blender 1 tsp. of sugar

A spot of salt or to taste

A couple of red bean stew drops to sprinkle 1 tsp. of oregano

Filling:

2 tbsp. oil

2 tsp. slashed garlic

2 onions slashed finely

2 capsicums slashed finely

2 cups of readymade heated beans A couple of drops of Tabasco sauce

1 cup disintegrated or generally crushed (curds) 1 cup ground cheddar

A touch of salt 1 tsp. oregano

½ tsp. pepper

1 ½ tsp. red stew drops or to taste 1 tbsp. of finely hacked jalapenos To serve:

1 cup ground pizza cheddar (blend mozzarella and cheddar cheeses)

Strategy:

Set up the flour tortillas.

Presently proceed onward to making the red sauce. In a skillet, pour around 2 tbsp. of oil and heat. Include some garlic. Include the remainder of the fixings referenced under the heading "For the sauce". Continue mixing. Cook until the sauce lessens and turns out to be thick.

For the filling, heat one tbsp. of oil in another container. Include onions and garlic and cook until the onions are caramelized or accomplish a brilliant dark colored shading. Include the remainder of the fixings required for the filling and cook for a few minutes. Take the dish off the fire and mesh some cheddar over the

sauce. Blend it well and let it sit for some time.

Let us begin collecting the dish. Take a tortilla and spread a portion of the sauce superficially. Presently place the filling at the inside in a line. Move up the tortilla cautiously. Do likewise for all the tortillas.

Presently place all the tortillas in a plate and sprinkle them with ground cheddar. Spread this with an aluminum foil.

Preheat the Air fryer cookerat 160° C for 4-5 minutes. Open the container and spot the plate inside. Save the fryer at a similar temperature for an additional 15 minutes. Turn the tortillas over in the middle of to get auniform cook.

Fixings: For batter:

Veg Momos

1   ½ cup generally useful flour

½ tsp. salt or to taste 5 tbsp. water

For filling:

2   cup carrots ground 2 cup cabbage ground 2 tbsp. oil

2 tsp. ginger-garlic glue 2 tsp. soya sauce

2 tsp. vinegar

Strategy:

Work the blend and spread it with stick wrap and put in a sheltered spot. Next, cook the components for the filling and endeavor to ensure that the vegetables are protected well with the sauce.

Overlap the hitter and cut it into a square. Recognize the filling in within. Wrap the hitter to cover the filling and crush the edges together.

Pre heat the air-fryer at 200° F for 5 minutes. Detect the gnocchis in the fry case and close it. Let thecook at a comparable temperature for an extra 20 minutes.

CORNFLAKES FRENCH TOAST

RECIPE INGREDIENTS:

Bread cuts (dark colored or white) 1 egg white for each 2 cuts 1 tsp. sugar for each 2 cuts Crushed cornflakes

Strategy:

Set up two cuts and cut them along the corner to corner.

Dunk the bread triangles into this blend and afterward cover them with the squashed cornflakes.

Pre-heat the Air-Fryer at 180° C for 4 minutes. Look for the covered bread triangles in the fry crate and close it. Let them cook at a similar temperature for an additional 20 minutes at any rate. Part of the way through the procedure, turn the triangles over with the goal that you get auniform cook. Serve these cuts with chocolate sauce.

COTTAGE CHEESE POPS

RECIPE INGREDIENTS:

1 cup curds cut into 2" 3D squares 1 ½ tsp. garlic glue

Salt and pepper to taste 1 tsp. dry oregano

1 tsp. dry basil

½ cup hung curd 1 tsp. lemon juice

1   tsp. red stew drops

Strategy:

Cut the curds into thick and long rectangular pieces.

Include the remainder of the fixings into a different bowl and blend them well to get aconsistent blend.

Plunge the curds pieces in the above blend and leave them aside for quite a while.

Pre-heat the air-fryer at 180° C for around 5 minutes. Spot the covered curds pieces in the fry crate and close it appropriately. Let them cook at a similar temperature for 20 additional minutes. Continue turning them over in the crate with the goal that they are cooked appropriately. Serve with tomato ketchup.

MINT GALETTE

RECIPE INGREDIENTS:

2cups mint leaves (Sliced fine)

2   medium potatoes bubbled and squashed 1 ½ cup coarsely squashed peanuts

3   tsp. ginger finely hacked

1-2 tbsp. new coriander leaves

2 or 3 green chilies finely hacked 1 ½ tbsp. lemon juice

Salt and pepper to taste

Strategy:

Mix the cut mint leaves in with the rest of the fixings in an ideal bowl. Structure this mix into round and level galettes.

Wet the galettes to some degree with water.

Pre heat the air-fryer at 160 Deg. Fahrenheit for 5 minutes. Detect the galettes in the fry case and let them cook for an extra 25 minutes at a comparable tem.

CURDS STICKS

RECIPE INGREDIENTS:

2 cups curds 1 major lemon-squeezed

1   tbsp. ginger-garlic glue

For flavoring, utilize salt and red bean stew powder in limited quantities

½ tsp. carom

A couple papadums 4 or 5 tbsp. corn flour 1 cup of water Method:

Take the curds. Cut it into long pieces.

Presently, make a blend of lemon juice, red bean stew powder, salt, ginger garlic glue and carom to use as a marinade. Let the curds pieces marinate in the blend for quite a while and afterward move them in dry corn flour. Leave them aside for around 20 minutes.

Take the papadum into a container and dish them. When they are cooked, smash them into little pieces. Presently take another holder and pour around 100 ml of water into it. Disintegrate 2 tbsp. of corn flour right now. Dunk the curds pieces right now corn flour and move them on to the bits of squashed papadum so that the papadum adheres to the curds. Pre heat the air fryer cooker for about 10 minutes at 290 Fahrenheit. At that point open the container of the fryer and spot the curds pieces inside it. Close the bin appropriately. Let the fryer remain at 160 degrees for an additional 20 minutes. Partially through, open the bushel and hurl the curds around a piece to take into account uniform cooking. When they are done, you can serve it either with ketchup or mint chutney. Another prescribed side is mint chutney.

PALAK GALETTE

RECIPE INGREDIENTS:

2tbsp. garam masala 2 cups palak leaves

1   ½ cup coarsely squashed peanuts 3 tsp. ginger finely cleaved

1-2 tbsp. new coriander leaves

2   or 3 green chilies finely cleaved 1 ½ tbsp. lemon juice

Salt and pepper to taste

Strategy:

Blend the fixings in a perfect bowl.

Structure this mix into round and level galettes.

Wet the galettes hardly with water. Coat each galette with the squashed peanuts.

Pre heat the air-fryer at 160 e.g. Fahrenheit for 5 minutes. Recognize the galettes in the fry compartment and let them cook for an extra 25 minutes at a comparative temperature. Keep surrendering them to get a uniform cook. Serve either with mint chutney or ketchup.

MASALA FRENCH FRIES

RECIPE INGREDIENTS:

2 medium measured potatoes stripped and cut into thick pieces longwise

Elements for the marinade:

1 tbsp. olive oil

1 tsp. blended herbs

½ tsp. red bean stew pieces A touch of salt to taste 1 tbsp. lemon juice Method:

Heat up the potatoes and brighten them. Cut the potato into fingers. Mix the components for the marinade and add the potato fingers to it guaranteeing that they are secured well.

Pre-heat the air-fryer for about 5 minutes at 300 Fahrenheit. Take out the holder of the fryer and detect the potato fingers in them. Close the bushel. By and by spare the fryer at 200 Fahrenheit for 20 or 25 minutes. In the method, fling the fries twice or thrice with the objective that they get cooked suitably.

DAL MINT KEBAB

Fixings:

1 cup chickpeas

Half inch ginger ground or one and a half tsp. of ginger-garlic glue 1-2 green chilies slashed finely

¼ tsp. red bean stew powder A spot of salt to taste

½ tsp. simmered cumin powder 2 tsp. coriander powder

1 ½ tbsp. slashed coriander

½ tsp. dried mango powder 1 cup dry breadcrumbs

¼ tsp. dark salt

1-2 tbsp. universally handy flour for covering purposes 1-2 tbsp. mint (finely cleaved)

1   onion that has been finely hacked

½ cup milk

Strategy:

Take an open vessel. Heat up the chickpeas in the vessel until their surface turns out to be delicate. Ensure that they don't get wet.

Presently bring this chickpeas into another holder. Include the ground ginger and the cut green chilies. Crush this blend until it turns into a thick glue. Continue including water as and when required. Presently include the onions, mint, the breadcrumbs and all the different masalas required. Blend this well until you get a delicate batter. Presently take little chunks of this blend (about the size of a lemon) and form them into the state of level and round kebabs.

Here is the place the milk becomes possibly the most important factor. Pour a limited quantity of milk onto every kebab to wet it. Presently roll the kebab in the dry breadcrumbs.

Pre-heat the air- fryer cooker for 5 minutes at 300 Fahrenheit. Take out the bin. Orchestrate the kebabs in the container leaving holes between them with the goal that no two kebabs are contacting one another. Save the fryer at 340 Fahrenheit for around thirty minutes. Part of the way through the cooking procedure, turn the kebabs over with the goal that they can be cooked appropriately. Prescribed sides for this dish are mint chutney, tomato ketchup or yogurt chutney.

Fixings:

Curds CROQUETTE

2   cups curds cut into somewhat thick and long pieces (like French fries)

1 major capsicum (Cut this capsicum into huge 3D shapes)

1   onion (Cut it into quarters. Presently isolated the layers cautiously.) 5 tbsp. gram flour

A touch of salt to taste

For chutney:

2   cup new green coriander

½ cup mint leaves 4 tsp. fennel

1   small onion

2   tbsp. ginger-garlic glue 6-7 garlic chips (discretionary) 3 tbsp. lemon juice

Salt

Strategy:

Take a spotless and dry compartment. Put the coriander in to it, mint, fennel, and ginger, onion/garlic, salt and lemon juice. Blend them. Empty the blend into a processor and mix until you get athick glue.

Presently proceed onward to the curds pieces. Cut these pieces nearly till the end and leave them aside. Presently stuff all the pieces with the glue that was gotten from the past advance. Presently leave the stuffed curds aside.

Add the chutney and to it the gram flour and some salt. Combine them appropriately. Rub this blend everywhere throughout the stuffed curds pieces. Presently leave the curds aside.

Presently, to the extra chutney, include the capsicum and onions. Apply the chutney liberally on every one of the bits of capsicum and onion. Presently take satay sticks and orchestrate the curds pieces and vegetables on discrete sticks.

Pre-heat the air-fryer cooker at 290 Fahrenheit for around 5 minutes. Open the crate. Organize the satay sticks appropriately. Close the container. Keep the sticks with the curds at 180 degrees for around 30 minutes at a similar temperature for just 7 minutes. Turn the sticks in the middle of with the goal that one side doesn't get scorched and furthermore to give a uniform cook.

Fixings:

Grill CORN SANDWICH

2 cuts of white bread 1 tbsp. relaxed spread

1 cup sweet corn bits 1 little capsicum

For Barbeque Sauce:

¼ tbsp. Worcestershire sauce

½ tsp. olive oil

½ drop garlic squashed

¼ cup slashed onion

¼ tbsp. red bean stew sauce

½ cup water

Technique:

Take the cuts of bread and clear the edges. Directly cut the cuts on a level plane.

Cook the components for the sauce and hold up till it thickens. By and by, add the corn to the sauce and blend till it obtains the flavors. Cook the capsicum and strip the skin off. Cut the capsicum into cuts. Apply the sauce on the cuts.

Pre-heat the Air-fryer for about 5 minutes at 300 Fahrenheit. Open the receptacle of the Fryer and recognize the prepared sandwiches in it with the ultimate objective that no two sandwiches are reaching each other. By and by spare the fryer at 250 degrees for around 15 minutes. Turn the sandwiches in the cooking system to cook the two cuts.

HONEY CHILI POTATOES

Fixings: For potato:

3 major potatoes (Cut into strips or 3D shapes) 2 ½ tsp. ginger-garlic glue

¼ tsp. salt

1 tsp. red stew sauce

¼ tsp. red stew powder/dark pepper

A couple of drops of eatable orange food shading

For sauce:

1 capsicum, then cut into thin and long pieces (longwise). 2 tbsp. olive oil

2   onions. Cut them into equal parts. 1 ½ tbsp. sweet stew sauce

1   ½ tsp. ginger garlic glue

½ tbsp. Red bean stew sauce. 2 tbsp. Tomato ketchup 2 tsp. soya sauce

2   tsp. vinegar

A touch of dark pepper powder 1-2 tsp. red stew pieces

Strategy:

Make the blend for the potato fingers and coat the chicken well with it.

Preheat the Air fryer at 250 Fahrenheit for 5 minutes or thereabouts. Open the container of the Fryer. Spot the fingers inside the bin. Presently let the fryer remain at

290   Fahrenheit for another   20   minutes.   Keep tossing the fingers occasionally through the cook to get a uniform cook.

BURGER CUTLET

RECIPE INGREDIENTS:

1 enormous potato bubbled and pounded

½ cup breadcrumbs

A spot of salt to taste

¼ tsp. Ginger finely slashed 1 green bean stew finely cleaved 1 tsp. lemon juice

1   tbsp. Crisp coriander leaves. Cleave them finely

¼ tsp. red bean stew powder

½ cup of bubbled peas

¼ tsp. cumin powder

¼ tsp. dried mango powder

Technique:

Combine the fixings and guarantee that the flavors are correct. You will presently make round cutlets with the blend and turn them out well.

Preheat the Air Fryer at 250 Fahrenheit for 5 minutes. Open the bin of the Fryer and mastermind the cutlets in the bushel. Close it cautiously. Save the fryer at 150 degrees for around 10 or 12 minutes. In the middle of the cooking procedure, surrender the cutlets to get a uniform cook. Serve hot with mint chutney.

PIZZA RECIPE INGREDIENTS:

One pizza base

Ground pizza cheddar (mozzarella cheddar ideally) for fixing Use cooking oil for brushing and fixing purposes

Elements for fixing:

2   onions hacked

2 capsicums hacked

2 tomatoes that have been deseeded and hacked 1 tbsp. (discretionary) mushrooms/corns

2 tsp. pizza flavoring

Some curds that have been cut into little 3D shapes (discretionary)

Strategy:

Put the pizza base in a pre-heated air-fryer cooker for around 5 minutes. (Preheated to 340 Fahrenheit).

Take out the base. Pour some pizza sauce on the base in the middle. Utilizing a spoon spread the sauce over the base, ensuring that you leave some hole around the circuit. Mesh some mozzarella cheddar and sprinkle it over the sauce layer.

Take all the vegetables referenced in the fixing list above and blend them in a bowl. Include some oil and flavoring. Likewise, include some salt and pepper as per taste. Blend them appropriately. Put this garnish over the layer of cheddar on the pizza. Presently sprinkle some more ground cheddar and pizza flavoring on this layer.

Preheat the Air Fryer at 250 Fahrenheit for around 5 minutes. Open the fry crate and spot the pizza inside. Close the crate and save the fryer at 170 degrees for an additional 10 minutes. In the event that you feel that it is undercooked, you may put it at a similar temperature for an additional 2 minutes or something like that.

Fixings:

Cheddar FRENCH FRIES

2 medium estimated potatoes stripped and cut into thick pieces the long way

Elements for the marinade:

1 tbsp. olive oil

1 tsp. blended herbs

½ tsp. Red bean stew chips A spot of salt to taste 1 tbsp. lemon juice

For the topping:

1 cup softened cheddar (You could place this into a channeling pack and make an example of it on the fries.)

Strategy:

Take all the fixings referenced under the heading "For the marinade" and blend them well.

Presently fill a holder 3 cups of water. Include a spot of salt into this water. Carry it to the bubble. Presently whiten the bits of potato for around 5 minutes. Channel the water utilizing a strainer.

Dry the potatoes on a towel and a while later spot them on another dry towel. Cover these potato fingers with the marinade made in the past development.

Pre-heat the Air Fryer cooker for about 5 minutes at 300 Fahrenheit. Take out the bushel of the fryer cooker and locate the potato fingers in them. Close the bushel. Presently save the fryer at 220 Fahrenheit for 20 or 25 minutes. In the middle of the procedure, hurl the fries twice or thrice with the goal that they get cooked appropriately.

Towards the finish of the cooking procedure (the most recent 2 minutes or something like that), Include the liquefied cheddar over the fries and serve hot.

3 BUFFET IDEAS FOR YOUR GUESTS WITH PREP TIPS AND SET-UP TIPS

A buffet is an extraordinary thought in case you're having many visitors over for a meal. This sort of meal permits the visitors to arrange and pick which foods they might want to eat, as they move from one finish of the serving station to the next. Setting up a buffet isn't overpowering on the off chance that you make it stride by-step and do a touch of planning. To set up a buffet, set up the space, set up the table, and put out food for the visitors.

Setting up the Space

1. Consider your financial limit. Choose the amount you need to spend inside and out, including food, flatware, plates, and beverages. Next, decrease the sum you need to spend by 15%. The staying 85% is the thing that you should really spend. The extra 15% permits you some additional cash for startling expenses and things like duties, tips, and potential crises.

•   Create a spending graph, either on a piece of paper or in a PC program, for example, Excel or Microsoft Word.

2. Start planning your buffet table ahead of time. Accumulate the entirety of your serving dishes together the night prior to the occasion and spot them on the table. Connect clingy notes to remind you which food goes in which dish.

•   Arranging your table ahead of time will guarantee that you are not settling on a minute ago choices and Prep.s.

•   If you have additional time, consider drawing the set-up on a piece of paper. Pick the one that you like the best. At that point, reproduce it utilizing your table and dishes.

3. Pick a live with a great deal of potential open space. Ten square feet is a perfect measure of space to fit all visitors easily with space for getting food and blending. Eight square feet takes into consideration some seating, seven and a half square feet can be agreeable for littler groups, and six square feet ought to be the base measure of room that you assign for the buffet.

•   If your area has numerous rooms, consider serving the food and beverages in a single room, at that point having the seating in another room.

4. Spot the table in the focal point of the space for the best stream. Clean the room you plan to use for your occasion, including all messiness, furniture, and enhancements. Spot the serving table in the room; at that point, place extra tables to either side for things like plates, flatware, and cups. This will permit the visitors to access the food from the two sides of the buffet table and will keep the line moving rapidly.

•   An eight-foot table should hold enough food for twenty to thirty individuals. You should assemble different tables in the event that you are having a bigger number of individuals than that over.

•   Make sure that you have a lot of serving spoons and tongs for each dish- - one for each side of the table.

5. Plan a different table for drinks. By arranging the refreshment table away from the food table, you allow your visitors to pick their food and pouring a beverage.

•   This limits the potential for spills. This is another approach to guarantee that your visitors can move the lines easily.

•   Consider having separate tables for alcoholic and non-mixed drinks.

•   Water ought to be served at its own table. Contingent upon what number of visitors you have, you might need to have numerous pitches. Along these lines, your visitors aren't holding up in line.

6. Plan the traffic stream. Assign a passageway and exit to the buffet. You can do this by just telling individuals as they approach the table, or by making a sign for each finish of the table. Leave a lot of room before and on the sides of the table, just in the event that individuals choose to stop briefly. This lessens the opportunity of swarming.

•   Keep the kinds of food as isolated as could be expected under the circumstances. For instance, keep dessert a long way from the primary course of the meal.

•   If you have veggie lovers as well as vegan choices, it may be a smart thought to keep those different from the non-vegan and non-vegan tables.

•   Consider having a little table saved for tidbits. You can put this closer to the wine or champagne table, even.

Setting up the Table

1. Recall any challenges you've encountered with past buffets. Consider what irritating or troublesome the last time you went to a buffet was. Consider what you would have enjoyed during a buffet and plan your table around that thought. For instance:

•   If you wished you had space to put a plate down immediately, leave enough additional room on the buffet table for individuals to do as such.

•   If you wished you had the choice of tasting the food first, leave toothpicks or little spoons by the dishes for your visitors with the goal that they can attempt the food.

•   If you run into issues with refuse, consider setting up more rubbish containers and making them progressively recognizable so visitors can without much of a stretch spot them.

2. Have a decent introduction. Consider what sort of plates, cups, utensils, holders, and tablecloth you might want to use for your table. You don't need to utilize you're fine china, yet a table is increasingly mouth-watering if the set up looks decent. It's alright to utilize plastic flatware, plates, and cups, as long as it is all new and clean. Try not to put your food out in oily, cardboard boxes. Rather, utilize plastic or metal compartments. You will likewise require a tablecloth. A costly tablecloth will conceivably get destroyed by the wreckage, however, search for one that adds cheer to the table.

• Decide on shading or a topic when putting out everything on the table. This will bring the appearance of the table together and make the meal look all the more engaging.

• As opposed to picking loads of hues and examples, stay with only a couple of strong hues.

• Many providing food spots will offer things like plates, cups, and flatware. Rental spots for tables and chairs will now and again have tablecloths that you can obtain too.

3. Place the plates toward the beginning of the line. Your visitors can't get to the food well without first having plates accessible. In the event that you are planning an occasion with many individuals, it is a smart thought to set up a buffet with a few piles of plates of around ten plates each. You don't, be that as it may, need to heap the plates excessively high, or they will be at risk for spills.

• Be sure to put sauces close to the kind of food they have a place with.

• If you have a separate tables for the things like hors d'oeuvres and treats, you should include tables for plates close to them too.

4. Put flatware toward the finish of the table. Finish the table with utensils and napkins. A typical mix-up made by numerous hosts when planning an occasion is to put utensils and napkins at the front of the table. It very well may be lumbering to attempt to clutch blades, forks, spoons, and cloths alongside a plate while your visitors are attempting to serve themselves.

• Make sure you put out a wide range of flatware that will be required. For instance, remember spoons if there will be soup.

5. Make names. Get ready names for each dish early. This can be on little bits of paper, clingy notes, or cardboard. Put the names beside each dish once the entirety of the food is out on the table. This will permit visitors to comprehend what the dish is before they put it on their plate, which takes out a ton of uneaten and discarded food.

- Make sure the names are written in striking, enormous, and clear composing that all visitors will have the option to peruse easily. Composed names will be more intelligible than transcribed marks.

- If a food contains a typical allergen, for example, peanuts, it would be a smart thought to include a notice mark too, for example, Contains Peanuts.

- If you realize that a portion of your visitors is veggie lover or vegan, it is pleasant to make reference to which dishes contain meat or dairy.

Putting Out Food

1. Give a fair meal. Plan a meal with a plate of mixed greens, protein, vegetable, starch, sugar and pastry, except if you are setting up a mixed drink party. Buffet meals can feel dissipated and lopsided. Once in a while, there are such a large number of canapés, side dishes, or principle plates. Planning a decent meal will assist you in maintaining a strategic distance from this issue. If you are hosting a mixed drink get-together, it is alright to just serve an assortment of starters and desserts.

- You can seldom turn out badly by including a vegetable and natural product plate.

- Make sure to put out a veggie lover or vegan alternative.

2. Plan the food as indicated by the season. The kind of food we eat for meals regularly changes with the seasons. During summer, it feels tiring to eat an overwhelming meal loaded up with potatoes and meats. While throughout the winter, a light serving of mixed greens and lean fish may feel too light.

-      Fruits that contain a ton of water are extraordinary for summer buffets, similar to watermelon.

-      Rich foods, as gooey pound potatoes, are useful for winter meals.

3. Choose six to eight things. You would prefer not to have excessively not many or such a large number of things to browse. Too hardly any things can leave a few visitors without food or decision on the off chance that they don't care for all that you've served. An excessive number of decisions may cause an increasingly tangled line with an excessive amount of extra food. Six to eight things are decent to add up to give everybody enough decisions. The serving size relies upon the measure of individuals you are expecting.

-      You can convey a rundown of thoughts for dishes and request input up to 14 days before the buffet.

-      Be sure to have an assortment of food. Try not to have six or eight all-meat things. Remember dishes with vegetables and grains for them also.

-      If you'll be serving meat, attempt to have two unique options, for example, chicken and fish, instead of two chicken dishes.

4. Line up the food as per temperature. The principal stop on the food line ought to be the hot foods. You need the visitors to find a workable pace before they chill off something over the top. Thusly, your visitors won't feast on cool primary courses when they discover their seats. The chilly foods ought to be toward the finish of the table. On the off chance that conceivable, it is ideal for picking room temperature.

-      Put out scraping dishes to keep foods hot, and ice platters to keep food cold.

5. Mastermind the food deliberately. Put the least expensive and the food you have the vast majority of toward the start of the table. Put the most costly and rare food toward the finish of the table. It is a smart thought to set it up along these lines on the grounds that the food toward the start of the table regularly goes the fastest.

• Consider exchanging foods over the span of the buffet. On the off chance that the carrots aren't being eaten enough, change them out with a food that is going quick.

• Some foods become unappetizing, the more they sit. For instance, if the serving of mixed greens is beginning to look disgusting or the dish is coagulating, change it out!

6. Include beautifications. When the table is set up, add beautifications to amp up the intrigue of the table. Try not to pick whatever will disrupt everything or square individuals. Huge candles on candles may not be a smart thought, yet setting little strips or retires from table won't hinder anybody going after food.

• If you have a buffet for a vacation, pick enrichments that relate with that occasion. Holy person Patrick's Day designs could be green, white, and gold. A Fourth of July buffet can be decked out in red, white, and blue.

• If you truly need candles, consider LED or battery-worked candles. They last more and you don't need to stress over fire perils.

• Don't escape with the embellishments. A disperse of confetti is better than huge decorations and figures that occupy an excess of room.

• If you need to have an announcement embellishment, consider putting it on a table that won't be frequented, for example, the cake table or beverages table.

How to Decorate a Buffet Table

Your buffet is the focal point of your occasion, so you should invest a great deal of time and energy into making it locks in. By picking a subject, getting a classy measure of adornments, making a coherent movement for your visitors, and doing a preliminary run, you can guarantee that your table will be embellished perfectly and helpfully for your occasion.

Choosing a Theme

1. Pick a shading topic. Your table will be significantly more strong if there is a subject to your beautifications. The topic can be either a shading or an occasion, for example, a birthday, a season, or a particular occasion. If the topic is a shading rather than an occasion, restrict yourself to 2-3 hues that go well together.

If the topic is an occasion, pick hues that compare with that occasion. For instance, in the event that it is a Christmas buffet, use adornments that are red, green, and gold.

2. Purchase or make things identified with your topic. Make a focal point that consolidates your subject utilizing the organic product, blossoms, props, or candles. You would then be able to pick things that allude to that topic for the remainder of the table, for example, palatable enhancement, blossoms, natural product, leaves, or cinnamon sticks.

• Some different thoughts for table beautifications, contingent upon your topic, are strips or shells.

3. Abstain from exaggerating the designs. You need the enrichments to be tasteful, not vainglorious or overpowering. In a perfect world, the food will be in plain view, and any style around the table will upgrade the appearance of the food, not shroud it or overpower it.

• Also, abstain from sprinkling the table with sparkle or other non-eatable improvements, as these frequently end up on individuals' plates or in their mouths.

4. Organize your tablecloth, a table cloth, napkins, and placemats. Pick either a tablecloth or table linen to put underneath the food on the buffet table. Napkins are an absolute necessity too. Placemats are discretionary, yet can be a pleasant touch to have underneath your serving dishes. While picking these things, be certain that they are inside your shading plan and that they work out positively for each other.

- Consider curiously large material napkins in hues that coordinate your subject. For a progressively easygoing buffet, paper napkins are okay. Regardless, supply a lot of extra napkins in the event of a wreck.

- Table sprinters should hang around 6 inches (15 cm) down the table on the two sides.

5. Set up a mark for every food thing. Make names for each dish that you will have on the table. Use cardstock or paper collapsed down the middle, with the name of the dish composed on one side. Compose or type in an intense, clear textual style that is huge enough for any visitor to peruse.

- Write whether a dish is veggie-lover, vegan, or gluten-free on the mark, underneath the name of the dish.

6. Consider making a menu to show. For an additional touch, you can make a menu of all the various foods that will be served. Show the menu either utilizing a little menu easel on the table or remain close to the start of the table. That way, visitors will recognize what they will discover further down the table and can settle on progressively educated food decisions.

Masterminding the Basics on the Table

1. Plan your game plan before you start putting the embellishments. This will keep you from sitting around revamping it. Choose which improvements you need to utilize, where they will go, and what course you need the visitors to follow.

2. Set up a consistent excursion down the table. Envision yourself beginning toward the start of the table, getting a plate, dishing up a starter and a serving of mixed greens, and afterwards descending to the primary course dish. Consider the request that you would eat a meal in, and mastermind the food dishes in a specific order.

3. Move your buffet table to a helpful area. It should be unmistakable, yet not in individuals' way. If you have many visitors and your room is huge, set the table away from any dividers with the goal that your visitors approach the table from the two sides. In the event that the room is littler, place the table against a divider, off the beaten path. In the event that conceivable, leave space for individuals to remain on either end of the table to stay away from an excessive amount of swarming in the front.

4. Set out your tablecloth or table linen. Both of these will make a beautiful base for the buffet table and can cover a table that you might not have any desire to have appeared. In the event that you utilize a table cloth, position it in the focal point of the table and ensure that it runs the full length of the table.

5. Put the plates and bowls toward the start of the buffet table. Plates are the principal thing your visitors will require, so they ought to be toward the start of the table. Set out a larger number of plates than you might suspect you'll require since visitors regularly take another plate each time that they come back to the table.

6. Spot the utensils toward the finish of the table. Having the utensils toward the finish of the table mitigates individuals from holding them while attempting to hold the plate. With just two hands, that can be a troublesome undertaking! You can likewise have utensils at both the start and the finish of the table, in the event that you would like.

• Provide the entirety of the utensils that will be required for the food you're serving. For instance, remember the soup spoons in case you're serving soup!

7.Set the napkins close to the utensils, or enclose the utensils by the napkins. Wrapping the utensils can make it simpler for your visitors to get the entire pack on the double, rather than getting every utensil exclusively.

8. Have various piles of plates, cups, utensils, and napkins. Since hungry individuals can be anxious to get what they require and plunk down, it is ideal to have different piles of plates, cups, utensils, and napkins. That way, numerous individuals can snatch one simultaneously without expecting to hold up in a line or drive into one another.

9. Leave space for individuals to immediately put their plates down. This progression is frequently missed yet is significant. In the event that a visitor needs to get another napkin or modify something, you need them to have space to put their plate down for a minute when orchestrating your table, attempt to leave little pockets of the room where a plate could fit.

10. Do a training run. This will assist you with visualizing the final product and check whether anything should be balanced. Ensure that the table isn't excessively packed and that your enrichments won't obstruct any food. Do a preliminary stroll down the buffet table too, claiming to serve yourself. Ensure that everything is put consistently and close enough.

•   At this stage, alter whatever should be fixed and evacuate any enhancements that are unwieldy or ugly.

Consolidating Your Decorations

1. Raise a portion of your dishes. Adding stature to certain dishes is tastefully engaging and adds life to your table—for example, boxes and topsy turvy holders with the material. Simply don't misrepresent the rise, as this looks tumultuous, yet it tends to be perilous. You table ought to have unpretentious ascents and plunges.

•   Place all the serving dishes that will be utilized on the table as you design. This will assist with guaranteeing that you have enough space for everything that should be on the table.

2. Organize your themed improvements. Since your dishes are set, feel free to occupy in the spaces with the embellishments that you've picked. Be aware of not setting things before food dishes, or in regions where they will get thumped over by elbows. Take a stab at setting bigger things at the rear of the table and littler things among dishes and around the edges of the table.

3. Set out candles. Candles are an awesome beautification for any buffet table. Consider putting tall candles at the rear of the table if the table is against the divider, with the goal that they won't get thumped over. Else, you can adorn little containers with candles inside and place them around the table. On the off chance that having blazes appears to be hazardous for your occasion, consider utilizing flashing electric candles.

The Making of a Beautiful and Easy Thanksgiving Dinner Table

Orchestrating a Thanksgiving table needn't be a mind-boggling venture. With a smidgen of time and creative mind, in addition to confidence in rich effortlessness, you'll have a great supper table set-up without whine.

Steps

1. Select a plain shaded tablecloth. White is a magnificent shading as it will set off anything you decide to add to the table; however, the decision is yours. Keep away from examples or structures, as these overpower the table too rapidly.

2. Pick a shading topic. Normal hues reflect fall - oranges, yellows, golds, reds and tans. Orange is additionally an impression of pumpkins, squash and different indications of collect abundance. Purchase serviettes (napkins) that mirror the picked subject - there are likewise different fall plans pre-imprinted on serviettes that may be reasonable for your topic.

3. Discover a Cornucopia container. This can be set on the table to speak to the abundance of gather. You can leave it unfilled, or fill it with natural products, for example, red apples and yellow pears.

4. Get shrewd! Make fall shaded paper things to give shading to the table:

•	Leaves - Choose an assortment of paper that reflects practical leaf hues and accommodates your picked shading subject, for example, reds and oranges. Cut the papers into straightforward leaf structures (draw a layout on the light card that you can follow with the scissors or art shaper). Cause the same number of paper leaves as you to feel you possess energy for. You may wish to transform some into game plans and utilize some free, so remember this when making them.

•	Make a little bunch of courses of action with a portion of the leaves. Spot these around the base of a glass flame holder and supplement an orange/gold and so forth light in the highest point of the holder.

•	Strew a couple of the single leaves around the table in an imaginative style. Guarantee that shading blends are coordinating and in the topic.

•	Napkin rings and labels - Use extra bits of paper to make napkin rings and informal IDs.

•	Cut flimsy portions of paper and change these strips to fit around your collapsed material napkins. Paste or tape set up. Fluctuate the hues on the off chance that you have a decent eye for coordinating structures.

•	Make unofficial IDs from similar shades of paper. Utilize a pleasant coordinating shade of dim mustard type paper to stamp the letters on, or spare time and utilize a Gel pen or like essentially compose the names.

•	Placemats - Place pieces of hued paper slantingly covering each other to make precious stones that fit the rectangular state of a placemat. You can likewise attempt round shapes whenever liked, or be truly brave and attempt shapes, for example, pumpkins, turkeys or Cornucopias. Paste set up.

5. Use nature for motivation. Adding regular components to the table underlines the reap topic.

• Purchase smaller than normal squash to enrich the table. These come previously bundled with their own amazing appeal and hues, so there truly is no compelling reason to do whatever else with them. Search for some that despite everything have wispy rings, as these include a fragile completing touch.

• If you approach clean fall leaves, you may get a kick out of the chance to add these to the table, or even make a showcase utilizing leaves, pine cones and twigs.

• Use natural product, for example, apples and pears, in little shows.

• Add a presentation of crisp roses in shades of yellow, oranges or quieted reds.

• Use nuts with the shells off. Either place them deliberately free on the table or add to a bowl, the Cornucopia crate or some other game plan. In the event that you have a little toy squirrel, place it alongside the walnut nuts.

6. Set the remainder of the table as you would consistently for an evening gathering. Utilize your best dinnerware and flatware and on the off chance that you haven't bought uniquely themed Thanksgiving serviettes, utilize plain-shaded fabric ones that coordinate the topic. Include fine quality dish sets and the set the unofficial ID set up.

How to Eat at a Buffet

A buffet is where individuals can serve themselves whatever they'd like. Buffets are an incredible decision for individuals who need numerous choices and have a sound craving. Regardless of whether you need to follow legitimate behaviour, figure out how to take advantagehe of your experience, eating at a buffet is really basic and regularly justified, despite all the trouble on the off chance that you eat enough to take care of the expense of food.

Taking advantage of a Buffet

1. Wear-free attire. Put on free, open to apparel when setting off to a buffet. A pair of tight pants or a perfectly sized dress may get awkward as you eat. Wear garments that are made of a delicate material that can without much of a stretch extend and dodge pants with catches if conceivable.

2. Eat costly foods first. Start with pricier foods, similar to steak or shrimp. In the event that you are vegan, start with gourmet foods or entangled dishes that you couldn't without much of a stretch make for yourself. Along these lines, you can guarantee that you are getting what you paid for or considerably more than what you paid for.

3. Utilize a plate of mixed greens or soup bowl for dessert. Sweet dishes are regularly little, so get more treat by utilizing a soup or serving of mixed greens bowl for pastries like frozen yoghurt. If you aren't getting frozen yoghurt, utilize a plate that is made for fundamental courses to get a bit of pie or cake. Try not to do this on the off chance that it is illegal by the buffet you are eating at.

4. Drink water the day preceding setting off to the buffet. Remaining hydrated will keep your stomach extended, which will permit you to eat more food. Notwithstanding, don't drink a ton of water not long before going into the buffet, or you may feel full.

5. Eat a nibble before the buffet. Being too ravenous can lead you to eat rapidly toward the start of your meal, which may cause you to feel full quicker. Eat a light nibble about an hour prior setting off to the buffet. A bunch of peanuts, an apple, or yoghurt would be a decent bite.

6. Start with lighter foods. Try not to stack up on pasta or bland foods when you start eating. Start with lighter foods so you will at present have space in your stomach. Start with a serving of mixed greens or shrimp as a starter before plunging into heavier food.

7. Eat gradually. Eating your food too quickly will cause you to feel too full to even think about eating as much as you would've had the option to eat on the off chance that you'd found a steady speed. Bite gradually as you eat and take breaths between nibbles. Hold up a moment or two preceding returning awake for seconds.

8. Stay away from pop. The carbonation in the soft drink may cause you to feel more full than water would. Rather, go for juice or water. In the event that you need pop, hold on to have it toward the finish of your meal.

9. Abstain from squandering food. Despite the fact that you might need to benefit from the buffet. It is smarter to get a ton of little plates and making various excursions as opposed to squandering food. Additionally, remember that some deal buffets will charge at the cost of the food you don't eat.

Following Buffet Etiquette

1. Stroll around before you eat. Try not to pick the main thing that looks tempting. Rather, go for a stroll around the whole buffet and look at what is being advertised. Observe the things that look best to you.

• Exploring the substance of the buffet will likewise assist you with avoiding eating food that you don't generally like or eating excessively.

2. Snatch a plate, plate, and utensils. You can't get the food you need without having a plate to put it on. Get one littler hors d'oeuvre plate in the first place. Keep in mind, and you can generally return for another plate when you need something different.

•   Check to ensure the plate is, in reality, clean before getting it. It shouldn't have any food particles or sleek buildups left on it. Get another plate if yours is grimy.

3. Perceive lines. There might be lines before the serving stations. On the off chance that you see different individuals arranged and they seem, by all accounts, to be pausing, get behind the last individual. In the event that you aren't sure on the off chance that it is a line, basic solicit one from the individuals in the event that they're pausing. A few buffets might be more formal than others so investigate perceive how others are carrying on before serving yourself.

4. Get a hors d'oeuvre. Start your meal with a hors d'oeuvre. This could be a serving of mixed greens, soup, breadsticks, or whatever you'd like. Take a little segment of it to spare space for the remainder of your meal. Beginning with a starter will likewise assist you with pacing yourself during the meal.

•   If you don't need a starter, you can start with the fundamental course.

5. Pick a fundamental course and side. Subsequent to completing the tidbit, put aside your plate or put it in a container for messy dishes. At that point, put a new plate on your plate. You don't need to supplant your utensils. Get the principle dish and side (or sides) of your decision. For instance, you can get a chicken bosom with pureed potatoes.

6. Return for quite a long time. In case you're as yet eager, return for a considerable length of time. This is flawlessly satisfactory at a buffet. Simply make a point to get a new plate each time you get another food. You can even go up for thirds in case you're as yet eager.

•   If you're at a buffet you haven't paid for, as at a gathering, be considerate of others before getting seconds or thirds. Leave some food for another person that hasn't gotten any food yet.

7. Eat dessert. Take a gander at each sweet alternative before picking one. You can have a go at something new, yet you ought to consider what you commonly like and abhorrence before taking something. For instance, don't get pumpkin pie on the off chance that you don't commonly like pumpkin dishes. If you can't choose, take a limited quantity of various treats.

Eating Well at a Buffet

1. Be wary about to what extent the food has been sitting out. It's hard to tell to what extent food has been out except if you ask, yet there are approaches to abstain from eating food that has conceivably turned sour. Frequently, it's a smart thought to keep away from foods that are hanging out in enormous tanks. Foods that are in huge tanks are bound to have been there for longer than different foods. Additionally, if the food gives off an impression of being stained, an unexpected surface in comparison to regular, or has a surprising smell, it is ideal to proceed onward to another dish.

- Tell a staff part on the off chance that you think any food has turned sour.

- You can ask to what extent a food has been out in the event that you are uncertain.

2. Pick little bits. It's enticing to take a gigantic part of the lasagna that looks flavorful, yet stay away from this. Take a little part of each food. It's even alright to get undesirable foods you wouldn't ordinarily eat as long as you take a limited quantity. If you choose, you need more, and you can generally return.

3. Pick foods you wouldn't cook for yourself. Buffets frequently offer foods like toast and fried eggs. While these are scrumptious, search for sound choices you wouldn't ordinarily cook for yourself with the goal that the meal feels like a treat. For instance, pick the smoked salmon or barbecued trout on the off chance that you don't regularly make it at home.

4. Maintain a distance from such a large number of boring foods. It's alright to have some bland foods. However, these foods are generally undesirable and will top you off rapidly. Boring foods will be foods like potatoes, rice, and pasta. Take a little part of these foods.

5. Try not to indulge. It's enticing to keep returning for food at a buffet essentially in light of the fact that it's there. Maintain a strategic distance from this allurement. Quit eating when you feel full.

- Sit confronting endlessly from the buffet. This is thought to assist you with making fewer outings to the serving station.

•   Skipping the plate will assist you with abstaining from indulging since you can not take as a lot of food during one excursion.

6. Pick solidified yoghurt or organic product as sweet. In the event that it's your lavish expenditure meal, it's alright to go for a bit of cake or dessert. If you need to remain sound, pick a pastry that isn't so stacked in calories. Solidified yoghurt or a bowl of the crisp natural product would be a smart thought.

How to Set Up a DIY Drink Station at a Party

Contingent upon the kind of gathering you want to have and the kind of visitors you plan to engage, there is a wide range of drink stations you might be planning to set up. You have a lot of choices, from a make-your-own-mixed drink bar to a top-if-off-yourself hot chocolate buffet. Whatever kind of drink station you plan to set up, make a point to stock and prepare it appropriately, and to keep up the station during your gathering.

Stocking Your Drink Station with Beverages

1. Select great or occasional drinks. If you as of now have a work of art or custom sort of drink as a primary concern, let it all out. In any case, in case you're considering what kinds of beverages to highlight at your gathering, the season can be an extraordinary wellspring of motivation. Perhaps you need to make hot buttered juice for a winter evening gathering. Then again, perhaps you're facilitating a mid-year garden get-together, and need to set up a DIY lemonade station.

•   Be sure to pick something that will take into account you and your visitors' inventiveness. Following the lemonade model, your station could highlight newly squeezed lemonade, some different squeezes or seasoned seltzer waters to include, and embellishing like new berries, mint leaves, and lavender petals.

2. Make a rundown of all that you plan to include. This incorporates both fluid fixings just as include ins. When you've chosen the sort of drink station you need to set up, consider the entirety

of the particular fixings you need to give. Look online for additional data, via scanning for various recipes of the beverage you're considering.

- Don't disregard foods grown from the ground herbs, as they can include visual intrigue and the smell they offer can make an incredible beverage far and away superior.

- Note that a wide range of kinds of beverages can be made with or without liquor. Permitting your visitors to settle on that decision themselves guarantees that their beverages are exactly what they were seeking after.

3. Cut and squeeze early. Many beverage recipes call for explicit fixings to be squeezed or cut into sizes fitting for decorating. For example, numerous mixed drinks call for lime juice or potentially a lime cut. Be certain set up any fixings that require hazardous or noteworthy Prep. beforehand.[2]

- Be sure to get sufficiently ready! It's ideal to abstain from utilizing blades or blenders during a gathering.

- Whenever you're utilizing a recipe that calls for the juice of any kind, consider squeezing new natural products the day of the gathering for the best flavour.

4. Post suggested recipes at the station. In this way, you've settled on a Bloody Mary bar. You plan to offer a couple of various kinds of tomato juice and pre-made Bloody Mary blends, a couple of various sorts of alcohol, plenty of vegetables and other include ins, and an ice chest entryway of various hot sauce. Your visitors have bounty to work with and will without a doubt, end up making some extraordinary beverages. All things considered, a few visitors may value a touch of direction.

- For case, record your prescribed recipe and make a sign that says something like "Sarah's Sassy Bloody Maria: 2 oz tequila, 2 stalks of cured asparagus, 2 pearl onions, in a glass rimmed with powdered hamburger jerky and filled to the overflow with McClure's Bloody Mary Mix."

5. Give various sorts of liquor. Regardless of whether you determine a great mixed drink station, you'll need to offer some assortment as far as the primary fixing. For example, possibly you'll concentrate on offering forte elements for the best martinis around, with a couple of decision jugs

of vodka and gin specifically. You should put out a container of whiskey and another of tequila too.

•   Don't overlook alcohols. Contingent upon the kinds of drink you need to offer, vermouths and certain cordials will be fundamental. Sharp flavoring is extraordinary as well, and come in a wide range of flavours.

•   Further, not every person who drinks liquor likes to drink alcohol. In the event that you need to ensure there are possibilities for everybody, it merits putting out a block of ice can with certain brews and a container of champagne.

6. Always offer a non-mixed drink alternative. In any event, when you're facilitating a grown-up get-together and anticipate that the liquor should be streaming, you ought to consistently ensure visitors can discover a non-alcoholic alternative when they're prepared to back off for the night. In the case of nothing else, a water pitcher is constantly a smart thought.

•   Another incredible choice to set out is carbonated water. Numerous individuals enjoy drinking shining water all alone, while others will probably use to it spritz beverages of assorted types.

7. Label everything plainly. Whatever you use to hold your various fixings, ensure they're marked plainly and accurately. This is significant for a few reasons, including advising the individuals who might be adversely affected by specific things. In case you're utilizing press bottles, essentially include a bit of concealing tape and compose the substance on the tape in indelible marker.

•   If you have bowls of a lot of dry fixings, particularly flavours, cause small signs you to can connect to toothpicks or sticks and stick into the bowl too.

Choosing Equipment for Your Drink Station

1. Provide the fitting serving hardware. A few factors ought to be considered to figure out what kind of cups or dishes you'll need to set out at your beverage station. For example, on the off chance that you've made an enormous group of hot chocolate, you'll likely need to keep it in a

vessel that will preserve its glow. A scoop would then be able to be utilized to give out single parts into mugs, and visitors can include alcohol, marshmallows, and so forth as they wish.

• Aside from temperature, different factors to consider are the age of your visitors. For example, if youngsters will utilize the beverage station, you might need to utilize plastic cups and utensils.

2. Include estimating hardware. Particularly if your beverage station will incorporate liquor, it's imperative to give something to assist individuals with deciding bits of specific fixings. For example, put out a shot glass or tablespoon and notice it explicitly in your posted recipes. For example, "Start with 1 shot glass of whichever alcohol you have… "

3. Ensure the best possible temperature. One of the most significant parts of a beverage station is ensuring the beverages you offer can be made at the correct temperature. More often than not, this will basically mean giving loads of ice. An ice pail can work, yet a cooler with a scoop is far and away superior. Make certain to have some reinforcement ice in your cooler as well.

• On the other hand, you may need to keep drinks warm. Right now, the base fluid -,, for example, hot apple juice - in a simmering pot. Turn the stewing pot on and set it to "low" or "keep warm."

4. Use hardware that will make self-administration simpler. One of the most widely recognized kinds of holders that barkeeps use, for example, are press bottles. These delicate plastic containers with cone-shaped spouts can help encourage simple beverage blending. Further, the top on a crush jug can remain on all through the gathering, lessening the danger of spills and shielding every fixing from defilement.

• Use press jugs to hold well known, regular fixings like lime juice or straightforward syrup.

• Other hardware that can make self-administration less difficult incorporates things like mixing utensils and drink strainers.

- Don't overlook a scoop for the ice, and a compartment to hold the scoop when it isn't being utilized.

Keeping up Your Drink Station During a Party

1. Inform visitors concerning the station upon appearance. As visitors show up, make certain to bring up both the area and topic of the beverage station. Shockingly better, let visitors think about your plans to have a beverage station when you welcome them, and urge them to bring whatever fixings they may support also.

- For case, remember something for your greeting along the lines of, "We'll have a make-your-own-mojito station set up with the necessities, yet don't hesitate to carry your own mystery fixings to share."

2. Clean the station intermittently. All through the gathering, attempt to watch out for the station or request that somebody assist you with doing as such. Above all, you'll need to swing through and clean up from consistently. Specifically, make a point to wipe up any spills each time you check the station.

- Make sure napkins or paper towel are still in acceptable stockpile during each check.

- Be sure to have obviously marked junk jars and reusing holders close by for visitors' utilization.

3. Check the stock occasionally. There are a couple of things you have to ensure your beverage station hosts all through the gathering. Watch out for your base fixings and principle increases, particularly if individuals appear to enjoy a specific contribution. Have reinforcements of all that you would prefer not to come up short on prepared to serve.[9]

- Make sure that nobody over-serves themselves. One great approach to do this is by just putting out a specific measure of alcohol at once. Each time you check the station, you can give more varying.

- You likely as of now have back up ice and extra cut limes. There are different things you may need to renew also. During planning, consider all that you may require a greater amount of - „ for example, cups and flatware - and have backups prepared.

How to Make a Green Candy Buffet

Candy buffets are an enjoyment approach to engage visitors who have a sweet tooth. It's an enjoyable approach to get ready for a gathering, and here are a few proposals to support you.

Steps

1. Select appropriate holders for the confections. There are heaps of compartment prospects, yet the most significant factor in guaranteeing that the holders will flaunt the green confections inside. Thusly, clear glass or plastic holders are an ideal decision, alongside compartments that lift up the confections and demonstrate them to further their best potential benefit.

- Try bowls, glasses, sundae glasses, containers (counting Mason containers), jars, dishes and platters. Tall stemmed glasses with wide overflows can be particularly viable, for example, those utilized for mixed drinks.

- Tins and other hazy items can likewise be utilized given it is clear to the visitor concerning what is inside.

2. Ensure that it is simple for visitors to get the confections. The best executes scoops and smaller than usual tongs, which will permit visitors to gather a couple of confections one after another without being enticed to utilize their fingers. Keeping up the cleanliness when numerous individuals are sharing the buffet is fundamental!

- Provide little plates, bowls, bins or different compartments for visitors to scoop their confections into.

3. Choose green confections. This is unquestionably the enjoyment part! When you are set to searching for just green shades of treats, you'll begin seeing them all over the place. A few thoughts include:

- Green jam beans and green sticky bears and other gel confections

- Green wrappers on any sort of treats

- Green wrapped chocolates and green chocolate; green Easter eggs if it's around Easter season.

- Green candies, suckers and some other candy on a stick

- Green boxes of confections – the confections inside shouldn't really be green if the bundling is green, as it will just look extraordinary on the buffet table.

- Green candy sticks, greenstone sweets

- Green licorice

- Green marzipan figures

- Green mints

- Green toffees, caramels

- Green taffy.

4.Set up the buffet table. Consider utilizing a green tablecloth for covering. On the off chance that this is excessively, however, utilize white as it's an easy-going foundation for each of the one-shading topics. Plan out how you will organize the compartments on the buffet table, alongside scoops, tongs and serving plates, and so forth. A few recommendations include:

- Keep the bigger things to the back and the little ones to the front

- Provide green napkins (serviettes) for clingy fingers

- Avoid having the tablecloth contact the ground or hinder the visitors; with numerous individuals processing around the table, there is a danger, all things considered, being pulled down.

- Place anything sensitive away from the edge of the buffet table.

- Encourage visitors to help themselves by making it clear where the plates and scoops are

- Consider having a region for sweet food that addresses the issues of diabetics, vegans, gluten-bigoted, and so forth visitors with the goal that they don't get a handle on left. Leave a little sign signifying the fixings or expressing that they are "sans gluten"/"without dairy", and so forth., things.

5. Try not to be reluctant to include a couple of non-candy green things that are still sweet. Green macaroons, green whoopie pies, green cupcakes, and so on., will all assist with making the green subject and add to the general sweetness.

6. Add other enlivening components to the buffet table. To finish the green topic, dress the table up with a couple of unappetizing green enhancements also. A few proposals include:

- Green strips around containers and different holders

- Green withdraws from the tablecloth.

•   Green puppets, for example, a little leprechaun or a tree.

•   Green decorative design (use bunches of leaves and roses which normally have green tinges)

•   Green dabs, glass rocks, moved up yarn, and so on inside a glass container with a tight top screwed or even stuck on (you don't need individuals confusing these with confections).

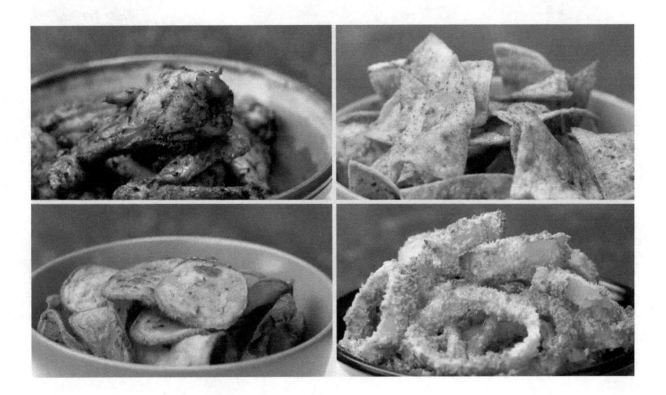

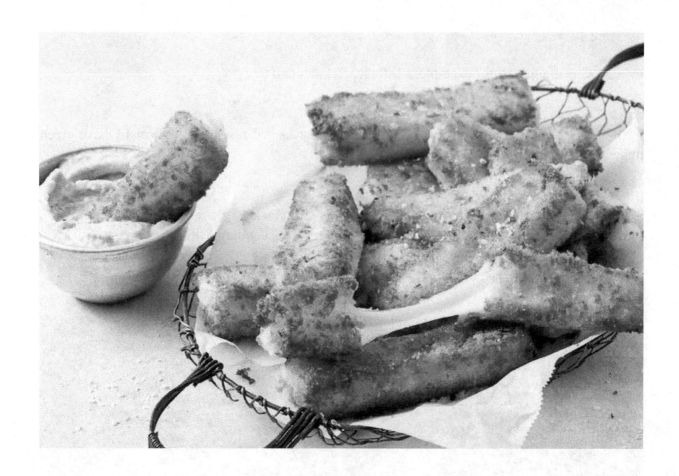

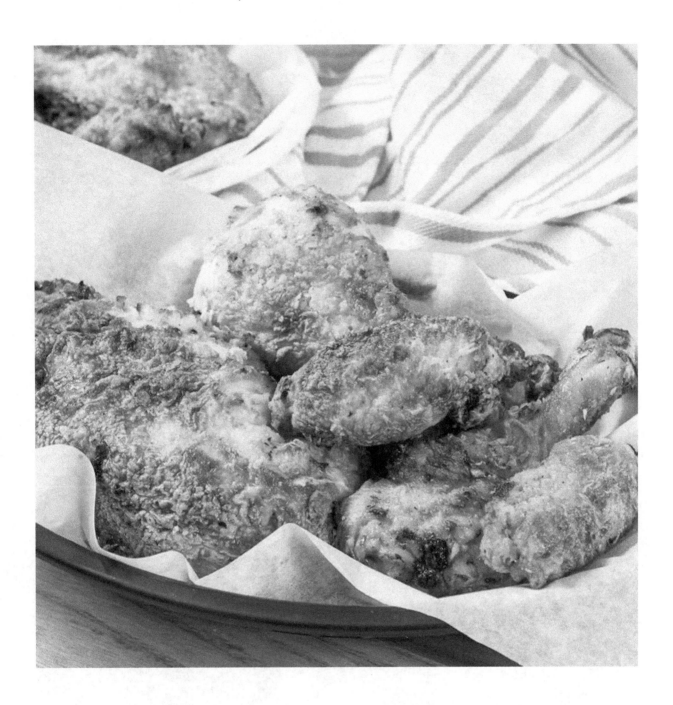

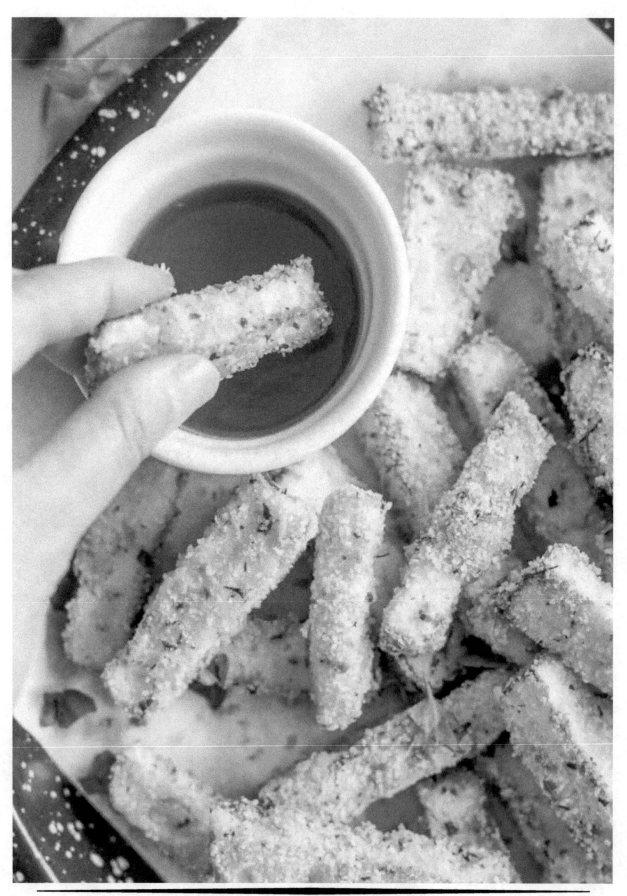

CPSIA information can be obtained
at www.ICGtesting.com
Printed in the USA
LVHW062312230521
688301LV00006B/268